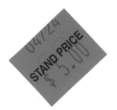

Techniques of
Working with Resistance

Techniques of
Working with Resistance

Edited by
Donald S. Milman, Ph.D.
and
George D. Goldman, Ph.D.

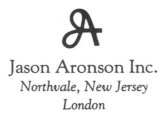

Jason Aronson Inc.
Northvale, New Jersey
London

Library of Congress Cataloging-in-Publication Data

Main entry under title:

Techniques in working with resistance.

  Includes bibliographies and index.
  1. Resistance (Psychoanalysis)   2. Psychotherapy.
3. Resistance (Psychoanalysis) — Addresses, essays,
lectures.   4. Psychotherapy — Addresses, essays, lectures.
I. Milman, Donald S., 1924–   .   II. Goldman, George D.
[DNLM: 1. Physician-Patient Relations.   2. Psychotherapy —
methods.   WM 420 T255]
RC489.R49T43   1986   616.89'14   85-18653
ISBN 0-87668-616-1

The editors gratefully acknowledge permission to use the following material:

Chapter 2: We acknowledge Sigmund Freud Copyrights, Ltd., The Institute of Psycho-Analysis, and The Hogarth Press, Ltd., for permission to quote from volumes 16 and 20 of *The Standard Edition of the Complete Psychological Works of Sigmund Freud*, translated and edited by James Strachey. Sigmund Freud, *Introductory Lectures on Psychoanalysis*, pp. 42–43, 157–160, 286–296, reprinted by permission of W. W. Norton & Company, Inc., and Allen & Unwin, Ltd.

Chapter 3: "On the Techniques of Resistance and Character Analysis," a selection from *Character Analysis*, by Wilhelm Reich, translated by Vincent R. Carfagno. Copyright © 1945, 1949, 1972 by Mary Boyd Higgins as Trustee of the Wilhelm Reich Infant Trust Fund. Reprinted with permission of Farrar, Straus & Giroux, Inc. First presented at the Tenth International Psychoanalytic Congress, Innsbruck, September 1927.

Chapter 4: Reprinted from *The Ego and the Mechanisms of Defense*, by Anna Freud, by permission of International Universities Press, Inc., copyright 1966 by International Universities Press, Inc. Reprinted by permission of Mark Paterson on behalf of the Executors of Anna Freud.

Chapter 5: Reprinted from *The Technique and Practice of Psychoanalysis*, by Ralph Greenson, by permission of International Universities Press, Inc., copyright 1967 by International Universities Press, Inc. Reprinted by permission of Hildegard Greenson.

Chapter 6: Reprinted from *The Search for the Self*, ed. by Heinz Kohut and Paul Ornstein, pp. 547–561, by permission of International Universities Press, Inc., copyright 1978 by International Universities Press, Inc. Reprinted by permission of Paul H. Ornstein, M. D. Originally presented as a lecture to the German Psychoanalytic Association in Berlin on October 10, 1970.

Manufactured in the United States of America.

To Our Grandchildren

Matthew and Ryan McNamara
Zachary and Joshua Goldman

May they overcome their resistances
to fully utilizing their potential.

Contributors

Peter L. Giovacchini, M.D., is a Clinical Professor of Psychiatry, University of Illinois College of Medicine. He is Director of the Center for Psychoanaytic Studies, Chicago, a former co-editor of the *Annals of Adolescent Psychiatry*, the author of 160 published articles, and the author, co-author, or editor of 17 books. He is in the private practice of psychoanalysis.

George D. Goldman, Ph.D., is a Clinical Professor of Psychology and the Director of Clinical Services, Postdoctoral Psychotherapy Center, Gordon F. Derner Institute of Advanced Psychological Studies, Adelphi University, Garden City, New York, and also maintains a private practice.

James S. Grotstein, M.D., obtained his M.D. from Western Reserve University. He is Training/Supervising Analyst at the Los Angeles Psychoanalytic Institute and Associate Clinical Professor of Psychiatry at UCLA. He is Director of the Interdisciplinary Group for Advanced Studies in Primitive Mental States. His publications have generally been about borderline, schizophrenic, and manic-depressive conditions.

Althea J. Horner, Ph.D., is currently in practice in Los Angeles. She is on the senior faculty of Wright Institute Los Angeles Postgraduate Center, and a member of the National Psychological Association for Psychoanalysis. Dr. Horner is the author of *Object Relations and the Developing Ego in Therapy* and the editor of *Treating the Oedipal Patient in Brief Psychotherapy*.

Morton Kissen, Ph.D., is an Associate Professor of Psychology and Supervisor of Psychotherapy, and Assistant Director, Postdoctoral Program in Psychotherapy, Adelphi University. He is also in private practice.

Robert Langs, M.D., is Program Director of the Lenox Hill Hospital Psycho-therapy Program and founder of The Society for Psychoanalytic Psychother-apy. He is Editor-in-Chief of *The Yearbook of Psychoanalytic Psychotherapy* and the author of more than fifteen volumes that center on the technique of psy-choanalytic psychotherapy, including the recent *Psychotherapy: A Basic Text, The Psychotherapeutic Conspiracy* and *Cure through Madness*. Dr. Langs is a member of the American Psychoanalytic Association and a graduate of the Downstate Psychoanalytic Institute at Brooklyn, now located at the Bellevue Medical Center of New York.

Helen Block Lewis, Ph.D., is Professor Emerita (adjunct) of Psychology at Yale University; Editor of *Psychoanalytic Psychology*, the official publication of the Division of Psychoanalysis of the American Psychological Association; and Past President of the Division of Psychoanalysis, American Psychological Association.

James F. Masterson, M.D., is Director of The Masterson Group and The Character Disorder Foundation, and also adjunct Clinical Professor of Psy-chiatry at Cornell University Medical College and The New York Hospital (Payne Whitney Clinic). He is the author of six books — *The Psychiatric Di-lemma of Adolescence; Psychotherapy of the Borderline Adolescent; From Border-line Adolescent to Functioning Adult: The Test of Time; Psychotherapy of the Borderline Adult: A Developmental Approach; The Narcissistic and Borderline Disorders: An Integrated Approach;* and *Countertransference and Psychotherapeu-tic Technique* — as well as sixty-one papers. He also does private practice in New York City.

Robert A. Mednick, Ph.D., received his psychoanalytic and supervisory training at the Postgraduate Center for Mental Health, and is training in child analysis and therapy at the Gordon F. Derner Institute of Advanced Psychological Studies, Adelphi University, Garden City, New York. Pres-ently he is the Dean of Training at the Institute for Mental Health Education, Englewood, New Jersey, in the programs for psychoanalysis and psychoana-lytic psychotherapy. He is a supervisor and on the faculty at the Long Island Consultation Center, Queens, New York. Topics of his recent publications include the ontogenesis of subjectivity, supervision of psychoanalytic ther-apy, narcissism, and developmental arrest.

Donald Meltzer, M.D., is affiliated with the Roland Harris Educational Trust and the Tavistock Clinic, Tavistock Centre, London, England.

Robert Mendelsohn, Ph.D., is an Associate Professor at the Gordon F. Derner Institute of Advanced Psychological Studies, Adelphi University, Garden City, New York, and practices individual and group psychotherapy in Port Washington, New York. He has a Ph.D. in Clinical Psychology from the University of Massachusetts and a Postdoctoral Certificate in both individual and group psychotherapy from Adelphi University. He is also a Diplomate in Clinical Psychology of the American Board of Professional Psychology.

Donald S. Milman, Ph.D., is a Professor of Psychology and Director, Postdoctoral Program in Psychotherapy, Gordon F. Derner Institute of Advanced Psychological Studies, Adelphi University, Garden City, New York. He also maintains a private practice.

Benjamin Wolstein, Ph.D., is a Clinical Professor of Psychology at the Gordon F. Derner Institute of Advanced Psychological Studies, Adelphi University, Garden City, New York, a Clinical Professor of Psychology at New York University, and a Training and Supervising Analyst at The William Alanson White Institute.

Contents

Acknowledgments   *xiii*

PART I
Basic Concepts of Resistance

1. Introduction to Resistance   *1*

2. Resistance and Repression   *25*
    Sigmund Freud

3. Character Resistances   *41*
    Wilhelm Reich

4. Technique and Resistance   *117*
    Anna Freud

5. Resistance Analysis   *133*
    Ralph Greenson

6. Narcissism as a Resistance and as a Driving Force in
    Psychoanalysis   *167*
    Heinz Kohut

PART II

Specific Techniques

7.   Resistances and the Basic Dimensions of Psychotherapy   *181*
      Robert Langs

8.   Resistance: A Misnomer for Shame and Guilt   *209*
      Helen Block Lewis

9.   Object Relations and Transference Resistance   *227*
      Althea J. Horner

10. Transference and Resistance as Psychic Experience   *249*
      Benjamin Wolstein

11. Resistance to Countertransference   *269*
      Robert Mendelsohn

12. Resistance to Dream Analysis   *279*
      Donald Meltzer

PART III

Resistance in Specific Diagnostic Categories

13. Resistance in Character Disorders   *289*
      Peter L. Giovacchini

14. An Object Relations Perspective on Resistance in Narcissistic
      Patients   *317*
      James S. Grotstein

15. Resistance of the Borderline Patient with a False Self   *339*
      James F. Masterson

16. Resistance in Psychotic Psychopathology   *363*
      Robert A. Mednick

17. The Reluctance to Experience Positive Affects   *381*
      Morton Kissen

Index   *405*

Acknowledgments

The editors wish to thank Mrs. Marge Burgard and Mrs. Mary Gentile-Hamilton for their professionalism and for always being there when we needed them. Dr. Carol Costello and Mr. Stephen Levine have also given invaluable contributions, and we particularly wish to thank them for their help in the initial chapter. In addition, Mr. Bruce Hillowe provided editorial expertise, and the summary material in Chapter 1 is essentially his. Dr. Michael Gorkin and Ms. Linda Nagel also gave very helpful editorial assistance for which we are most grateful.

Dr. Jason Aronson has always been patient and helpful, encouraging us to do the book and patient in waiting to receive the final copy. For this we thank Dr. Aronson, Joan Langs, and the staff of Jason Aronson Inc. In particular, we are grateful to Barbara Sonnenschein, Director of Editorial Production, for that rare combination of personal interest and professional expertise that made the final editing so much easier.

Both editors of this book are Institute of Advanced Psychological Studies professors, and almost everything that has happened in the Institute has, in some way, been touched by Dr. Gordon F. Derner, our late Dean. We are indeed fortunate to have had the privilege of his friendship and professional leadership for these many years at Adelphi University. He will remain alive in our memories.

PART I

Basic Concepts of Resistance

CHAPTER 1

Introduction to Resistance

As the title of this book suggests, our aim is to discuss the elusive topic of resistance and, further, to offer some techniques for dealing with resistance as it emerges in dynamic psychotherapy. We have gathered what we consider to be some of the major contributions of the past, and we have added a considerable number of new contributions from some of today's prominent theorists and clinicians.

In this introductory chapter, we offer some preliminary remarks about the concept of resistance. Here we seek merely to orient the reader in the rather sprawling terrain of resistance theory. We leave the more detailed map to be drawn by the book's contributors. We also offer an outline of the book's contents. The main thesis of each contribution is briefly sketched, highlighting some of the clinical applications that are explicit or implicit in each author's approach. We believe this kind of overview may prove useful as an initial guide to the book.

Resistance, we may say, following other investigators (Greenson 1967, Sandler, Dare, and Holder 1973), comprises all those forces within the patient that oppose the treatment process. This is a simple, comprehensive, and useful definition—one that most clinicians (though not everyone, including some of the contributors to this book) would accept. Inherent in this definition are two important ideas. First, resistance is a *clinical* or *technical* concept. Although the same forces within the patient that oppose treatment certainly may manifest themselves in the patient's day-to-day life outside of treatment, we do not speak of resistance unless these forces exert an impact within the therapy process itself. In a word, resistance is a technical, treatment-specific notion. Second, because the patient's resistance occurs during treatment, it reflects an internal conflict or difficulty that comes into play with a given therapist. In short, all resistances have both an intrapersonal and an interpersonal component.

But why does the patient resist at all? What motivates resistance? The simple and generally accepted answer is that the patient resists in order to avoid pain—real or imagined. Perhaps Shakespeare said it best in *Hamlet*: "[We] rather bear those ills we have than to fly to others that we know not of." Thus, in spite of the patient's wish to cooperate (the "working alliance"), and in spite of the type or extent of his suffering or distress, the patient will nonetheless also bring to bear various forces that oppose the treatment. Dynamically oriented clinicians are aware of this fact, and it is well known that successful treatment hinges upon an effective grappling with and resolution of the patient's resistance(s).

This awareness among psychoanalytically oriented clinicians is about as old as psychoanalysis itself. From his earliest work with hysterics, Freud was concerned with the problem of resistance. It was a subject that he continually returned to in his writings, always adding new and seminal insights which have informed all subsequent work on resistance theory.

Freud introduced the term *resistance* in *Studies in Hysteria* (1893–1895) to describe a phenomenon he had observed during the treatment of a 24-year-old patient, Fräulein Elisabeth von R. In language that catches the excitement of his discovery, Freud describes how he first stumbled across the notion of resistance. It seems that his patient, Elisabeth von R., was not always able or willing to cooperate in reporting her thoughts and memories, as Freud had instructed her to do. At times, though Freud would sit with his hands pressed firmly upon her head, Elisabeth von R. would declare insouciantly that she could think of nothing—her mind was a blank. In turn, Freud found himself wondering why she was failing to remember, failing to cooperate. Freud's eventual and excited conclusion: "A new understanding seemed to open before my eyes when it occurred to me that this must no doubt be the same psychical force that had played a part in the generating of the hysterical symptom and had at that time prevented the pathogenic idea from becoming conscious" (p. 268). The therapeutic task, Freud continued, was to coax the patient into giving up this resistance.

From this early discovery, Freud was gradually to widen his understanding of resistance and the many guises under which it appeared. In his monumental work *The Interpretation of Dreams* (1900), there are numerous references to resistance, particularly resistance that is due to dream censorship. It is in the latter part of this work, during a discussion on why dreams may be forgotten, that Freud enunciates one of the "rules" of psychoanalysis: "*Whatever interrupts the progress of analytic work is a resistance*" (p. 517; italics in original).

Freud's initial emphasis regarding the source of resistance is on those forces that he referred to, generally, as "repression." He was soon to emphasize the notion of transference as the source of some of the most powerful and pervasive resistances. Having adumbrated a notion of transference in the early writings on hysteria, he more fully developed the concept in "Fragment of an Analysis of a Case of Hysteria," or the Dora case (1905). Courageously, he made it clear in that report that his failure to understand the impact of Dora's transference (he had treated Dora in 1900) had undermined the treatment. From this time on, Freud steadily refined his understanding of transference resistances, an understanding that received clear and concise expression in his two technical papers on transference (1912, 1915).

There is a tone of caution and a plea for therapeutic stamina in all these papers: resistances that find their source in repression and transference do not easily fade. The analyst must be patient. He must observe and work through these resistances with the patient slowly and surely. But work through them he *can*. In some of his later work on resistance, however, Freud's optimism begins to wane. In 1914, in one of his technical papers, "Remembering, Repeating and Working Through," Freud had introduced the notion of the repetition compulsion, or the "compulsion to repeat" (p. 150)—a particularly sticky resistance which leads to a kind of psychological stasis. By 1920, in *Beyond the Pleasure Principle*, Freud linked this repetition compulsion to the death instinct—that is, to the individual's instinctive self-destructiveness. What Freud was saying, in part, is that there is a basic, biological undertow within human beings that allows a neurotic pattern, once established, to go on repeating itself compulsively and destructively.

To this already pessimistic note, Freud adds in one of his last papers, "Analysis Terminable and Interminable" (1937), a further bit of therapeutic skepticism. Some of the roots of neurosis, he indicates, are constitutional and immutable. He presents two unresolvable problems relating to the castration complex: a woman's unrealizable wish for a penis, and a man's feeling that his passivity vis-à-vis other men signifies castration. These, Freud believes, are "bedrock" issues that cannot be changed and that lead to resistances that *may* prove unresolvable.

In the span of some 45 years of clinical observation we have just described, Freud approached the topic of resistance in a variety of ways. He never attempted to systematize his ideas on resistance in a paper; the closest he came to providing any overall schema was in an addendum to his book *Inhibitions, Symptoms and Anxiety* (1926), in which he categorizes resistances according to their source. An excerpt from this work is included in the present volume.

Two other early efforts at categorization that deserve mention are those of Deutsch (1939) and Glover (1955). In her paper "A Discussion of Certain Forms of Resistance" (1939), Deutsch suggested a threefold systematization of resistances: (1) transference resistances, (2) resistances that serve as defenses against the recollection of childhood material, and (3) intellectualizing resistances. Her focus was, in essence, on those categories that Freud had referred to as repression-resistances and transference-resistances. In short, Deutsch's effort was clear and concise but did not offer much that was new.

A more descriptive, useful (albeit somewhat simplistic) approach toward categorizing resistances was suggested by Glover in his *Technique of Psycho-Analysis* (1955). There, he differentiated between "crass" and "unobtrusive" resistances. The former included such obvious resistances as rejection of everything the analyst says, assumed stupidity, and circumlocution, as well as lateness, missed appointments, or the breaking off of treatment (i.e., maneuvers that we would today refer to as breaks in the therapeutic frame). The "unobtrusive" resistances comprise those resistances that hide behind a surface compliance with the analyst and the treatment—for example, a repetitious recitation of dream material session after session, or superficial agreement with all of the analyst's interpretations. (Such unobtrusive resistances can remain unnoticed by the analyst for quite some time.)

In addition to those early efforts to categorize resistances, there is one other investigator whose work we would like to mention: namely, Greenson. In his textbook *The Technique and Practice of Psychoanalysis*

(1967), Greenson presents a useful categorization of resistances, as well as some basic rules for working with resistances. Because Greenson's work has probably had the widest impact in the last two decades on analysts in training, a brief outline of some of his main points seems warranted here.

Greenson points out that precisely because resistance theory covers the gamut of technical issues, any single attempt to classify resistances will be incomplete. Instead, he suggests a multifaceted approach, with full awareness that there is overlap among the various classification schemas. He presents five varieties of classification. Resistances, he says, may be classified according to: (1) *source*—that is, Freud's schema (1926) whereby resistances are seen as emanating from the ego, superego, or id; (2) *fixation point*—whether resistances principally reflect oral, anal, phallic, latency, or adolescent concerns; (3) *type of defense*—for example, repression, isolation; (4) *diagnostic category*—those resistances typical in hysterias, obsessional neuroses, depressive neuroses, and so on; and (5) *degree of ego-syntonicity*—the extent to which a resistance is experienced as syntonic or alien by the patient.

In keeping with his overall tendency to focus on practical rather than theoretical concerns, Greenson finds the fifth and last manner of classifying resistances perhaps the most helpful. He points out that resistances need to be made ego-alien before effective analysis can be accomplished. In the beginning of treatment—that is, until a reliable working alliance is established—it is advisable to work only with ego-alien resistances. Later in the treatment it becomes possible to clarify, confront, and interpret ego-syntonic resistances, with the aim of rendering them ego-alien and ultimately working them through.

Greenson's discussion of resistance is replete with such helpful procedural guides. Of special use are three rules of technique that Greenson sets forth (pp. 136–145), rules that he intends "not [as] commands or laws but rather guideposts." These rules are: analyze resistance before content, analyze ego before id, and begin with the surface. Familiar to all analysts, these rules have been stated or implied by a number of previous investigators, such as A. Freud and Reich (selections from their writings are included in this volume). The strength of Greenson's work is the clear and instructive manner in which he delineates how these rules may be applied in actual clinical situations with patients.

Since Greenson's 1967 volume, there has been a widening of our understanding of resistances that occur in the treatment of certain categories of patients. The focus of Greenson's volume is on the psychoanalytic treatment of neuroses and higher-level character disorders. Today, with the "widening scope of psychoanalysis," there is a focus on more disturbed and difficult patients—those with borderline and narcissistic conditions. Precisely what technical procedures are most efficacious in treating these conditions is a subject of much debate, and this debate can be heard repeatedly in many of the chapters in this volume. Indeed, one of the aims of our book is to provide some of the current approaches to resistance theory and technique in the treatment of these more primitive disorders. The reader is directed, specifically, to the chapters of Kohut, Giovacchini, Grotstein, Masterson, and Mednick.

Along with the more current material, we have provided some of the classic literature on resistance theory from S. Freud, A. Freud, and Reich. There are also chapters that focus on specific aspects of resistance, such as transference (Horner), countertransference (Mendelsohn), affective components (Kissen), and the technical problems in dream analysis (Meltzer). Finally, there are provocative and challenging approaches to resistance theory (Lewis, Langs, and Wolstein).

The following section contains outlines of each of the chapters in this book.

SIGMUND FREUD:
RESISTANCE AND REPRESSION

In *Inhibitions, Symptoms and Anxiety* (1926), Freud suggests a classification of resistances according to source. Employing a structural model, he distinguishes five types of resistances—three of which emanate from the ego, one from the superego, and one from the id. Those from the ego are *repression-resistances*—those due to the ego's defenses; *transference-resistances*—those due to the various types of transference displacements from past to present objects; and *gains from illness*—those resistances that issue from advantages or secondary gains from illness. From the id come *id-resistances*—those that derive from impulses of the libido and that necessitate "working through." The superego spawns *superego-resistances*, which derive from guilt and the need for punishment.

Clinical Applications

1. Resistance will be apparent when the fundamental technical rule to "say everything" is not followed.

2. Expect resistance to alter in intensity during an analysis, to become more intense as a new topic is broached and to fade when the topic has been resolved.

3. Ego-resistances, to the extent that they are unconscious, should be directly brought to consciousness by the therapist.

4. When conscious, ego resistances can be overcome through logical argument, by promising the ego rewards for, and explaining the advantages of, giving them up.

5. Id-resistance, or the compulsion to repeat, can be overcome only by an extensive working-through process.

6. Freud was least optimistic about overcoming superego-resistance, which he later ascribed to an unconscious sense of guilt, primary masochism, and, ultimately, the death instinct.

WILHELM REICH: CHARACTER RESISTANCES

Reich's contribution to modern theories of resistance is second only to Freud's. In this chapter, from *Character Analysis* (1933), Reich outlines the concepts of character resistance, such as character armor and the layering of resistances, and introduces the technique of character analysis. When the technique of character analysis is used consistently and systematically, character resistances — manifested in a patient's specific mannerisms and enacted in the transference — become not an obstruction but, rather, the most powerful vehicle of analysis. Only after the hierarchy of resistances has been confronted, revealed, and resolved can affect-laden infantile experiences be spontaneously recalled and constructively interpreted. Character analysis is a provocative, sometimes dangerous process. Character resistances must be consistently and persistently stressed, a process as disagreeable and unpleasant for the patient as it is powerful. Patients should be made aware at the out-set of analysis of the foreseeable difficulties.

Clinical Applications

1. The sequence of character analysis is as follows: first, the patient is simply made aware *that* he is resisting; second, he is told *how* he is resisting; finally, when character resistances are resolved, the patient gains insight into *what* he is resisting, that is, the underlying id impulse.

2. The principal resistance usually proceeds from a specific character trait (for example, deceptiveness, incoherence, emotional blockage), and it is this trait, as it is exhibited in the transference, that the analyst should isolate and repeatedly put before the patient until it becomes ego-alien.

3. Character resistances are affectively evident in the negative transference. These strong resistances are often founded in a defense against the person of the analyst himself. One technique Reich uses to relieve their blockage is to urge the patient to give a description of the analyst's "person."

4. Affect, not content, gives the analyst the correct order for uncovering the layered resistances.

ANNA FREUD: TECHNIQUE AND RESISTANCE

Anna Freud's classic work *The Ego and the Mechanisms of Defense* (1936), an excerpt from which is included in this volume, contributed significantly to the understanding of resistance. In this work, she adds to our understanding of both the defenses and their functions and the nature of resistance and resistance analysis. She suggests that we can-not interpret the content of the id without understanding the resis-tances and the ego defenses used to keep the id content hidden. Con-versely, exclusive analysis of the resistances increases understanding of the ego but sacrifices knowledge of the content of the id. Anna Freud disputes Reich's (1933) concept of "consistent analysis of resis-tance." The consistent analysis of resistance—the character armor—is of primary importance, she states, "only when we can detect no trace at all of the present conflict between ego, instinct and affect" (p. 33). She adds that analysis of the resistance need not refer only to analysis of the armor plating but, rather, "should apply to that of all resistances."

Clinical Applications

1. Ego defenses may become transference resistances. This "transference of defense" occurs when the patient repeats in therapy defensive measures that he employed in childhood to ward off threatening id impulses.

2. Patients oppose interpretations of resistance to the transference more than they do interpretations of the transference of libidinal impulses because the former are ego-syntonic, whereas the latter are readily experienced as ego-alien.

3. Acting out, observed when the patient ceases to obey the rules of treatment or when he enacts in his daily life the instinctual impulses and defensive reactions aroused in the transference, should be restricted as far as possible by interpretations and, if necessary, by the imposition of nonanalytic prohibitions.

4. Resistance in children is revealed not so much by inhibitions in their play during play therapy, as by transformations of affect (for example, reversal, displacement, repression). With children, free association is not a useful way to arrive at a clear conceptualization of their individual internal world. Other methods of observing the id impulses in children exist, however, such as interpretations of their drawings, dreams, and play.

RALPH GREENSON: RESISTANCE ANALYSIS

Ralph Greenson's basic and influential text, *The Technique and Practice of Psychoanalysis*, contains valuable insights and illustrations that elucidate how analysts—above all, classical analysts—work with resistances. In the sections excerpted here, Dr. Greenson discusses such topics as the concepts of resistance and defense, and the function of transference as resistance, and provides some helpful rules for working with resistance. The underlying theme is that resistance analysis (and, particularly, transference resistance analysis) comprise the heart and soul of psychoanalytic treatment. A master of technique, Greenson provides numerous case vignettes that highlight the various and intricate forms that resistances take.

Clinical Applications

Greenson's thumbnail sketch for working with resistance is: recognize the resistance, demonstrate it to the patient, clarify it, interpret it, and then work it through. The case vignettes give a brief but revealing sense of how a skilled analyst in the classical tradition might work with a given resistance, in a given patient, at a given moment.

HEINZ KOHUT: NARCISSISM AS A RESISTANCE AND AS A DRIVING FORCE IN PSYCHOANALYSIS

In expanding the applicability of psychoanalysis, Heinz Kohut has also reformulated many of its concepts, including resistance. Issues involving the patient's narcissistic vulnerability may arise as *nonspecific* resistances in any analysis, since treatment as a whole, regardless of pathology, may offend the pride of the analysand by contradicting his fantasy of independence. In patients with narcissistic personality disorders, *specific* resistances against the formation and continuation of a narcissistic transference often emerge: the patient anticipates and fears a reenactment during the analysis of the rejection of his narcissistic needs, as occurred with the original early childhood self-objects.

Clinical Applications

1. Even in analyses with neurotic patients who develop classical transference neuroses, a negative transference may be more indicative of feelings of narcissistic injury than of the reactivation of infantile conflicts involving oedipal issues.

2. In the early stages of treatment, the analyst should not focus on the unconscious repressed conflict revealed by the content of a patient's parapraxis. Instead he should focus on the patient's narcissistic injury, explaining to him that the mere fact that he committed a parapraxis constituted a narcissistic injury and aroused feelings of relative helplessness.

3. The analyst should admit (or at least not deny) that a patient's attempt to hurt him emotionally has succeeded, and should then express his sincere understanding of the patient's feelings of vulnerability and helplessness that motivated the attack.

ROBERT LANGS:
RESISTANCES AND THE
BASIC DIMENSIONS OF PSYCHOTHERAPY

Robert Langs's original theoretical and technical contribution encompasses a redefinition of resistance to include anything done by either patient or therapist that does not promote the growth of a meaningful communicative network between them. This approach distinguishes gross *behavioral* resistances—for example, lateness— from *communicative* resistances, which involve the patient's failure to provide meaningful communications for interpretation. In general, resistances and counterresistances arise when therapist or patient distorts critical areas of the psychotherapeutic relationship by the following: deviating from the therapeutic frame; relating in a pathologically symbiotic or autistic form, or parasitically; attempting cure through action, evacuation, or merger rather than insight; failing to establish a communicative network; failing to recognize dynamic and genetic issues, particularly in the transference and countertransference; and failing to attend to narcissistic needs.

Clinical Applications

1. Gross behavioral resistances call for (a) rectification of any break in the therapeutic frame that may be contributing to the resistance, and (b) interpretation of the behaviors as indirect communications.

2. With communicative resistances, the therapist should remain silent, hold the patient, rectify any counterresistance, and wait until the patient relaxes his communicative defensiveness.

3. Resistances may be analyzed only when patient and therapist are relating in a healthy symbiotic way. It is only when the therapist offers this kind of relatedness that he is not supporting on an unconscious level the resistant tendencies of the patient.

HELEN BLOCK LEWIS: RESISTANCE: A MISNOMER FOR SHAME AND GUILT

Helen Block Lewis takes the iconoclastic position that the classical concept of resistance should be abandoned as a therapeutic dead end, and as a vestige of Freud's individualistic and instinctual metapsychology. Clinical phenomena called resistances are more constructively analyzed by looking at the affective states of shame and guilt that underlie them. So-called resistances are interpersonal communications and represent an attempt by the patient to remain affectionally related to the therapist in the face of some threatened breakage of the interpersonal bond.

Clinical Applications

1. Resistances should be analyzed as states of shame and guilt, and as natural reactions that accompany the breaking of affectional bonds, rather than as the patient's attempt to resist the forces of health.
2. The patient's feelings of shame toward the therapist (for example, at being helped) give rise to retaliatory, hostile, and derogatory thoughts about therapy and the therapist ("therapy does not work"), which in turn lead to "shameful" images of the self as patient ("I'm too sick to be helped").
3. A patient's indifference to an interpretation may cover shame, and may succeed in evoking shame in the therapist.

ALTHEA J. HORNER: OBJECT RELATIONS AND TRANSFERENCE RESISTANCE

Although Althea Horner's view of resistance, like that of Lewis, includes interpersonal and affective components, she nonetheless believes the primary source of resistance is the transference. Early object relational issues, and the psychic dangers and infantile wishes associated with the inner representational world, will be relived in the transference; it is the working through of transference issues that constitutes the heart of therapy. And this is so, she indicates, in the treatment of more disturbed patients, just as with patients with oedipally based disorders.

Clinical Applications

1. Because of severe separation anxiety and panic that accompanies loss, some borderline patients may protect their connection with the therapist with a pervasive transference resistance marked by an assiduous clinging to a positive attitude, and by an attempt to avoid any change in the status quo.

2. In patients with a false-self organization, a positive transference may be both an aspect of the therapeutic alliance and a manifestation of transference resistance. If the therapist participates in an alliance with the false self by, for instance, playing the role of helper, rescuer, or encourager, he will be colluding with the resistance.

3. A positive transference becomes contaminated and the source of resistance when a patient maintains, often secretly, the fantasy of a special preferred relationship with the therapist.

4. Dangers to the boundaries of the self must not be ignored and resistances overridden by an exhortive struggle or an indiscriminate therapeutic attitude of "going for affect." If structural deficits are not tended to first, adverse reactions to treatment are possible.

BENJAMIN WOLSTEIN: TRANSFERENCE AND RESISTANCE AS PSYCHIC EXPERIENCE

Benjamin Wolstein provides a metapsychological framework broad enough to encompass classical, ego-interpersonal or object-relational, and contemporary experiential theories of resistance. He finds in the opposition of transference and resistance a self-creating dialectical movement. Transference is the emergence of an individual's unique unconscious experience into conscious, social, ego-interpersonal behavior, and active movement outward from within. It represents a spontaneous striving of the psychic center of the self to individuate its uniqueness in human relations, to make itself known to self and other together. Resistance is the turning of the dynamic of transference back on itself, a reactive movement inward from without. Whereas transference is an attempt to see others through the self and evokes the anxiety of self-individuation, resistance indicates a conflict in seeing the self through others and evokes the anxiety of other-relatedness. Transference and resistance, along with anxiety, constitute the self-defining core of psychoanalytic experience.

Clinical Applications

Wolstein's thought-provoking metapsychological – indeed, philosophical – speculations may be transformed by the practicing psychoanalyst for direct and specific clinical application to the individual case. They provide a frame of reference for processing the patient–therapist interaction in a concrete way.

ROBERT MENDELSOHN:
RESISTANCE TO COUNTERTRANSFERENCE

Robert Mendelsohn investigates the topic of countertransference resistance. For him, all countertransference reactions have objective as well as subjective aspects. Thus, countertransference, like transference, is inherent in the treatment process; moreover, it is not simply a hindrance to this process. Countertransference resistance, however, is a hindrance, inasmuch as it involves the analyst's resistance to experiencing the totality of the therapeutic interaction, including the totality of his reactions to his patient.

Clinical Applications

1. Because of the dual subjective-objective nature of countertransference, even so-called objective countertransferences – responses realistically induced in the analyst by the patient's transference – will differ from analyst to analyst.

2. The analyst will resist countertransference reactions in his own characteristic ways, using his own specific character defenses. Thus, for example, a patient's attempt to cure the analyst may be misperceived (and perhaps seen as the patient's resistance) due to the influence of the analyst's own character, resistances, and transferences.

3. By creating an "internal work-space" where he holds and molds his patient, the analyst can protect both himself and his patient from destructive resistances as they arise in the therapy.

DONALD MELTZER:
RESISTANCE TO DREAM ANALYSIS

Donald Meltzer explores resistances to dream analysis on the part of patients and therapists. Drawing on the works of Klein and Bion, Meltzer views dreams as an actual visual record of the transactions of narcissism and object relations in the depths of the mind. The patient's resistance to dream analysis is manifested in an inability to remember dreams and is due to either the evacuation or the acting out of psychoanalytic experiences. Therapists resist understanding dreams because of fear of invasion by the patient's projective identifications, fear of confusion, or an intolerance of the inherently impotent role of psychotherapist.

Clinical Applications

1. In analyses where patient and analyst are frequently at loggerheads or where the patient perceives basic differences between himself and the analyst (e.g., sex, culture, education, interests, therapeutic intentions), the patient may fail to report *remembered* dreams, and come up with an adolescent-like rationalization for the secrecy ("You would only misunderstand").

2. The evacuation of thought and memory in some psychotic and borderline patients is also evident in their inability to remember dreams.

3. Forgetting the manifest content of a patient's dream, veering off the dream and following only the associations, or finding the dream so powerful that associations cannot be attended to are all signs of the analyst's resistance to dream analysis.

4. The therapist's expectation that he can use dreams to persuade his patient or as a source of "mutative interpretations" will inevitably be disappointed, especially when the patient has a tendency to deny psychic reality, or the therapist has not accepted his fundamental impotence vis-à-vis the patient's psychic structures. Sometimes this diappointment may dampen the analyst's interest in working with dreams.

5. The appearance of a particular patient in the analyst's own dreams may indicate that the patient has forced the analyst to deal

with personality issues that have not been resolved in his personal analysis.

PETER L. GIOVACCHINI:
RESISTANCE IN CHARACTER DISORDERS

Central to Peter Giovacchini's chapter is the notion that resistance may emerge from different psychic levels, depending upon the degree of pathology; and, further, that the analytic setting should be adjusted to accommodate resistances that are essential for the patient's self-cohesion.

The primary attributes of analysis should not be compromised (that is, an intrapsychic deterministic focus with resolution of the transference and repetition compulsion through interpretation), but resistances to the secondary, formal attributes of analysis (that is, a patient who lies on the couch and free associates while a neutral, nonjudgmental, and calm analyst does not give advice or necessarily answer questions) should be respected.

Clinical Applications

1. Initially accepting the resistances to formal psychoanalytic procedures of a character-disordered patient may be crucial to establishing a holding environment.

2. Schizoid patients may balk at using a couch due to a need to maintain control and a fear of being in someone else's power. They may not see a difference between symbolic submission and the actual act of lying down.

3. Narcissistic patients, whose fragile sense of self is maintained by constant attention and attentiveness, may resist lying on the couch where they cannot see the analyst. They will often criticize the analyst's neutrality and relative lack of identity, too, due to their fears of isolation and abandonment.

4. Patients whose mothers were emotionally passive and uninvolved may suffer the same infantile deprivation in an ordinary analytic relationship, which is characterized by toned-down responses from the analyst. To prevent these patients from withdrawing, and to

make a transference possible by setting up a contrast to the infantile environment, a more active therapeutic approach is required.

JAMES S. GROTSTEIN: AN OBJECT RELATIONS PERSPECTIVE ON RESISTANCE IN NARCISSISTIC PATIENTS

James Grotstein uses an object-relational model to explain the manifestations and intrapsychic determinants of resistance in narcissistic patients. These patients develop resistances when they feel in danger of being overwhelmed by fears of dependency, and when they try to regain states of bonding with the object. Resistances may take several forms, such as attempts to destroy, alter, or render unintelligible inner thought processes or the communicative link to the therapist; the personification of resistance as a powerful inner alien being to whom the patient is held hostage; group resistances such as cult allegiance; and encapsulation and confusion.

Clinical Applications

1. When the therapist has difficulty thinking about his patient, or perhaps even feels he is being driven crazy by the patient's elliptical associations, it may be the result of the patient's fragmenting attack on his own thoughts and feelings.

2. Chronic resistance in the form of personification emerges as a split-off inner companion, or twin-self, that knows the patient best and soothes and pities him but also fights for its own life, fearing the patient's hope, progress, and happiness. Confrontation with this resistance will ensue once the therapist defines and isolates it.

3. Resistance may take the form of intense loyalty to an internal family, group, powerful personages, or a cult. In the patient's mind, to get well equates with forswearing vows of eternal bonding and therefore will result in death or persecution.

4. Obsessive compulsive, phobic, paranoid, anorectic, and narcissistic patients tend to "encapsulate" their resistances into autistically protective selves. Hysteric, borderline, and depressed patients tend to intertwine with the object in "confusional" resistances.

JAMES F. MASTERSON: RESISTANCE OF THE BORDERLINE PATIENT WITH A FALSE SELF

James Masterson examines resistances arising from both character and narcissistic psychopathologies in borderline patients. The resistances of the borderline patient with a false self defend against thoughts, wishes, and feelings that might lead to individuation and expression of the true self. Such individuation would lead to abandonment by the withdrawing object relations unit (WORU) and a consequent deep depression. Instead of having formed a true self through experimentation and interplay between an evolving self and the environment, the borderline patient has compensated by developing a false self in order to meet the early expectations of a maternal object who was hostile to any separation-individuation and rewarded clinging and compliance. Thus, to adapt and defend against the abandonment depression, the false self has entered into a pathologic ego alliance with the rewarding object relations unit (RORU).

Clinical Applications

1. The therapist must avoid conveying therapeutic expectations that may become a vehicle for the development by the borderline patient of a new false self based on the perceived wishes of the therapist.
2. As the RORU–pathologic ego alliance that emerges in the subtle but pervasive clinging in the transference is confronted by the therapist, the patient shifts his clinging and acting-out behavior elsewhere — usually to love relationships in his life.
3. Acting out of the RORU fantasy will revolve around the patient's fantasy that "They [the therapist or outside love partners] want me; I want to be wanted; I don't want me but they do."
4. As he begins to individuate, the patient may project the WORU onto a love partner by inducing the partner to criticize or demean him. Thus, he avoids the abandonment depression that would ensue if the negative feelings of the WORU were internalized.
5. When the negative feelings of the WORU are exposed and contained, the patient's abandonment depression and inability to accept himself will emerge, and early memories will be recaptured.

ROBERT A. MEDNICK:
RESISTANCE IN PRESTRUCTURAL (PSYCHOTIC) PSYCHOPATHOLOGY

With Robert Mednick's chapter we move to a different theoretical framework, self-psychology, and to an examination of resistance in the most severe psychopathological category: psychosis. Using Stolorow's and Kohut's theory, Mednick identifies two psychic patterns that are the primary sources of resistance in psychoses. The first source is the patient's dread of repeating the loss of the archaic self-object — a dread that is activated as the therapist becomes established as a self-object in the patient's mental life. The second source of resistance is due to prestructural weakness and involves the patient's feeling of disequilibrium when he experiences too intense or too rapid mergers and/or separations from the self-object bond. Thus, resistances occur as part and parcel of the progressive internalization of the therapist as self-object and serve to avoid threats of self-dissolution or loss of the self-object bond.

Clinical Applications

1. Whereas in neuroses the therapist interprets what the patient is trying to ward off defensively, in psychoses he should instead focus on the state the patient is trying to achieve, and verbally empathize with this striving. The essential task is to make the therapist–patient self-object tie more a source of strength than of danger.

2. Resistances in the form of action may be viewed as a type of organizing metaphor. For instance, pacings between the door of the consultation room and the chair may represent attraction to the therapeutic re-creation of the archaic self-object tie alternating with terrifying dread of its reexperienced loss.

3. Ruptures in the self-object tie between therapist and patient, and consequent resistances, may be caused by even simple comments that impose a sense of separateness on the patient, for instance, "How are *you* doing?"

4. When the therapist accurately empathizes with and articulates the psychotic patient's experience, this may be felt by the patient as a disequilibrating merger.

MORTON KISSEN: THE RELUCTANCE TO EXPERIENCE POSITIVE AFFECTS

Morton Kissen discusses a pervasive, underlying resistance that may be seen across the diagnostic spectrum. A reluctance to experience positive affects is an ego-syntonic and characterological form of resistance in all patients but it is especially evident in those who are more primitively fixated. Viewed structurally, the source of the resistance is superego pathology. In an object-relational context, its source is an identification with, and fear of separation from, a damaged parental introject. The resistance plays a significant role in eating disorders, anhedonia, and paranoid-masochistic character pathology. And, in general, it appears in the seeking of unpleasant experiences, in discomfort following personal compliments, and in certain negative therapeutic reactions.

Clinical Applications

1. Whereas neurotic patients manifest negative therapeutic reactions toward the end of psychotherapy, more primitive patients manifest such reactions continuously throughout treatment.

2. The therapist's task is to remind the patient repeatedly of the resistive and defensive nature of his painful self-experiences since most patients have never considered that their depressive affect might be an anhedonic avoidance of positive pleasurable affects. The reminders will eventually allow the patient to internalize the therapist's optimistic attitudes.

3. Masochistic characters should be denied expressions of pity which would, in effect, join them in their demonstrations of inadequacy. Paradigmatic interventions of a humorous, playful, or ironic nature can aid in resolving masochistic resistances; they can also serve as a constructive means of utilizing and containing the unpleasant countertransference feelings (projective identifications) induced by masochistic patients.

CONCLUSION

Since Freud's initial work in the 1890s, a somewhat scattered approach has tended to characterize the bulk of writings on resistance theory.

There has been a lack of central, coherent, and organized models which can be used as a single frame of reference for understanding resistances. Indeed, nearly 100 years later, a single agreed-upon perspective still does not exist. To be sure, almost all writing on technique involves a discussion of *some* resistances. Transference resistances, for instance, have been discussed at great length, both in Freud's era and among present-day analysts. And, in the last three decades, countertransference factors which contribute to resistances have received considerable attention. Overall schemas, however, attempting to categorize all types of resistance, have been in short supply.

Of necessity, therefore, we do not attempt that approach in this volume. However, this compilation of papers and essays on resistance is the first of its kind in print. Both theoretical and technical concerns are addressed, and it is our aim and hope that the dynamically oriented clinician will find these chapters both thought-provoking and useful in his or her daily work with a wide variety of patients.

REFERENCES

Breuer, J., and Freud, S. (1893–1895). Studies on hysteria. *Standard Edition* 2. London: Hogarth Press, 1955.

Deutsch, H. (1939). A discussion on certain forms of resistance. *International Journal of Psycho-Analysis* 20:72–83.

Freud, A. (1936). *The Ego and the Mechanisms of Defense.* New York: International Universities Press, 1946.

Freud, S. (1900). The interpretation of dreams. *Standard Edition* 4/5.

_____ (1905). Fragment of an analysis of a case of hysteria. *Standard Edition* 7:1–122.

_____ (1912). The dynamics of transference. *Standard Edition* 12:97–108.

_____ (1914). Remembering, repeating and working-through. *Standard Edition* 12:145–186.

_____ (1915). Observations on transference-love. *Standard Edition* 12:157–171.

_____ (1920). Beyond the pleasure principle. *Standard Edition* 18:3–64.

_____ (1926). Inhibitions, symptoms and anxiety. *Standard Edition* 20:77–175.

_____ (1937). Analysis terminable and interminable. *Standard Edition* 23:209–253.

Glover, E. (1955). *The Technique of Psycho-Analysis*. London: Balliere, Tindall and Cox.

Greenson, R. (1967). *The Technique and Practice of Psychoanalysis*. New York: International Universities Press.

Reich, Wilhelm (1933). *Character Analysis*. 2nd ed. New York: Orgone Institute Press, 1945.

Sandler, J., Dare, C., and Holder, A. (1973). *The Patient and the Analyst*. New York: International Universities Press.

CHAPTER 2

Resistance and Repression

Sigmund Freud

Although some aspects of the theory of resistance have evolved over time, as we've seen from the previous chapter, the fundamental structure of resistance has remained basically unaltered from the beginning. Resistance is part and parcel of psychoanalytic work. Freud's indication that resistance goes step-by-step with the analytic process is clearly shown in the following excerpt from his Introductory Lectures on Psycho-Analysis *(1916–1917). In this presentation the basic guidelines that still exist today are considered: the crucial place of resistance in psychoanalytic work, its relation to and difference from defense, and the fundamental problem of resistance as it is manifested and dealt with in transference.*

RESISTANCE AND REPRESSION[1]

Ladies and gentlemen,—Before we can make any further progress in our understanding of the neuroses, we stand in need of some fresh observations. Here we have two such, both of which are very remarkable and at the time when they were made were very surprising. Our

---

[1][The essence of Freud's views on repression is already given in his contribution to *Studies on Hysteria* (1895d), *Standard Ed.*, 2, 268–70. He gave a similar description of his discovery in his history of the psychoanalytic movement (1914d), ibid., 14, 16. An account of the development of Freud's theory of repression will be found in the Editor's Note to his metapsychological paper on the subject (1915d), *Standard Ed.*, 14, 143 ff. – a paper which, together with Section IV of the paper on 'The Unconscious' (1915e), ibid, 180 ff., contains Freud's deepest reflections on the question.]

discussions of last year will, it is true, have prepared you for both of them.[2]

In the first place, then, when we undertake to restore a patient to health, to relieve him of the symptoms of his illness, he meets us with a violent and tenacious resistance, which persists throughout the whole length of the treatment. This is such a strange fact that we cannot expect it to find much credence. It is best to say nothing about it to the patient's relatives, for they invariably regard it as an excuse on our part for the length or failure of our treatment. The patient, too, produces all the phenomena of this resistance without recognizing it as such, and if we can induce him to take our view of it and to reckon with its existence, that already counts as a great success. Only think of it! The patient, who is suffering so much from his symptoms and is causing those about him to share his sufferings, who is ready to undertake so many sacrifices in time, money, effort and self-discipline in order to be freed from those symptoms—we are to believe that this same patient puts up a struggle in the interest of his illness against the person who is helping him. How improbable such an assertion must sound! Yet it is true; and when its improbability is pointed out to us, we need only reply that it is not without analogies. A man who has gone to the dentist because of an unbearable toothache will nevertheless try to hold the dentist back when he approaches the sick tooth with a pair of forceps.

The patient's resistance is of very many sorts, extremely subtle and often hard to detect; and it exhibits protean changes in the forms in which it manifests itself. The doctor must be distrustful and remain on his guard against it.

In psycho-analytic therapy we make use of the same technique that is familiar to you from dream-interpretation. We instruct the patient to put himself into a state of quiet, unreflecting self-observation, and to report to us whatever internal perceptions he is able to make—feelings, thoughts, memories—in the order in which they occur to him. At the same time we warn him expressly against giving way to any motive which would lead him to make a selection among these associations or to exclude any of them, whether on the ground that it is too *disagreeable* or too *indiscreet* to say, or that it is too *unimportant* or *irrelevant*, or that it is *nonsensical* and need not be said. We urge him always to follow only the surface of his consciousness and to leave aside any criticism of

---

[2][The concept of resistance had been introduced in Lecture VII.]

what he finds, whatever shape that criticism may take; and we assure him that the success of the treatment, and above all its duration, depends on the conscientiousness with which he obeys this fundamental technical rule of analysis.[3] We already know from the technique of dream-interpretation that the associations giving rise to the doubts and objections I have just enumerated are precisely the ones that invariably contain the material which leads to the uncovering of the unconscious. [Cf. Lecture VII.]

The first thing we achieve by setting up this fundamental technical rule is that it becomes the target for the attacks of the resistance. The patient endeavours in every sort of way to extricate himself from its provisions. At one moment he declares that nothing occurs to him, at the next that so many things are crowding in on him that he cannot get hold of anything. Presently we observe with pained astonishment that he has given way first to one and then to another critical objection: he betrays this to us by the long pauses that he introduces into his remarks. He then admits that there is something he really cannot say — he would be ashamed to; and he allows this reason to prevail against his promise. Or he says that something has occurred to him, but it concerns another person and not himself and is therefore exempt from being reported. Or, what has now occurred to him is really too unimportant, too silly and senseless: I cannot possibly have meant him to enter into thoughts like that. So it goes on in innumerable variations, and one can only reply that 'to say everything' really does mean 'to say everything'.

---

[3][Freud had already stated the rule in connection with the interpreting of dreams in Lecture VII. He first laid it down in Chapter II of *The Interpretation of Dreams* (1900a), *Standard Ed.*, 4, 100–2, and again in his contribution to a book of Löwenfeld's (Freud, 1904a [1903], *Standard Ed.*, 7, 251). The actual term 'fundamental rule' was first used in the technical paper on 'The Dynamics of Transference' (1912b), *Standard Ed.*, 12, 107, where an Editor's footnote gives some other early references. Perhaps the fullest account is in another technical paper, 'On Beginning the Treatment' (1913c), ibid., 134–6. Among later mentions may be noted a passage near the beginning of Chapter IV of the *Autobiographical Study* (1925d), ibid., 20, 40–1, and an interesting allusion to the deeper reasons for the obstacles to obeying the rule, towards the end of Chapter VI of *Inhibitions, Symptoms and Anxiety* (1926d), ibid., 121. In the latter passage, in the course of a discussion of the part played by the defensive process of 'isolation' in ordinary directed thinking, Freud mentions especially the difficulties felt by obsessional neurotics in this connection.]

One hardly comes across a single patient who does not make an attempt at reserving some region or other for himself so as to prevent the
treatment from having access to it. A man, whom I can only describe
as of the highest intelligence, kept silence in this way for weeks on end
about an intimate love-affair, and, when he was called to account for
having broken the sacred rule, defended himself with the argument
that he thought this particular story was his private business. Analytic
treatment does not, of course, recognize any such right of asylum. Suppose that in a town like Vienna the experiment was made of treating a
square such as the Hohe Markt, or a church like St. Stephen's, as
places where no arrests might be made, and suppose we then wanted to
catch a particular criminal. We could be quite sure of finding him in
the sanctuary. I once decided to allow a man, on whose efficiency
much depended in the external world, the right to make an exception
of this kind because he was bound under his oath of office not to make
communications about certain things to another person. He, it is true,
was satisfied with the outcome; but I was not. I determined not to repeat an attempt under such conditions.

Obsessional neurotics understand perfectly how to make the technical rule almost useless by applying their over-conscientiousness and
doubts to it.[4] Patients suffering from anxiety hysteria occasionally succeed in carrying the rule *ad absurdum* by producing only associations
which are so remote from what we are in search of that they contribute
nothing to the analysis. But it is not my intention to induct you into
the handling of these technical difficulties. It is enough to say that in
the end, through resolution and perseverance, we succeed in extorting
a certain amount of obedience to the fundamental technical rule from
the resistance—which thereupon jumps over to another sphere.

It now appears as an *intellectual* resistance, it fights by means of arguments and exploits all the difficulties and improbabilities which normal but uninstructed thinking finds in the theories of analysis. It is
now our fate to hear from this single voice all the criticisms and objections which assail our ears in a chorus in the scientific literature of the
subject. And for this reason none of the shouts that reach us from outside sound unfamiliar. It is a regular storm in a tea-cup. But the patient
is willing to be argued with; he is anxious to get us to instruct him,
teach him, contradict him, introduce him to the literature, so that he
can find further instruction. He is quite ready to become an adherent

---

[4][Cf. the end of the last footnote.]

of psycho-analysis—on condition that analysis spares him personally. But we recognize this curiosity as a resistance, as a diversion from our particular tasks, and we repel it. In the case of an obsessional neurotic we have to expect special tactics of resistance. He will often allow the analysis to proceed on its way uninhibited, so that it is able to shed an ever-increasing light upon the riddle of his illness. We begin to wonder in the end, however, why this enlightenment is accompanied by no practical advance, no diminution of the symptoms. We are then able to realize that resistance has withdrawn on to the doubt belonging to the obsessional neurosis and from that position is successfully defying us. It is as though the patient were saying: 'Yes, that's all very nice and interesting, and I'll be very glad to go on with it further. It would change my illness a lot if it were true. But I don't in the least believe that it *is* true; and, so long as I don't believe it, it makes no difference to my illness.' Things can proceed like this for a long time, till finally one comes up against this uncommitted attitude itself, and the decisive struggle then breaks out.[5]

Intellectual resistances are not the worst: one always remains superior to them. But the patient also knows how to put up resistances, without going outside the framework of the analysis, the overcoming of which is among the most difficult of technical problems. Instead of remembering, he *repeats* attitudes and emotional impulses from his early life which can be used as a resistance against the doctor and the treatment by means of what is known as 'transference'.[6] If the patient is a man, he usually extracts this material from his relation to his father, into whose place he fits the doctor, and in that way he makes resistances out of his efforts to become independent in himself and in his judgements, out of his ambition, the first aim of which was to do things as well as his father or to get the better of him, or out of his unwillingness to burden himself for the second time in his life with a load of gratitude. Thus at times one has an impression that the patient has entirely replaced his better intention of making an end to his illness by the alternative one of putting the doctor in the wrong, of making him realize his impotence and of triumphing over him. Women

---

[5][The part played by doubt in cases of obsessional neurosis is referred to in Lecture XVII. The necessity for special technical methods in dealing with such cases was mentioned by Freud a little later in his Budapest Congress paper (1919*a*), *Standard Ed.*, 17, 166.]

[6][Lecture XXVII is devoted to a full discussion of this phenomenon.]

have a masterly gift for exploiting an affectionate, erotically tinged transference to the doctor for the purposes of resistance. If this attachment reaches a certain height, all their interest in the immediate situation in the treatment and all the obligations they undertook at its commencement vanish; their jealousy, which is never absent, and their exasperation at their inevitable rejection, however considerately expressed, are bound to have a damaging effect on their personal understanding with the doctor and so to put out of operation one of the most powerful motive forces of the analysis.

Resistances of this kind should not be one-sidedly condemned. They include so much of the most important material from the patient's past and bring it back in so convincing a fashion that they become some of the best supports of the analysis if a skilful technique knows how to give them the right turn. Nevertheless, it remains a remarkable fact that this material is always in the service of the resistance to begin with and brings to the fore a *façade* that is hostile to the treatment. It may also be said that what is being mobilized for fighting against the alterations we are striving for are character-traits, attitudes of the ego. In this connection we discover that these character-traits were formed in relation to the determinants of the neurosis and in reaction against its demands, and we come upon traits which cannot normally emerge, or not to the same extent, and which may be described as latent. Nor must you get an impression that we regard the appearance of these resistances as an unforeseen risk to analytic influence. No, we are aware that these resistances are bound to come to light; in fact we are dissatisfied if we cannot provoke them clearly enough and are unable to demonstrate them to the patient. Indeed we come finally to understand that the overcoming of these resistances is the essential function of analysis[7] and is the only part of our work which gives us an assurance that we have achieved something with the patient.

If you further consider that the patient makes all the chance events that occur during his analysis into interferences with it, that he uses as reasons for slackening his efforts every diversion outside the analysis, every comment by a person of authority in his environment who is

---

[7][That this was a relatively late development in analytic technique is shown, for instance, by a paragraph in Freud's Nuremberg Congress paper (1910d), *Standard Ed.*, 11, 144.]

hostile to analysis, any chance organic illness or any that complicates his neurosis and, even, indeed, every improvement in his condition – if you consider all this, you will have obtained an approximate, though still incomplete, picture of the forms and methods of the resistance, the struggle against which accompanies every analysis.[8]

I have treated this point in such great detail because I must now inform you that this experience of ours with the resistance of neurotics to the removal of their symptoms became the basis of our dynamic view of the neuroses. Originally Breuer and I myself carried out psychotherapy by means of hypnosis; Breuer's first patient[9] was treated throughout under hypnotic influence, and to begin with I followed him in this. I admit that at that period the work proceeded more easily and pleasantly, and also in a much shorter time. But results were capricious and not lasting; and for that reason I finally dropped hypnosis.[10] And I then understood that an insight into the dynamics of these illnesses had not been possible so long as hypnosis was employed.[11] That state was precisely able to withhold the existence of the resistance from the doctor's perception. It pushed the resistance back, making a certain area free for analytic work, and dammed it up at the frontiers of that area in such a way as to be impenetrable, just as doubt does in obsessional neurosis. For that reason I have been able to say that psycho-analysis proper began when I dispensed with the help of hypnosis.[12]

If, however, the recognition of resistance has become so important, we should do well to find room for a cautious doubt whether we have not been too light-heartedly assuming resistances. Perhaps there really are cases of neurosis in which associations fail for other reasons, per-

---

[8][The present description of the forms taken by resistance in general is as full as any by Freud. But the special case of transference-resistance is discussed in greater detail in his paper on 'The Dynamics of Transference' (1912b).]

[9][See Lecture XVIII.]

[10][Fairly exact dates for Freud's use of hypnotism (1887–1896) will be found in an Editor's footnote to the case of Lucy R. in *Studies on Hysteria* (1895d), *Standard Ed.*, 2, 110–11.]

[11][Freud tells us that he first realized the great importance of resistance during his analysis of Elisabeth von R. He was at that time using the 'pressure' technique, without hypnosis. See *Studies on Hysteria* (1895d), *Standard Ed.*, 2, 154.]

[12][Cf. Freud's statement in very similar words in his history of the psycho-analytic movement (1914d), *Standard Ed.*, 14, 16. Earlier he had not been inclined to draw such a clear-cut line (cf. ibid., 7–8).]

haps the arguments against our hypotheses really deserve to have their content examined, and perhaps we are doing patients an injustice in so conveniently setting aside their intellectual criticisms as resistance. But, Gentlemen, we did not arrive at this judgement lightly. We have had occasion to observe all these critical patients at the moment of the emergence of a resistance and after its disappearance. For resistance is constantly altering its intensity during the course of a treatment; it always increases when we are approaching a new topic, it is at its most intense while we are at the climax of dealing with that topic, and it dies away when the topic has been disposed of. Nor do we ever, unless we have been guilty of special clumsiness in our technique, have to meet the full amount of resistance of which a patient is capable. We have therefore been able to convince ourselves that on countless occasions in the course of his analysis the same man will abandon his critical attitude and then take it up again. If we are on the point of bringing a specially distressing piece of unconscious material to his consciousness, he is extremely critical; he may previously have understood and accepted a great deal, but now it is just as though those acquisitions have been swept away; in his efforts for opposition at any price, he may offer a complete picture of someone who is an emotional imbecile. But if we succeed in helping him to overcome this new resistance, he recovers his insight and understanding. Thus his critical faculty is not an independent function, to be respected as such, it is the tool of his emotional attitudes and is directed by his resistance. If there is something he does not like, he can put up a shrewd fight against it and appear highly critical; but if something suits his book, he can, on the contrary, show himself most credulous. Perhaps none of us are very different; a man who is being analysed only reveals this dependence of the intellect upon emotional life so clearly because in analysis we are putting such great pressure on him.

How, then, do we account for our observation that the patient fights with such energy against the removal of his symptoms and the setting of his mental processes on a normal course? We tell ourselves that we have succeeded in discovering powerful forces here which oppose any alteration of the patient's condition; they must be the same ones which in the past brought this condition about. During the construction of his symptoms something must have taken place which we can now reconstruct from our experiences during the *resolution* of his symptoms. We already know from Breuer's observation that there is a precondition for the existence of a symptom: some mental process must not have been brought to an end normally—so that it could become conscious. The symptom is a substitute for what did not happen at that point. We now know the point at which we must locate the operation of the force which we have surmised. A violent opposition must have started against the entry into consciousness of the questionable mental process, and for that reason it remained unconscious. As being something unconscious, it had the power to construct a symptom. This same opposition, during psycho-analytic treatment, sets itself up once more against our effort to transform what is unconscious into what is conscious. This is what we perceive as resistance. We have proposed to give the pathogenic process which is demonstrated by the resistance the name of *repression*.

We must now form more definite ideas about this process of repression. It is the precondition for the construction of symptoms; but it is also something to which we know nothing similar. Let us take as our model an impulse, a mental process that endeavours to turn itself into an action. We know that it can be repelled by what we term a rejection or condemnation. When this happens, the energy at its disposal is withdrawn from it; it becomes powerless, though it can persist as a memory. The whole process of coming to a decision about it runs its course within the knowledge of the ego. It is a very different matter if we suppose that the same impulse is subjected to repression. In that case it would retain its energy and no memory of it would remain behind; moreover the process of repression would be accomplished unnoticed by the ego. This comparison, therefore, brings us no nearer to the essential nature of repression.

I will put before you the only theoretical ideas which have proved of service for giving a more definite shape to the concept of repression. It is above all essential for this purpose that we should proceed from the purely descriptive meaning of the word 'unconscious' to the systematic meaning of the same word.[13] That is, we will decide to say that the fact of a psychical process being conscious or unconscious is only one of its attributes and not necessarily an unambiguous one. If a process of this kind has remained unconscious, its being kept away from consciousness may perhaps only be an indication of some vicissitude it has gone

---

[13][The spatial analogy to resistance and repression, which follows here, is similar to the one in the second of his *Five Lectures* (1910*a*), *Standard Ed.*, 11, 25-7.]

through, and not that vicissitude itself. In order to form a picture of this vicissitude, let us assume that every mental process—we must admit one exception, which we shall mention at a later stage[14]—exists to begin with in an unconscious stage or phase and that it is only from there that the process passes over into the conscious phase, just as a photographic picture begins as a negative and only becomes a picture after being turned into a positive. Not every negative, however, necessarily becomes a positive; nor is it necessary that every unconscious mental process should turn into a conscious one. This may be advantageously expressed by saying that an individual process belongs to begin with to the system of the unconscious and can then, in certain circumstances, pass over into the system of the conscious.

The crudest idea of these systems is the most convenient for us—a spatial one. Let us therefore compare the system of the unconscious to a large entrance hall, in which the mental impulses jostle one another like separate individuals. Adjoining this entrance hall there is a second, narrower, room—a kind of drawing-room—in which consciousness, too, resides. But on the threshold between these two rooms a watchman performs his function: he examines the different mental impulses, acts as a censor, and will not admit them into the drawing-room if they displease him. You will see at once that it does not make much difference if the watchman turns away a particular impulse at the threshold itself or if he pushes it back across the threshold after it has entered the drawing-room. This is merely a question of the degree of his watchfulness and of how early he carries out his act of recognition. If we keep to this picture, we shall be able to extend our nomenclature further. The impulses in the entrance hall of the unconscious are out of sight of the conscious, which is in the other room; to begin with they must remain unconscious. If they have already pushed their way forward to the threshold and have been turned back by the watchman, then they are inadmissable to consciousness;[15] we speak of them as *repressed*. But even the impulses which the watchman has allowed to cross the threshold are not on that account necessarily conscious as well; they can only become so if they succeed in catching the eye of

---

[14][The exception, which seems to have escaped mention, must no doubt be the case of external perception.]

[15]['*Bewusstseinsunfähig.*' The term is due to Breuer, who constructed it on the model of '*hoffähig*' ('admissible to Court', 'having the *entrée*'). See Section 5 of his contribution to *Studies on Hysteria* (1895d), *Standard Ed.*, 2, 225 n.]

consciousness. We are therefore justified in calling this second room the system of the *preconscious*. In that case becoming conscious retains its purely descriptive sense. For any particular impulse, however, the vicissitude of repression consists in its not being allowed by the watchman to pass from the system of the unconscious into that of the preconscious. It is the same watchman whom we get to know as resistance when we try to lift the repression by means of the analytic treatment.

The concepts of transference and transference resistance are central to psychoanalysis as treatment structure. The centrality of transference resistance is emphasized in the following short excerpt from Freud's Autobiographical Study *(1925).*

I now come to the description of a factor which adds an essential feature to my picture of analysis and which can claim, alike technically and theoretically, to be regarded as of the first importance. In every analytic treatment there arises, without the physician's agency, an intense emotional relationship between the patient and the analyst which is not to be accounted for by the actual situation. It can be of a positive or of a negative character and can vary between the extremes of a passionate, completely sensual love and the unbridled expression of an embittered defiance and hatred. This *transference* – to give it its short name – soon replaces in the patient's mind the desire to be cured, and, so long as it is affectionate and moderate, becomes the agent of the physician's influence and neither more nor less than the mainspring of the joint work of analysis. Later on, when it has become passionate or has been converted into hostility, it becomes the principal tool of the resistance. It may then happen that it will paralyse the patient's powers of associating and endanger the success of the treatment. Yet it would be senseless to try to evade it; for an analysis without transference is an impossibility. It must not be supposed, however, that transference is created by analysis and does not occur apart from it. Transference is merely uncovered and isolated by analysis. It is a universal phenomenon of the human mind, it decides the success of all medical influence, and in fact dominates the whole of each person's relations to his human environment. We can easily recognize it as the same dynamic factor which the hypnotists have named 'suggestibility', which is the agent of hypnotic *rapport* and whose incalculable behaviour led to difficulties with the cathartic method as well. When there is no inclination to a transference of emotion such as this, or when it has become entirely negative, as happens in dementia praecox or paranoia, then there is also no possibility of influencing the patient by psychological means.

It is perfectly true that psycho-analysis, like other psychotherapeutic methods, employs the instrument of suggestion (or transference). But the difference is this: that in analysis it is not allowed to play the decisive part in determining the therapeutic results. It is used instead to induce the patient to perform a piece of psychical work – the overcoming of his transference-resistances – which involves a permanent alteration in his mental economy. The transference is made conscious to the patient by the analyst, and it is resolved by convincing him that in his transference-attitude he is *re-experiencing* emotional relations which had their origin in his earliest object-attachments during the repressed period of his childhood. In this way the transference is changed from the strongest weapon of the resistance into the best instrument of the analytic treatment. Nevertheless its handling remains the most difficult as well as the most important part of the technique of analysis.

As we have previously indicated, the consideration of different aspects of resistance as they are manifested in analysis was considered by Freud in a number of different theoretical, technical, and case study presentations. Very frequently, then, issues of resistance were embedded in other material and not often brought together for a systematic perusal and appraisal. However, one of the most concise, and at the same time far-reaching, considerations of this concept was Freud's Inhibitions, Symptoms and Anxiety (1926), *a landmark in the development of psychoanalysis. While the classification scheme prescribed therein is not all-encompassing, it does provide a fairly extensive perspective on the focus of resistance.*

MODIFICATIONS OF EARLIER VIEWS

Resistance and Anticathexis

An important element in the theory of repression is the view that repression is not an event that occurs once but that it requires a permanent expenditure [of energy]. If this expenditure were to cease, the repressed impulse, which is being fed all the time from its sources, would on the next occasion flow along the channels from which it had been forced away, and the repression would either fail in its purpose or would have to be repeated an indefinite number of times.[1] Thus it is because instincts are continuous in their nature that the ego has to make its defensive action secure by a permanent expenditure [of energy]. This action undertaken to protect repression is observable in analytic treatment as *resistance*. Resistance presupposes the existence of what I have called *anticathexis*. An anticathexis of this kind is clearly seen in obsessional neurosis. It appears there in the form of an alteration of the ego, as a reaction-formation in the ego, and is effected by the reinforcement of the attitude which is the opposite of the instinctual trend that has to be repressed—as, for instance, in pity, conscientiousness and cleanliness. These reaction-formations of obsessional neurosis are essentially exaggerations of the normal traits of character which develop during the latency period. The presence of an anticathexis in hysteria is much more difficult to detect, though theoretically it is equally indispensable. In hysteria, too, a certain amount of alteration of the ego through reaction-formation is unmistakable and in some circumstances becomes so marked that it forces itself on our attention as the principal symptom. The conflict due to ambivalence, for instance, is resolved in hysteria by this means. The subject's hatred of a person whom he loves is kept down by an exaggerated amount of tenderness for him and apprehensiveness about him. But the difference between reaction-formations in obsessional neurosis and in hysteria is that in the latter they do not have the universality of a character-trait but are confined to particular relationships. A hysterical woman, for instance, may be specifically affectionate with her own children whom at bottom she hates; but she will not on that account be more loving in general than other women or even more affectionate to other children. The reaction-formation of hysteria clings tenaciously to a particular object and never spreads over into a general disposition of the ego, whereas what is characteristic of obsessional neurosis is precisely a spreading-over of this kind—a loosening of relations to the object and a facilitation of displacement in the choice of object.

There is another kind of anticathexis, however, which seems more suited to the peculiar character of hysteria. A repressed instinctual impulse can be activated (newly cathected) from two directions: from

---

[1] [Cf. the paper on 'Repression' (1915*d*), *Standard Ed.*, 14, 151.]

within, through reinforcement from its internal sources of excitation, and from without, through the perception of an object that it desires. The hysterical anticathexis is mainly directed outwards, against dangerous perceptions. It takes the form of a special kind of vigilance which, by means of restrictions of the ego, causes situations to be avoided that would entail such perceptions, or, if they do occur, manages to withdraw the subject's attention from them. Some French analysts, in particular Laforgue [1926], have recently given this action of hysteria the special name of 'scotomization'.[2] This technique of anticathexis is still more noticeable in the phobias, whose interest is concentrated on removing the subject even further from the possibility of the occurrence of the feared perception. The fact that anticathexis has an opposite direction in hysteria and the phobias from what it has in obsessional neurosis—though the distinction is not an absolute one—seems to be significant. It suggests that there is an intimate connection between repression and external anticathexis on the one hand and between regression and internal anticathexis (i.e. alteration in the ego through reaction-formation) on the other. The task of defence against a dangerous perception is, incidentally, common to all neuroses. Various commands and prohibitions in obsessional neurosis have the same end in view.

We showed on an earlier occasion[3] that the resistance that has to be overcome in analysis proceeds from the ego, which clings to its anticathexes. It is hard for the ego to direct its attention to perceptions and ideas which it has up till now made a rule of avoiding, or to acknowledge as belonging to itself impulses that are the complete opposite of those which it knows as its own. Our fight against resistance in analysis is based upon this view of the facts. If the resistance is itself unconscious, as so often happens owing to its connection with the repressed material, we make it conscious. If it is conscious, or when it has become conscious, we bring forward logical arguments against it; we promise the ego rewards and advantages if it will give up its resistance. There can be no doubt or mistake about the existence of this resistance on the part of the ego. But we have to ask ourselves whether it covers the whole state of affairs in analysis. For we find that even after the ego

---

[2][Freud discussed this term at some length in his later paper on 'Fetishism' (1927c) in connection with the concept of disavowal (*Verleugnung*).]
[3][Towards the end of Chapter I of *The Ego and the Id* (1923b).]

has decided to relinquish its resistances it still has difficulty in undoing the repressions; and we have called the period of strenuous effort which follows after its praiseworthy decision, the phase of 'working through'.[4] The dynamic factor which makes a working-through of this kind necessary and comprehensible is not far to seek. It must be that after the ego's resistance has been removed the power of the compulsion to repeat – the attraction exerted by the unconscious prototype upon the repressed instinctual process – has still to be overcome. There is nothing to be said against describing this factor as the *resistance of the unconscious*. There is no need to be discouraged by these emendations. They are to be welcomed if they add something to our knowledge, and they are no disgrace to us so long as they enrich rather than invalidate our earlier views – by limiting some statement, perhaps, that was too general or by enlarging some idea that was too narrowly formulated.

It must not be supposed that these emendations provide us with a complete survey of all the kinds of resistance that are met with in analysis. Further investigation of the subject shows that the analyst has to combat no less than five kinds of resistance, emanating from three directions – the ego, the id and the super-ego. The ego is the source of three of these, each differing in its dynamic nature. The first of these three ego-resistances is the *repression* resistance, which we have already discussed above and about which there is least new to be added. Next there is the *transference* resistance, which is of the same nature but which has different and much clearer effects in analysis, since it succeeds in establishing a relation to the analytic situation or the analyst himself and thus re-animating a repression which should only have been recollected.[5] The third resistance, though also an ego-resistance, is of quite a different nature. It proceeds from the *gain from illness* and is based upon an assimilation of the symptom into the ego. It represents an unwillingness to renounce any satisfaction or relief that has been obtained. The fourth variety, arising from the *id*, is the resistance which, as we have just seen, necessitates 'working-through'. The fifth,

[4][See 'Remembering, Repeating and Working-Through' (1914g) *Standard Ed.*, 12, 155-6. Freud returned to the subject in Section VI of his late technical paper 'Analysis Terminable and Interminable' (1937c).]
[5][CF. 'Remembering, Repeating and Working-Through' (1914g), *Standard Ed.*, **12,** 151 f.f.]

coming from the *super-ego* and the last to be discovered, is also the most obscure though not always the least powerful one. It seems to originate from the sense of guilt or the need for punishment; and it opposes every move towards success, including, therefore, the patient's own recovery through analysis.[6]

---

[6][This was discussed in the earlier part of Chapter V of *The Ego and the Id.*]

CHAPTER 3

Character Resistances

Wilhelm Reich

INTRODUCTION

Our therapeutic method is contingent upon the following basic theoretical concepts. The *topographical* point of view determines the principle of technique to the effect that the unconscious has to be made conscious. The *dynamic* point of view dictates that this making conscious of the unconscious must not proceed directly, but by way of resistance analysis. The *economic* point of view and the knowledge of *structure* dictate that, in resistance analysis, each individual case entails a definite plan which must be deduced from the case itself.

As long as the making conscious of the unconscious, i.e., the *topographical* process, was regarded as the sole task of analytic technique, the formula was justified that the patient's unconscious manifestations had to be translated into the language of the conscious in *the sequence in which they appeared*. In this process, the *dynamics* of the analysis were left largely to chance, that is, whether the act of becoming conscious actually released the germane affect and whether the interpretation had anything more than an intellectual influence on the patient. The very inclusion of the dynamic factor, i.e., the demand that the patient had not only to remember but also to experience what he remembered, complicated the simple formula that "the unconscious had to be made conscious." Since the dynamic effect of analysis depends not on the

41

material which the patient produces but on the resistances which he brings into play against this material and on the emotional intensity with which they are mastered, the task of analysis undergoes no insignificant shift. Whereas it is sufficient, from the topographical point of view, to make the patient conscious of the clearest and most easily interpretable elements of the unconscious in the sequence in which they appear, in other words, *to adhere to the pattern of the contents of the material*, it is necessary, when the dynamic factor is taken into consideration, to relinquish this plan as a means of orientation in the analysis. Instead, another must be adopted which embraces both the content of the material and the affect, namely, *the pattern of successive resistances*. In pursuing this plan, however, a difficulty arises in most cases, a difficulty which we have not considered in the foregoing presentation.

CHARACTER ARMORING AND CHARACTER RESISTANCE

The Inability to Follow the Basic Rule

Our patients are seldom capable of analysis at the outset. Only a very small number of patients are prepared to follow the basic rule and to open themselves completely to the analyst. First of all, it is not easy for the patient to have immediate trust in the analyst, if only because he is a stranger. Added to this, however, is the fact that years of illness, the unrelenting influence of a neurotic milieu, bad experiences with mental specialists—in short, the entire secondary fragmentation of the ego—have created a situation that is adverse to the analysis. The elimination of this difficulty becomes a precondition of the analysis, and it could be accomplished easily if it were not complicated by the characteristic, indeed character of the patient, which is itself a part of the neurosis and has developed on a neurotic basis. It is known as the "narcissistic barrier." Fundamentally, there are two ways of getting at these difficulties, especially at the difficulty entailed by the resistance to the basic rule. The first way, and the one usually pursued, I believe, is to prepare the patient for analysis through instruction, reassurance, challenge, exhortation, persuasion, and more of the same. In this case, by establishing a kind of positive transference, the analyst seeks to convince the patient of the necessity of being open and honest in the analysis. This roughly corresponds to the technique suggested by Nunberg. Vast experience has taught us, however, that this pedagogic or active approach is highly uncertain, is dependent upon uncontrollable contingencies, and lacks the secure basis of analytic clarity. The analyst is constantly at the mercy of the oscillations of the transference and treads on uncertain terrain in his efforts to make the patient capable of analysis.

The second method is more complicated, and not yet feasible for all patients. It is a far more secure approach. Here the attempt is made *to replace the instructional measures by analytic interpretations*. There is no question that this is not always possible, yet it remains the ideal goal toward which analysis strives. Instead of inducing the patient to enter into the analysis by persuasion, suggestion, transference maneuvers, etc., the analyst takes a more passive attitude and attempts to get an insight into the *contemporary* meaning of the patient's behavior, *why* he or she doubts, arrives late, speaks in a ranting or confused manner, communicates only every third idea or so, criticizes the analysis, or produces deep material, often in uncommon amounts. In other words, the analyst can do one of two things: (1) attempt to persuade a narcissistic patient who speaks in grandiloquent technical terminology that his behavior is detrimental to the analysis and that he would do better to rid himself of analytic terminology and to come out of his shell; or (2) dispense with any kind of persuasion and wait until he understands why the patient behaves as he does. It may turn out, for instance, that the patient's ostentatious behavior is an attempt to cover up a feeling of inferiority toward the analyst. In this case, the analyst will endeavor to influence him through a consistent interpretation of the meaning of his actions. In contrast to the first, this second approach is entirely in keeping with the principles of analysis.

From this endeavor to use purely analytic interpretations wherever possible in place of all the instructional or otherwise active measures which become necessary as a result of the patient's characteristics, a method of analyzing the *character* emerged in an unsought and unexpected way.

Certain clinical considerations make it necessary for us to designate as "*character resistances*" a special group of the resistances that we encounter in the treatment of our patients. *These derive their special character not from their content but from the specific mannerisms of the person analyzed.* The compulsive character develops resistances whose form is specifically different from that of the hysterical character, the form of whose resistances, in turn, is different from that of the genital narcissistic, impulsive, or neurasthenic character. *The form of the ego's reactions, which differs from character to character even where the contents of the experiences are the same, can be traced back to infantile experiences in the same way as the content of the symptoms and fantasies.*

Where Do the Character Resistances Come From?

Some time ago, Glover made an effort to discriminate between character neuroses and symptom neuroses. Alexander also operated on the basis of this distinction. I adhered to it in earlier works, but it turned out, on closer comparison of the cases, that this distinction makes sense only insofar as there are neuroses with circumscribed symptoms ("symptom neuroses") and neuroses without them ("character neuroses"). In the former, understandably, the symptoms are more conspicuous; in the latter, the neurotic character traits stand out. But are there symptoms which do not have a neurotic reaction basis, which, in other words, are not rooted in a neurotic character? The only difference between character neuroses and symptom neuroses is that, in the case of the latter, the neurotic character also produces symptoms, has become, so to speak, concentrated in them. That the neurotic character is at one time exacerbated in circumscribed symptoms and at another time finds other ways of discharging the libido stasis requires more detailed investigation. . . . But if it is acknowledged that the symptom neurosis is always rooted in a neurotic character, then it is clear that, in *every* analysis, we are dealing with resistances that are manifestations of a neurotic character. The individual analysis will differ only with respect to the importance ascribed to the analysis of the character in each case. However, a retrospective glance at analytic experiences cautions us against underestimating this importance in any one case.

From the point of view of character analysis, the differentiation between neuroses which are chronic, i.e., have existed since childhood, and those which are acute, i.e., appeared later, has no importance whatever; it is of no great moment whether the symptoms appear in childhood or later. What matters is that the neurotic character, i.e., the reaction basis for the symptom neurosis, is formed, at least in its principal features, by the time the Oedipal stage comes to a close. We have ample clinical experience to show that the boundary which the

patient draws between health and the outbreak of sickness always van-
ishes in the analysis.

Since the symptom formation does not hold up as a descriptive
characteristic, we have to look for others. Two which readily come to
mind are *illness insight* and *rationalizations*.

A *lack of insight into the illness* is not, of course, absolutely reliable but
it is certainly an essential indication of character neurosis. The neurotic symptom is sensed as something alien, and it engenders a feeling
of being ill. On the other hand, the neurotic character trait, e.g., the
exaggerated sense of order of the compulsive character or the anxious
shyness of the hysterical character, is organically incorporated into the
personality. One might complain of being shy, but one does not feel
sick for that reason. Not until the characterological shyness becomes a
pathological blushing or until the compulsive-neurotic sense of order
becomes a compulsive ceremony, not until, in other words, the neurotic character exacerbates symptomatically, does one feel that one is
sick.

Naturally, there are symptoms for which no insight, or insufficient
insight, exists. They are regarded by patients as bad habits or something which has to be accepted (e.g., chronic constipation, mild
ejaculatio praecox). Then there are some character traits which are
sometimes felt to be pathological, e.g., irrational, violent fits of anger,
gross negligence, a penchant for lying, drinking, splurging, and other
such. Generally, however, an insight into the sickness is indicative of a
neurotic symptom, whereas lack of insight points to a neurotic character trait.

In practical terms, the second important difference consists in the
fact that symptoms never exhibit such complete and credible *rationalizations* as neurotic character traits. Neither hysterical vomiting nor
abasia; neither compulsive counting nor compulsive thinking can be
rationalized. There is no question about the senselessness of a symptom, whereas the neurotic character trait has a sufficiently rational
motivation so as not to appear pathological or senseless.

Furthermore, there is a justification for neurotic character traits
which is immediately rejected as absurd when it is applied to symptoms. We often hear it said: "That's simply the way I am." The implication here is that the person concerned was born that way; he simply
cannot behave differently—that's his character. However, this does
not tally with the facts, for the analysis of its development shows that

the character had to become what it is, and not something else, for very specific reasons. Fundamentally, therefore, it is capable of analysis and of being changed, just like the symptom.

Occasionally, symptoms have become so ingrained in the personality that they are like character traits. An example is compulsive counting that is wholly absorbed within the framework of one's need to be orderly, or compulsive methodicalness that is fulfilled in the rigid subdivisions of each day. The latter is especially true of the compulsion to work. Such modes of behavior are held to be indicative more of eccentricity or excessiveness than of pathology. Hence, we see that the concept of illness is highly flexible, that there are many shades, ranging from the symptom as an isolated foreign body through the neurotic character trait and the "wicked habit" to rationally sound behavior. However, in view of the fact that these shades are not very much help to us, the differentiation between symptom and neurotic character trait recommends itself, even insofar as rationalizations are concerned, notwithstanding the artificiality of all divisions.

With this reservation, another differentiation occurs to us with respect to the structure of the symptom and of the character trait. in the process of analysis, it is shown that, in terms of its meaning and origin, the symptom has a very simple structure compared with that of the character trait. True enough, the symptom too is indeterminate; but the more deeply we penetrate into its reasons, the more we move away from the actual compass of the symptom and the more clearly we perceive its basis in the character. Hence, theoretically, the reaction basis in the character can be worked out from any symptom. The symptom is directly determined by a limited number of unconscious attitudes; hysterical vomiting, for example, is based on a repressed fellatio desire or an oral desire for a child. Each of them is expressed in the character, the former in a kind of childishness, the latter in a maternal attitude. But the hysterical character, which determines the hysterical symptom, is based on a multiplicity of — to a large extent antagonistic — strivings, and is usually expressed in a specific *attitude* or *mode of existence*. It is not nearly so easy to analyze the attitude as it is to analyze the symptom; fundamentally, however, the former, like the latter, can be traced back to and understood on the basis of drives and experiences. Whereas the symptom corresponds solely to one definite experience or one circumscribed desire, the character, i.e., the person's specific mode of existence, represents an expression of the person's entire past. So a symptom can emerge quite suddenly, while the development of each individual character trait requires many years. We must also bear in mind that the symptom could not have suddenly emerged unless a neurotic reaction basis already existed in the character.

In the analysis, the neurotic character traits as a whole prove to be a compact *defense mechanism* against our therapeutic efforts, and when we trace the origin of this character "armor" analytically, we see that it also has a definite economic function. Such armor serves on the one hand as a defense against external stimuli; on the other hand it proves to be a means of gaining mastery over the libido, which is continuously pushing forward from the id, because libidinal and sadistic energy is used up in the neurotic reaction formations, compensations, etc. Anxiety is continually being bound in the processes which are at the bottom of the formation and preservation of this armor in the same way that, according to Freud's description, anxiety is bound in the compulsive symptoms. We shall have more to say about the economy of the character formation.

Since, in its economic function as defensive armor, the neurotic character trait has established a certain, albeit *neurotic balance*, analysis constitutes a danger to this balance. It is from this narcissistic defense mechanism of the ego that the resistances originate which give the analysis of the individual case its special features. If, however, a person's mode of behavior represents the result of a total development which is capable of analysis and resolution, then it must also be possible to deduce the technique of character analysis from that behavior.

On the Technique of Analyzing the Character Resistance

In addition to the dreams, associations, slips, and other communications of the patients, the *way in which* they recount their dreams, commit slips, produce associations, and make their communications, in short their bearing, deserves special attention.[1] Adherence to the basic rule is something rare, and many months of character-analytic work are required to instill in the patient a halfway sufficient measure of can-

---

[1]Footnote, 1945: The *form* of expression is *far more important* than the ideational *content*. Today we use only the form of expression to arrive at the *decisively* important experiences of childhood. It is the form of expression and not the ideational content that leads us to the biological reactions which lie at the basis of the psychic manifestations.

didness. The way the patient speaks, looks at and greets the analyst, lies on the couch, the inflection of the voice, the degree of conventional politeness which is maintained, etc., are valuable cues in assessing the secret resistances with which the patient counters the basic rule. And once they have been understood, they can be eliminated through interpretation. It is not only *what* the patient says but *how* he says it that has to be interpreted. Analysts are often heard to complain that the analysis is not progressing, that the patient is not producing any "material." By material, what is usually meant is merely the content of the associations and communications. But the nature of the patient's silence or sterile repetitions is also material which has to be used fully. There is scarcely a situation in which the patient does not produce *any* material, and we have to lay the blame upon ourselves if we can't make use of the patient's bearing as material.

There is of course nothing new in the statement that behavior and the form of the communications are of analytic importance. What we are concerned with here, however, is the fact that they give us access to the analysis of the character in a very definite and relatively complete way. Bad experiences in the analysis of some neurotic characters have taught us that, *at the outset* of such cases, the form of communications is of greater importance than the content. We want merely to allude to the concealed resistances produced by the emotionally paralyzed, by the "good" men and women, the excessively polite and correct patients; by those patients, moreover, who always give evidence of a deceptive positive transference or, for that matter, by those who raise a passionate and monotonous cry for love; those who conceive of analysis as a kind of game; the eternally "armored" who laugh in their sleeve at anything and everything. The list could be extended indefinitely. Hence, one has no illusions about the painstaking work which the innumerable individual problems of technique will entail.

To allow what is essential in character analysis to stand out more clearly in contrast to symptom analysis, and to give a better idea of our thesis in general, let us consider two pairs of cases. The first pair consists of two men being treated for ejaculatio praecox: one is a passive-feminine character, the other a phallic-aggressive character. Two women suffering from an eating disturbance constitute the second pair: one is a compulsive character, the other a hysteric.

Let us further assume that the ejaculatio praecox of the two male patients has the same unconscious meaning: fear of the (paternal) phallus assumed to be in the woman's vagina. On the basis of the castration anxiety which lies at the root of the symptom, both patients produce a negative father transference in the analysis. They hate the analyst (father) because they perceive in him the enemy who limits their pleasure, and each of them has the unconscious desire to dispose of him. While the phallic-sadistic character will ward off the danger of castration by means of vituperations, disparagements, and threats, the passive-feminine character will become more and more confiding, more and more passively devoted, and more and more accommodating. In both of them the character has become a resistance: the former wards off the danger aggressively; the latter gets out of its way by compromising his standards, by deceptiveness and devotion.

Naturally, the character resistance of the passive-feminine type is more dangerous, for he works with devious means. He produces material in abundance, recalls infantile experiences, appears to adapt himself beautifully—but at bottom he glosses over a secret obstinacy and hate. As long as he keeps this up, he will not have the courage to show his true nature. If the analyst does not pay any attention to his manner and merely enters into *what* the patient produces, then, according to experience, no analytic effort or elucidation will change his condition. It may even be that the patient will recall his hatred of his father, but he will not *experience* it unless the meaning of his deceptive behavior is consistently pointed out to him in the transference, *before* a deep interpretation of the father-hatred is begun.

In the case of the second pair, let us assume that an acute positive transference has developed. In both women, the main content of this positive transference is the same as that of the symptom, namely an oral fellatio fantasy. However, the transference resistance ensuing from this positive transference will be wholly different in form. The woman suffering from hysteria, for example, will be *apprehensively* silent and behave timidly; the woman having a compulsive neurosis will be *obstinately* silent or behave in a cold, haughty way toward the analyst. The transference resistance employs various means in warding off the positive transference: in the one instance, aggression: in the other, anxiety. We would say that in both cases the id conveyed the same wish, which the ego warded off differently. And the form of this defense will always remain the same in both patients; the woman suffering from hysteria will always defend herself in a way expressive of anxiety, while the woman suffering from a compulsive neurosis will always defend herself aggressively, no matter what unconscious content is on the verge of breaking through. In other words, *the character resistance always remains the same in the same patient and disappears only when the neurosis has been uprooted.*

The character armor is the molded expression of *narcissistic* defense chronically embedded in the psychic structure. In addition to the known resistances which are mobilized against each new piece of unconscious material, there is a constant resistance factor which has its roots in the unconscious and pertains not to content but to *form*. Because of its origin in the character, we call this constant resistance factor "character resistance."

On the basis of the foregoing statements, let us summarize the most important features of character resistance.

Character resistance is expressed not in terms of content but formally, in the way one typically behaves, in the manner in which one speaks, walks, and gestures; and in one's characteristic habits (how one smiles or sneers, whether one speaks coherently or incoherently, *how* one is polite and *how* one is aggressive).

It is not what the patient says and does that is indicative of character resistance, but *how* he speaks and acts; not what he reveals in dreams, but *how* he censors, distorts, condenses, etc.

The character resistance remains the same in the same patient, regardless of content. Different characters produce the same material in a different way. The positive father transference of a woman suffering from hysteria is expressed and warded off differently than that of a woman suffering from a compulsive neurosis. Anxiety is the defense mechanism in the former; aggression in the latter.

The character resistance which is manifested in terms of form is just as capable of being resolved, with respect to its content, and of being traced back to infantile experiences and instinctual interests as the neurotic symptom is.[2]

In given situations, the patient's character becomes a resistance. In everyday life, in other words, the character plays a role similar to the one it plays as a resistance in the treatment: that of a psychic defense apparatus. Hence, we speak of the "character armoring" of the ego against the outer world and the id.

---

[2]In light of this clinical experience, the element of form has been incorporated into the sphere of psychoanalysis, which, until now, has focused predominantly on content.

If we trace the formation of the character into early childhood, we find that, in its time, the character armor ensued for the same reasons and for the same purposes the character resistance serves in the contemporary analytic situation. The resistive projection of the character in the analysis mirrors its infantile genesis. And those situations which seem to appear by chance but actually are brought about by the character resistance in the analysis are exact duplicates of those childhood situations which caused the formation of the charcter. Thus, in the character resistance, the function of defense is combined with the projection of infantile relationships to the outer world.

Economically, the character in everyday life and the character resistance in the analysis serve as a means of avoiding what is unpleasant (*Unlust*), of establishing and preserving a psychic (even if neurotic) balance, and finally of consuming repressed qualities of instinctual energy and/or quantities which have eluded repression. The binding of free-floating anxiety or—what amounts to the same thing—the absorbing of dammed-up psychic energy, is one of the cardinal functions of the character. Just as the historical, i.e., the infantile, element is embodied and continues to live and operate in the neurotic symptom, so too it lives and operates and is embodied in the character. This explains why the consistent loosening of the character resistance provides a sure and direct approach to the central infantile conflict.

How do these facts bear upon the analytic technique of character analysis? Is there an essential difference between character analysis and the usual resistance analysis?

There are differences and they relate to:

a. the sequence in which the material is to be interpreted
b. the technique of resistance interpretation itself

With respect to (*a*): In speaking of "selection of material," we shall have to be prepared to encounter an important objection. It will be said that any selection is in contradiction to the basic principle of psychoanalysis, namely that the analyst must follow the patient, must allow himself to be led by him. Every time the analyst makes a selection, he runs the risk of falling prey to his own inclinations. First of all, we have to point out that, in the kind of selection we are speaking of here, it is not a matter of neglecting analytic material. The whole point here is *to insure* that the material is interpreted in a *legitimate sequence*, in

keeping with the structure of the neurosis. All material is in turn interpreted; it is only that one detail is momentarily more important than
another. We also have to realize that the analyst always selects anyhow, for in the very act of singling out individual details of a dream instead of interpreting them successively, he has made a selection. And
as far as that goes, the analyst has also made a biased selection when he
considers only the content and not the form of the communications.
Hence, the very fact that the patient produces material of the most diverse kinds in the analytic situation forces the analyst to make selections in interpreting this material. It is merely a question of selecting
correctly, i.e., in keeping with the analytic situation.

With patients who, because of a particular character development,
repeatedly disregard the fundamental rule, as well as with all cases in
which the character is obstructing the analysis, it will be necessary to
single out the germane *character resistance from the welter of material and
to work it through analytically by interpreting its meaning*. Naturally, this
does not mean that the rest of the material is neglected or disregarded.
On the contrary, everything is valuable and welcome which gives us
an insight into the meaning and origin of the recalcitrant character
trait. The analyst merely puts off the analysis, and, above all, the interpretation of the material which does not have an immediate bearing
upon the transference resistance, until the character resistance has
been understood and broken through, at least in its basic features.
[Elsewhere] I tried to point out the dangers of giving deep interpretations before the character resistances have been resolved.

With respect to (b): Now we turn our attention to some special problems of the technique of character analysis. First, we must anticipate a
likely misunderstanding. We stated that character analysis begins with
the singling out and consistent analysis of the character resistance.
This does not mean that the patient is enjoined not to be aggressive,
not to be deceptive, not to speak in an incoherent manner, to follow
the basic rule, etc. Such demands would not only be contrary to analytic procedure, they would be fruitless. It cannot be sufficiently
stressed that what we are describing here has nothing whatever to do
with the so-called education of the patient and similar matters. In character analysis, we ask ourselves why the patient is deceptive, speaks in
an incoherent manner, is emotionally blocked, etc.; we endeavor to
arouse his interest in the peculiarities of his character in order to elucidate, with his help, their meaning and origin through analysis. In

other words, we merely single out from the orbit of the personality the character trait from which the cardinal resistance proceeds, and, if possible, we show the patient the surface relation between the character and the symptoms. But for the rest, we leave it up to him whether or not he wants to make use of his knowledge to change his character. Fundamentally, our procedure in this is not different from the one followed in the analysis of a symptom; the one exception is that, in character analysis, we have to *isolate* the character trait and put it before the patient *again and again* until he has succeeded in breaking clear of it and in viewing it as he would a vexatious compulsive symptom. In breaking clear of and objectifying the neurotic character trait, the patient begins to experience it as something alien to himself, and ultimately gains an insight into its nature.

In this process, it becomes apparent, surprisingly, that the personality changes—at least temporarily. And as the character analysis progresses, that impetus or disposition which gave rise to the character resistance in the transference automatically comes to the surface in an unconcealed form. Applying this to our example of the passive-feminine character, we can say that the more thoroughly the patient objectifies his inclinations to passive devotion, the more aggressive he will become. For, of course, his feminine, deceptive behavior was, in the main, an energetic reaction against repressed aggressive impulses. Hand in hand with the aggressiveness, however, the infantile castration anxiety also reappears which, at one time, caused the aggression to be transformed into a passive-feminine attitude. Thus, through the analysis of the character resistance, we arrive at the center of the neurosis, the Oedipus complex.

Let there be no illusions, however: the isolation and objectification as well as the analytic working through of such a character resistance usually take many months, demand great effort and, most of all, steadfast patience. Once the breakthrough has been achieved, the analytic work usually proceeds by leaps and bounds, borne by *affective* analytic experiences. If, on the other hand, such character resistances are left untended; if the analyst merely follows the patient, continually interpreting the content of his material, such resistances will, as time goes on, form a ballast that will be almost impossible to remove. When this happens, the analyst begins to feel in his bones that all his interpretations of content were wasted, that the patient continues to doubt everything. In later stages of the analysis, after the essential interpretations of the Oedipus complex have already been given, the analyst will find himself embroiled in a hopeless situation, if he has neglected to clear away these resistances right from the beginning.

I have already tried to refute the objection that resistances cannot be taken up until their *infantile* determinants are known. In the beginning of the treatment, it is merely necessary for the analyst to discern the *contemporary* meaning of the character resistance, for which purpose the infantile material is not always required. This material we need for the *dissolution* of the resistance. If, at the beginning, the analyst contends himself with putting the resistance before the patient and interpreting its contemporary meaning, it is not long before the infantile material emerges and, with its help, the resistance can then be eliminated.

When stress is laid upon a previously neglected fact, the impression is unwittingly created that other facts are being deprived of their importance. If in this work we lay such strong emphasis on the analysis of the *mode* of reaction, this does not mean that we neglect the content. We merely add something which had not been properly appreciated before this. Our experience teaches us that the analysis of the character resistance must be given absolute precedence; but this does not mean that the analysis is confined solely to character resistance until a certain date, when the analyst then takes up the interpretation of content. To a large extent, the two phases, resistance analysis and analysis of the early infantile experiences, overlap one another. It is merely that the analysis of the character is given priority at the beginning of the treatment ("preparing the analysis through analysis"), while the main accent in the later stages falls upon the interpretation of content and infantile experiences. This, however, is not a rigid rule; its application will depend upon the behavior pattern of the individual patient. The interpretation of infantile material will be taken up early with one patient, later with another. There is one rule, however, which must be strictly adhered to, namely that deep analytic interpretations have to be avoided, even in the case of fairly clear material, until the patient is prepared to assimilate them. This is of course nothing new. Yet, in view of the many different ways in which analysts work, it is obviously important to know what is meant by "prepared for analytic interpretation." In deciding this, we shall doubtless have to differentiate those contents which pertain directly to the character resistance and those which pertain to other spheres of experience. Normally, in the beginning of analysis, the analysand is prepared to take cognizance of the former but not of the latter. On the whole, the main idea behind character analysis is to gain the greatest possible security both in the preparatory work of the analysis and in the interpretation of infantile material. At this point, we are confronted with the important task of investigating and systematically describing the various forms of character transference resistances. The technique of dealing with them will emerge of itself from their structure.

The Technique of Dealing with Individual Situations as Derived from the Structure of the Character Resistance (Technique of Interpreting Ego Defense)

We now turn to the problem of the character-analytic technique of dealing with individual situations, and how this technique is derived from the structure of the character resistance. To illustrate this, we shall take a patient who develops resistances right at the outset, the structure of which, however, is far from immediately clear. In the following case, the character resistance had a very complicated structure; there were many determining factors, intermingled with one another. An attempt will be made to set forth the reasons which induced me to begin my interpretation precisely with one particular element of the resistance. Here, too, it will become apparent that a consistent and logical interpretation of the ego defense and of the mechanism of the "armor" leads into the very heart of the central infantile conflicts.

A CASE OF MANIFEST FEELINGS OF INFERIORITY

A thirty-year-old man turned to analysis because he "didn't really enjoy life." He could not really say whether or not he felt sick. Actually, he didn't think that he was really in need of treatment. Yet he felt that he should do whatever he could. He had heard of psychoanalysis — perhaps it could help him gain insight into himself. He was not aware of having any symptoms. It turned out that his potency was very weak; he seldom engaged in sexual intercourse, approached women only with great reluctance, did not derive any gratification from coitus, and, moreover, suffered from ejaculatio praecox. He had very little insight into his impotence. He had—so he said—reconciled himself to his meager potency; there were so many men who "didn't need it."

His demeanor and behavior betrayed at a glance that he was a severely inhibited and oppressed man. He didn't look into one's eyes while speaking, spoke softly, in a muffled way, with many hesitations and embarrassed clearings of the throat. In all this, however, one detected that he was making a strenuous effort to suppress his shyness and to appear bold. Nonetheless, his nature bore all the earmarks of severe feelings of inferiority.

Familiarized with the basic rule, the patient began to speak softly and hesitatingly. The first communications included the recollection of two "horrible" experiences. While driving a car, he had once run over a woman, who had died from the effects of the accident. Another time he had gotten into a situation where he had to perform a tracheotomy on a person who was suffocating (the patient had been a medical orderly in the war). He could think of these two experiences only with horror. During the first sessions, he spoke about his home in an unvaried, somewhat monotonous, soft, and muffled way. As the second youngest of several brothers and sisters, he had a second-rate position in the household. The oldest brother, some twenty years his senior, was the darling of the parents. He had traveled a great deal and he knew his way around "in the world." At home he vaunted his experiences, and when he returned from a trip, "the entire household revolved around him." Though the envy and hatred of his brother were clearly evident from the content of the communication, the patient vehemently denied having any such feelings when I made a cautious inquiry in this direction. He had, he said, never felt any such thing against his brother.

Then he talked about his mother, who had been very good to him and who had died when he was seven years old. While speaking about her, he began to cry softly, was ashamed of his tears, and didn't say anything for a long time. It seemed clear that the mother had been the only person who had given him a bit of attention and love, that her demise had been a severe shock to him, and he could not hold back his tears in remembering her. After the death of his mother, he had spent five years in the house of his brother. It was not from what he said but from the way he said it that his enormous animosity toward the domineering, cold, and unfriendly nature of his brother became evident.

Then, in short, not very pregnant sentences, he related that he had a friend now who very much loved and admired him. Following this communication, there was a prolonged silence. A few days later he reported a dream: *he saw himself in a strange city with his friend, except that the face of his friend was different.* Since, for the purpose of the analysis, the patient had left the town in which he had been living, it was reasonable to assume that the man in the dream represented the analyst. The fact that the patient identified him with his friend could be interpreted as an indication of an incipient positive transference; but the situation as a whole militated against conceiving of this as a positive transference, and even against its interpretation. The patient himself recognized the analyst in the friend but had nothing to add to this. Since he was either silent or monotonously expressing doubts about *his* ability to carry out the analysis, I told him that he had something against me but lacked the courage to articulate it. He vehemently denied this, whereupon I told him that he had also never dared to express his hostile emotions toward his older brother, indeed had not even dared to think of them consciously. I also pointed out that he had obviously established some kind of connection between me and his older brother. This was true, but I committed the error of interpreting his resistance too deeply. The interpretation did not achieve its purpose, so I waited a few days, observing his demeanor the while, to see what relevance the resistance had for the contemporary situation. This much was clear to me: in addition to the transference of the hatred of the brother, there was a strong defense against a feminine attitude (the dream about the friend). Naturally, I couldn't risk an interpretation in this direction. So I continued to point out that, for one reason or another, he was fighting shy of me and the analysis. I told him that his whole manner was indicative of a block against the analysis. He agreed with this and went on to say that this had always been his way in life—rigid, inaccessible, defensive. While I constantly and consistently, in every session and at every opportunity, called his attention to his recalcitrance, I was struck by the monotonous tone in which he expressed his complaints. Every session began with the same remarks: "What's this all leading to, I don't feel a thing, the analysis has no influence on me, will I be able to go through with it, I can't, nothing comes to mind, the analysis has no influence on me," and so on. I couldn't understand what he was trying to express. And yet it was clear that here lay the key to the understanding of his resistance.[3]

This offers us a good opportunity to study the difference between the character-analytic and the active-suggestive preparation of the patient for analysis. I could have urged the patient in a nice way and endeavored to exercise a kind of comforting influence to get him to produce additional communications. It is even possible that, by so doing, I might have brought about an artificial positive transference; but experiences with other cases had taught me that one does not get very far with this approach. Since his entire demeanor left no room for doubt that he opposed the analysis in general and me in particular, there was no reason why I should not continue in this interpretation and wait for further reactions. One time, when we returned to the dream, he said the best proof that he did not reject me was the fact that he identified me with his friend. I took this opportunity to suggest that perhaps he had expected me to have the same liking and admiration for him that his friend had, that he had been disappointed, and now very much resented my reserve. He had to admit that he had harbored such thoughts but had not had the courage to tell me. Subsequently he told me that he had always merely demanded love and especially recognition and that he had always behaved very *defensively*, especially toward manly-looking men. He felt that he was not on a par with them, and in his relationship with his friend he played the feminine role. Again he offered me material toward the interpretation of his feminine transference, but his demeanor as a whole cautioned me against making such a disclosure. The situation was difficult, for the elements of his resistance which I already understood, the transference of the hatred he felt for his brother and the narcissistic-feminine attitude toward his superiors, had been sharply rejected. Hence, I had to be very careful if I did not want to risk the abrupt termination of the analysis at that time. Moreover, in each session, he complained almost without letup and always in the same way that the analysis was not having any effect on him, etc. Even after some four weeks of analysis, I still did not under-

---

[3]Footnote, 1945: While this explanation is psychologically correct, it is not the whole story. We understood now that such complaints are the direct expression of vegetative, i.e., muscular, armor. The patient complains of an affect-paralysis because his plasmatic currents and sensations are blocked. In short, this defect is essentially of a purely *biophysical* nature. In orgone therapy, the motility block is loosened by means of biophysical methods and not by means of psychological methods.

stand this attitude, though it appeared to me as an essential and momentarily acute character resistance.

I fell ill at this time and had to interrupt the analysis for two weeks. The patient sent me a bottle of cognac as a tonic. He seemed pleased when I resumed the analysis, but continued to complain in the same way, and told me that he was tortured by thoughts of death. He couldn't get it out of his mind that something had happened to someone in his family, and while I was sick he couldn't stop thinking that I might die. One day, when he was especially tortured by this thought, he made up his mind to send me the cognac. It was a very tempting opportunity to interpret his repressed death wishes. There was more than ample material for such an interpretation, yet I was held back by the consideration and the definite feeling that it would have been sterile, merely ricocheting from the wall of his complaints: "Nothing gets through to me"; the "analysis has no affect on me." In the meantime, of course, the concealed ambiguity of the complaint that "nothing gets through to me" had become clear. This was an expression of his deeply repressed passive-feminine transference desire for anal intercourse. But would it have been sensible and justified to interpret his homosexual desire, however clearly manifested, while his ego continued to protest against the analysis? First, the meaning of his complaint about the fruitlessness of the analysis had to become clear. I might have shown him that his complaint was unfounded. He always had new dreams to report, the thoughts of death became more pronounced, and many other things were taking place in him. I knew from experience that telling him this would not have eased the situation, despite the fact that I clearly felt the armor which stood between the analysis and the material offered by the id. Moreover, in all probability, I had to assume that the existing resistance would not allow any interpretation to pass through to the id. Thus, I continued to dwell on his behavior—interpreting it to him as an expression of his strong defense—and told him we both had to wait until the meaning of this behavior became clear to us. He had already grasped that the thoughts of death which he had had on the occasion of my illness did not necessarily have to be an expression of his loving concern for me.

In the course of the following weeks, the impressions of his behavior and his complaints multiplied. It became more and more clear that these complaints were intimately related to the defense of his feminine transference, but the situation was still not ripe for exact interpretation. I lacked a tight formulation of the meaning of his behavior as a whole. Let us summarize the fundamental aspects of the solution which followed later:

a. He wanted recognition and love from me as well as from all other men who appeared masculine to him. The fact that he wanted love and had been disappointed by me had already been interpreted repeatedly, without success.

b. His attitude toward me, the transference of his unconscious attitude toward his brother, was clearly full of hate and envy; to avoid the danger of having the interpretation fizzle out, it was best not to analyze this attitude at this point.

c. He warded off his feminine transference; the defense could not be interpreted without touching upon the forbidden femininity.

d. He felt inferior to me because of his femininity — and his continuous complaints could only be an expression of his inferiority complex.

I now interpreted his feelings of inferiority toward me. At first, this had no success. After several days of consistently dwelling upon his nature, however, he finally produced some communications on his inordinate envy, not of me but of other men he also felt inferior to. And now I was suddenly struck by the idea that his continual complaints that "the analysis has no effect on me" could have no other meaning than, "It's worthless." It follows, therefore, that the analyst is inferior, impotent, and could not achieve anything with him. Thus *the complaints were to be understood partially as a triumph over and partially as a reproach against the analyst.* Now I told him how I viewed his continual complaints; even I was amazed at the success. He accepted my interpretation as quite plausible. He immediately came up with a large number of examples which revealed that he always acted this way when someone wanted to influence him. He said that he could not endure another person's superiority and always endeavored to disparage those toward whom he felt inferior. He went on to say that he had always done the exact opposite of what a superior had demanded of him. He brought forward a wealth of recollections about his insolent and deprecatory attitude toward teachers.

Here, then, lay his pent-up aggressiveness, the most extreme expression of which, until this point, had been the death wish. But our joy was short-lived. The resistance returned in the same form — the same complaints, the same depression, the same silence. But now I knew that my disclosure had very much impressed him and, as a consequence, his feminine attitude had become *more pronounced*. The immediate result of this, naturally, was a renewed warding off of the effeminacy. In the analysis of this resistance, I again proceeded from his feelings of inferiority toward me, but I enlarged upon the interpretation by pointing out that he not only felt inferior but also, indeed precisely for this reason, felt himself cast in a feminine role toward me, a fact which was too much of an insult to his manly pride.

Notwithstanding the fact that he had, before this, produced a great deal of material about his feminine behavior toward manly men and had also showed complete understanding of it, he no longer wanted to know anything about it. This was a new problem. Why did he refuse to admit something he himself had described earlier? I continued to interpret the meaning of his acute behavior, namely that he felt so inferior toward me, that he refused to accept what I explained to him, though this refusal constituted reversal of his earlier position. He admitted that this was true, and went on to give a detailed account of his relationship to his friend. It turned out that he had indeed played the feminine role; there had often been intercourse between the thighs. I could now show him that his defensive behavior was nothing other than the expression of a struggle against the surrender to analysis which, for his unconscious, was obviously related to the idea of surrendering to the analyst in a feminine way. This too, however, was an insult to his pride and was the reason for his tenacious opposition to the influence of the analysis. He reacted to this with a confirmatory dream: he is lying on a sofa with the analyst and is kissed by him. However, this clear dream released a new wave of resistance, again in the old form of complaints (the analysis was not having any affect on him, couldn't have any influence on him, what was it leading to anyhow, he was completely cold, etc.). I interpreted his complaints as a deprecation of the analysis and a defense against surrendering to it. At the same time, I began to explain to him the economic meaning of his block. I told him that, even on the basis of what he had related about his childhood and adolescence, it was clear he had immured himself against all the disappointments which he had experienced in the outside world and against the rough, cold treatment on the part of father, brother, and teachers. This had been his only salvation, even if a salvation which entailed many restrictions upon his enjoyment of life.

He immediately accepted this explanation as plausible and followed it up with remembrances of his behavior toward teachers. He had always found them so cold and alien (a clear projection of his own feelings), and even if he were outwardly agitated when they beat or scolded him, he remained inwardly indifferent. In this connection, he told me that he had often wished I were more strict. At first, the meaning of this desire did not appear to fit into the situation; much later it became clear that at the bottom of his obstinacy lay the intent to put me and my prototypes, the teachers, in the wrong.

For several days the analysis proceeded free of resistances; now he went on to relate that there had been a time in his early childhood when he had been very wild and aggressive. At the same time, curiously, he produced dreams which revealed a strong feminine attitude toward me. I could only surmise that the recollection of his aggressiveness had simultaneously mobilized the guilt feeling which was expressed in these dreams of a passive-feminine nature. I avoided an analysis of the dreams not only because they were not directly related to the existing transference situation but also because he did not appear prepared to grasp the connection between his aggression and dreams expressing a guilt feeling. I assume that some analysts will regard this as an arbitrary selection of material. Against this, however, I have to defend the clinically tested position that the optimum in therapy will be achieved when a direct connection has been established between the contemporary transference situation and the infantile material. So I merely voiced the supposition that his recollection of the wild conduct of his childhood indicated he had once been wholly different, the exact opposite of what he was today, and the analysis would have to uncover the time and the circumstances that led to the transformation of his character. Presumably, his present effeminacy was a moving out of the way of aggressive masculinity. The patient did not react to this disclosure at all; instead, he sank back into the old resistance: he couldn't manage it, he didn't feel anything, the analysis had no effect on him, etc.

I again interpreted his feelings of inferiority and his repeated attempt to show up the powerlessness of the analysis or, more to the point, of the analyst; but I also endeavored now to work out the transference of the attitude he held toward his brother. He himself had said that the brother had always played the dominant role. He entered into this only with great hesitation, evidently because it concerned the central conflict situation of his childhood. He repeated that the mother had paid a great deal of attention to the brother, without, however, going into his subjective attitude toward this preference. As was brought out by a cautious inquiry in this direction, he was completely closed to an insight into his envy of his brother. This envy, it had to be assumed, was so intimately associated with an intensive hate and repressed out of fear that not even the feeling of envy was permitted to enter consciousness. An especially strong resistance resulted from my attempt to draw out his envy of his brother; it lasted many days and was marked by stereotyped complaints about his powerlessness. Since the resistance did not give way, it had to be assumed that we were dealing with a very immediate defense against the person of the analyst. I again urged him to speak openly and without fear about the analysis and particularly about the analyst and to tell what impression the analyst had made on him on first encounter.[4] After a long hesitation, he told me in a faltering voice that the analyst had appeared crudely masculine and brutal to him, as a man who would be absolutely ruthless toward women in sexual matters. How did this fit in with his attitude toward men who appeared potent?

We were at the end of the fourth month of analysis. Now, for the first time, that repressed relationship to the brother broke through which was intimately related to the most disruptive element of the existing transference, envy of potency. Revealing strong affects, he suddenly remembered that he had always condemned his brother in the most rigorous manner because he (the brother) chased after all the girls, seduced them, and, moreover, made a show of it. My appearance had immediately reminded him of his brother. Given greater confidence by his last communication, I again explained the transference situation and showed him that he identified me with his potent brother and, precisely for this reason, could not open himself to me; that is, he condemned me and resented my alleged superiority, as he had once condemned and resented his brother's alleged superiority. I told him, furthermore, that it was clearly evident now that the basis of his inferiority was a feeling of impotence.

After this explanation, *the central element of the character resistance*

---

[4]Since then, I am in the habit of urging the patient to give me a description of my person. This always proves to be a fruitful measure for the removal of blocked transference situations.

emerged spontaneously. In a correctly and consistently carried out analysis, this will happen every time, *without the analyst having to push matters or give anticipatory conceptions*. In a flash he remembered that he had repeatedly compared his own small penis with his brother's big penis, and had envied his brother because of it.

As was to be expected, a powerful resistance again ensued; again he complained, "I can't do anything," etc. Now I was able to go a step further in my interpretations and show him that these complaints were a verbalization of his feeling of impotence. His reaction to this was completely unexpected. After my interpretation of his distrust, he declared for the first time that he had never believed any man, that he believed nothing at all, probably not even the analysis. Naturally, this was a big step forward. But the meaning of this communication, its connection to the preceding situation, was not immediately clear. He spoke for two hours on the many disappointments which he had experienced in his life, and was of the opinion that his distrust could be rationally traced back to these disappointments. The old resistance reappeared. Since I was not sure what lay behind it this time, I decided to wait. For several days the situation remained unchanged—the old complaints, the familiar behavior. I continued to interpret the elements of the resistance which had already been worked through and were very familiar to me, when suddenly a new element emerged. He said that *he was afraid of the analysis because it might deprive him of his ideals*. Now the situation was clear again. He had transferred to me the castration anxiety which he felt toward his brother. He was afraid of me. Naturally, I made no mention of the castration anxiety, but again proceeded from his inferiority complex and his impotence and asked him whether he did not feel himself superior to all people on the basis of his high ideals, whether he did not regard himself as better than all the others. This he readily admitted; indeed, he went even further. He asserted that he really was superior to all the others, who chased after women and were like animals in their sexuality. With less certitude he added that, unfortunately, this feeling was frequently disturbed by his impotence. Evidently, he had not yet entirely come to terms with his sexual debility. Now I was able to elucidate the neurotic manner in which he was attempting to deal with his feeling of impotence and to show him that he was seeking to regain a feeling of potency in the sphere of ideals. I showed him the compensation and again drew his attention to the resistances to the analysis which stemmed from his secret feeling of superiority. It was not only that he secretly thought of himself as better and more intelligent; it was precisely for this reason that he had to resist the analysis. For if it turned out to be a success, then he would have needed someone's help and the analysis would have vanquished his neurosis, the secret value of which we had just uncovered. From the point of view of the neurosis, this constituted a defeat and, in the terms of his unconscious, this also meant becoming a woman. In this way, moving forward from his ego and its defense mechanisms, I prepared the ground for the interpretation of the castration complex and the feminine fixation.

Thus, using the patient's demeanor as its point of departure, character analysis had succeeded in penetrating directly to the center of the neurosis, his castration anxiety, the envy of his brother stemming from the mother's preference of the brother, and the concomitant disappointment in her. The outlines of the Oedipus complex were already coming into view. Here, however, what is important is not that these unconscious elements emerged — this often happens spontaneously. What is important is the legitimate sequence in which they emerged and the intimate contact they had with the ego defense and the transference. Last but not least, it is important that this happened without pushing but through pure analytic interpretation of the patient's bearing and with accompanying affects. This constitutes what is specific to consistent character analysis. It means a thorough working through of the conflicts assimilated *by the ego.*

Let us compare this with what might have resulted if we had not consistently focused on our patient's ego defense. Right at the beginning, the possibility existed of interpreting both his passive homosexual relationship to his brother and the death wish. We have no doubt that dreams and subsequent associations would have yielded additional material for interpretation. However, unless his ego defense had been systematically and thoroughly worked through beforehand, no interpretation would have evoked an affective response; instead, we would have obtained an intellectual knowledge of his passive desire on the one hand and a narcissistic, highly affective defense against these desires on the other hand. The affects pertaining to the passivity and murder impulses would have remained in the function of defense. The result would have been a chaotic situation, the typical bleak picture of an analysis rich in interpretation and poor in success. Several months of patient and persistent work on the ego resistance, with particular reference to its form (complaints, inflection, etc.), lifted the ego to the level necessary to assimilate what was repressed, loosened the affects, and brought about a shifting in their direction to the repressed ideas.

Thus, it cannot be said that there were *two* techniques which could have been applied in this case; there was only one, if the intent was to change the case *dynamically*. I hope that this case has made sufficiently clear the predominant difference in the conception of the application of theory to technique. The most important criterion of effective analysis is the use of *few* (but accurate and consistent) interpretations, instead of many unsystematic interpretations which fail to take the dynamic and economic moment into account. If the analyst does not allow himself to be tempted by the material but correctly assesses its dynamic position and economic role, the result is that, though he will receive the material later, it will be that much more thorough and affect-laden. The second criterion is the maintaining of a continuous connection between the contemporary situation and the infantile situation. The initial disconnectedness and confusion of the analytic material is transformed into an orderly sequence, that is, the succession of the resistances and contents is now determined by the special dynamics and structural relations of the particular neurosis. When the work of interpretation is not performed systematically, the analyst must always make a fresh start, search about, divine more than deduce. When the work of interpretation proceeds along character-analytic lines, on the other hand, the analytic process develops naturally. In the former case, the analysis runs smoothly in the beginning only to become more and more entangled in difficulties; in the latter case, the most serious difficulties present themselves in the first weeks and months of the treatment, only to give way to smoother work, even in the deepest material. Hence, the fate of each analysis depends upon the introduction of the treatment, i.e., upon the correct or incorrect unraveling of the resistances. Thus, the third criterion is the unraveling of the case, not arbitrarily from any position which happens to be conspicuous and intelligible, but from those positions where the strongest ego resistance is concealed, followed by the systematic expansion of the initial incursion into the unconscious and the working through of the important infantile fixations, which are affect-laden at any given time. An unconscious position which manifests itself in dreams or in an association, at a certain point in the treatment and notwithstanding the fact that it is of central importance for the neurosis, can play a completely subordinate role, i.e., have no contemporary importance with respect to the technique of the case. In our patient, the feminine relationship to the brother was the central pathogen; yet in the first months the fear of losing the compensation for impotence provided by the fantasized ego ideals constituted the problem with respect to technique. The error which is usually made is that the analyst attacks the central element in the neurotic formation (which usually manifests itself in some way right at the outset), instead of first attacking those positions which have a specific contemporary importance. Systematically worked through in succession, these positions *must* eventually lead to the central pathogenic element. In short, it is important, indeed decisive for the success of many cases, *how, when,* and from which side the analyst penetrates to the core of the neurosis.

It is not difficult to fit what we are describing here as character analysis into Freud's theory of resistance formation and resistance resolution. We know that every resistance consists of an id impulse which is warded off and an ego impulse which wards off. Both impulses are unconscious. In principle, it would seem to be a matter of choice whether the striving of the id or the striving of the ego is interpreted first. For example: if a homosexual resistance in the form of silence is encountered right at the outset of an analysis, the striving of the id can be taken up by telling the patient that he is presently engaged in tender intentions toward the person of the analyst. His positive transference has been interpreted and, if he does not take flight, it will be a long time before he becomes reconciled to this hideous idea. Hence, the analyst must give precedence to that aspect of the resistance which lies closer to the conscious ego, namely *the ego defense,* by merely telling the patient, to begin with, that he is silent because he rejects the analysis *"for one reason or another,"* presumably because it has become dangerous to him in some way. In short, the resistance is attacked without entering into the striving of the id. In the former case, that aspect of the resistance which pertains to the id (in the above instance, the love tendency) has been attacked through interpretation; in the latter case, that part of the resistance pertaining to the ego, i.e., the rejection, is attacked through interpretation.

By using this procedure, we simultaneously penetrate the negative transference, in which every defense finally ends, and also the character, the armor of the ego. The surface layer of *every* resistance, i.e., the layer closest to consciousness, must of necessity be a negative attitude toward the analyst, whether the id striving is based on hate or love. The ego projects onto the analyst its defense against the striving of the id. Thus, the analyst becomes an enemy and is dangerous because, by his imposition of the irksome basic rule, he has provoked id strivings and has disturbed the neurotic balance. In its defense, the ego makes use of very old forms of defensive attitudes. In a pinch it calls upon hate impulses from the id for help in its defense, even when it is warding off a love striving.

Thus, if we adhere to the rule of tackling that part of the resistance which pertains to the ego, we also resolve a part of negative transference in the process, a quantity of affect-laden hate, and thereby avoid the danger of overlooking the destructive tendencies which are very often brilliantly concealed; at the same time the positive transference is strengthened. The patient also comprehends the ego interpretation more easily because it is more related to his conscious feelings; in this way, he is also more prepared for the id interpretations which follow later.

No matter what kind of id strivings we are dealing with, the ego defense always has the same form, namely one that corresponds to the patient's character; and the same id striving is warded off in various ways in various patients. Thus, we leave the character untouched when we interpret only the striving of the id; on the other hand, we include the neurotic character in the analysis when we tackle the resistances fundamentally from the defense, i.e., from the ego side. In the former case, we tell the analysand immediately *what* he is warding off; in the latter case, we first make it clear to him *that* he is warding off "something," then *how* he is going about it, what means he is employing to do it (character analysis), and only much later, when the analysis of the resistance has progressed sufficiently, he is told or finds out for himself what the defense is directed against. In this very roundabout way to the interpretation of the id strivings, all the germane attitudes of the ego are taken apart analytically, thus precluding the grave danger that the patient will learn something too soon, or that he will remain unemotional and unconcerned.

Analyses in which the attitudes are accorded so much analytic attention proceed in a more orderly and more effective manner, without the least detriment to the theoretical research work. It is only that the important events of childhood are learned later than usual. However, this is amply compensated for by the emotional freshness with which the infantile material springs forth *after* the character resistances have been worked through analytically.

Yet, we must not fail to mention certain unpleasant aspects of consistent character analysis. Character analysis subjects the patient to far more psychic strain; the patient suffers much more than when the character is left out of consideration. This has, to be sure, the advantage of a weeding out: those who don't hold out would not have been cured anyhow, and it is better to have a case fail after four or six months than to have it fail after two years. But experience shows that if the character resistance does not break down, a satisfactory success cannot be counted on. This is especially true of cases having concealed character resistances. The overcoming of the character resistance does not mean that the patient has changed his character; this is possible only after the analysis of its infantile sources. He must merely have objectified it and have gained an analytic interest in it. Once this has been accomplished, a favorable continuation of the analysis is very probable.

The Breaking Down of the Narcissistic Defense Apparatus

As we already mentioned, the essential difference between the analysis of a symptom and that of a neurotic character trait consists in the fact that, from the very outset, the former is isolated and objectified, whereas the latter must be continually singled out in the analysis so that the patient gains the same attitude toward it as toward a symptom. It is only seldom that this happens easily. There are patients who show very little inclination to take an objective view of their character. This is understandable, for it is a question of the breaking down of the narcissistic defense mechanism, and the working through of the libido anxiety which is bound in it.

A twenty-five-year-old man sought analytic help because of a few minor symptoms and a disturbance in his work. He exhibited a free, self-confident bearing, yet one sometimes had the vague impression that his behavior required great strain and that he did not establish a genuine relationship with the person with whom he happened to be speaking. There was something cold in his manner of speaking; his voice was soft and subtly ironic. Once in a while he smiled, but it was hard to know whether it was a smile indicative of embarrassment, superiority, or irony.

The analysis commenced with violent emotions and a vast amount of enactment. He cried when he spoke of his mother's demise and swore when he described the usual upbringing of children. He divulged only very general information about his past: his parents had had a very unhappy marriage; his mother had been very strict with him; and it wasn't until he had reached maturity that he established a rather superficial relationship with his brothers and sisters. All his communications sharpened the original impression that neither his crying nor his swearing nor any of his other emotions was sincere and natural. He himself stated that it really wasn't so bad as all that, and indeed he was forever smiling at everything he said. After several sessions, he took to provoking the analyst. When I had concluded the session, for example, he would continue to lie on the couch ostentatiously for a while; or he would strike up a conversation afterwards. Once he asked me what I would do if he seized me by the throat. Two sessions later he tried to frighten me by a sudden movement of his hand toward my head. I shrank back instinctively and told him that the analysis required of him only that he say everything, not that he do everything. Another time, he stroked my arm on taking leave. The deeper but inexplicable meaning of this behavior was an incipient homosexual transference which was expressing itself sadistically. When I translated these actions superficially as provocations, he smiled to himself and immured himself even more. The actions as well as the communications ceased; only the stereotyped smile remained. He began to immerse himself in silence. When I called his attention to the resistive character of his behavior, he merely smiled again and repeated, after a period of silence, the word "resistance" several times, in a clearly ironic tone of voice. In this way, his smiling and his tendency to treat everything ironically became the fulcrum of the analytic task.

The situation was difficult enough. Apart from the scanty information about his childhood, I knew nothing about him. So I had to concentrate on his mode of behavior in the analysis. For the time being, I withdrew into a passive position and waited to see what would come, but there was no change in his behavior. About two weeks elapsed in this way. Then it struck me that, in point of time, the intensification of his smiling coincided with my warding off his aggression. So, to begin with, I tried to make him understand the contemporary reason for his smiling. I told him that there was no doubt his smiling meant many different things, but at the moment it was his reaction to my cowardice as testified by my instinctive drawing back. He said that this was very likely true, but he would continue to smile nonetheless. He spoke little and on matters of subsidiary importance, treated the analysis ironically, and stated that he couldn't believe anything I told him. Gradually, it became more and more clear that his smiling served as a defense against the analysis. I repeatedly pointed this out to him throughout several sessions, but several weeks elapsed before he had a dream, the content of which was that a pillar made of brick was cut down into individual bricks by a machine. What relation this dream had to the analytic situation was all the more difficult to fathom inasmuch as he did not produce any associations at first. Finally, he stated that the dream was altogether quite clear; obviously, it dealt with the castration complex — and he smiled. I told him that his irony was merely an attempt to disavow the sign that the unconscious had given him through the dream. This evoked a screen memory, which was of the greatest importance for the future development of the analysis. He remembered that once, when he was about five, he had "played horsy" in the courtyard of his parents' home. He had crawled about on all fours, letting his penis hang out of his pants; his mother had caught him in the act and asked him what he was doing — he had merely smiled. For the time being, there was nothing else to be gotten out of him. Yet, some clarity had been gained; his smiling was a part of the mother transference. When I now told him that, obviously, he was acting here as he had acted toward his mother and that his smiling must have a definite meaning, he merely smiled. All this was of course very nice, he said, but its meaning eluded him. For several days we had the same smiling and silence on his part and, on my part, consistent interpretation of his behavior as a defense against the analysis and of his smiling as the conquering of a secret fear of this interpretation. Yet he warded off this interpretation of his behavior with his typical smile. This, too, was consistently interpreted as a block against my influence, and I pointed out to him that he evidently was always smiling in life. He admitted that this was the only possibility of holding one's own in the world. In admitting this, however, he had unwittingly concurred with my interpretation. One day he came into the analysis wearing his usual smile and said, "You'll be happy today, Doctor. I was struck by something funny. In my mother tongue, bricks mean the testicles of a horse. That's pretty good, isn't it? You see, it is the castration complex." I told him that this might or might not be the case, but as long as he persisted

in his defensive attitude, it was out of the question to think of
analyzing his dream. He would be sure to nullify every association and
every interpretation with his smiling. We have to append here that his
smile was hardly more than a suggestion of a smile; it expressed, rather,
a sense of mockery. I told him that he had no need to be afraid to laugh
heartily and loudly at the analysis. From then on, he came out much
more clearly with his irony. But the verbal association, so ironically
communicated, was a very valuable cue toward an understanding of
the situation. It seemed very probable that, as is often the case, the
analysis had been conceived of as a castration threat and had been
warded off in the beginning with aggression and later with smiling. I returned to the aggression he had expressed at the beginning of the analysis and supplemented my earlier interpretation by pointing out
that he had used his provocation to test to what extent he could trust
me, to see how far he could go. In short, his lack of trust was very likely
rooted in a childhood fear. This explanation made an evident impression on him. He was momentarily shaken, but quickly recovered and
began once again to deride the analysis and the analyst. Well aware,
from the few indications derived from the reactions to his dream, that
my interpretations were hitting home and were undermining his ego
defense, I refused to be diverted. Unfortunately, he was not too happy
about this, and he stuck to his smiling just as tenaciously as I stuck to
my explanatory work. Many sessions elapsed without any apparent
progress. I intensified my interpretations not only by becoming more
insistent but also by more closely relating his smiling to the supposed
infantile fear. I pointed out that he was afraid of the analysis because it
would arouse his childhood conflicts. He had, I said, at one time come
to terms with these conflicts, even if not in a very satisfactory way, and
now he recoiled from the possibility of having again to go through all
that he thought he had mastered with the help of his smile. But he was
deceiving himself, for his excitement in telling of his mother's death
had certainly been genuine. I also ventured the opinion that his relationship to his mother had not been unambiguous; surely he had not
only feared her and derided her but also loved her. Somewhat more seriously than usual, he related details of his mother's loveless attitude
toward him. Once, when he had been naughty, she had even injured
his hand with a knife. To this, however, he added, "Right, according to
analytic theory, this is again the castration complex?" But something
serious seemed to be preparing itself inside of him. On the basis of the

analytic situation, I continued to interpret the contemporary and latent meaning of his smile. During this time, additional dreams were reported. Their manifest content was rather typical of symbolic castration fantasies. Finally, he produced a dream in which horses appeared, and another dream in which the fire department was mobilized and out of a truck rose a high tower from which a powerful column of water was discharged into the flames of a burning house. At this time, occasional bed-wettings were also reported. He himself recognized, albeit still with a smile, the connection between the "horse dream" and his playing "horsy." He recalled, indeed, that the long genital of horses had always been of special interest to him, and added spontaneously that he had no doubt imitated such a horse in the childish game. Micturition had also afforded him great pleasure. He did not remember whether he had wet his bed as a child.

Another time when we were discussing the infantile meaning of his smile, he put a different interpretation on the smile of the childhood incident in which he had been playing "horsy." It was quite possible, he said, that it had been intended not as a sneer but as an attempt to disarm his mother, out of fear that she would scold him. In this way, he came closer and closer to what, on the basis of his behavior in the analysis, I had been interpreting to him for months. Thus, the function and meaning of the smile had changed in the course of his development: *at first it had been an attempt to propitiate, later it had become a compensation for inner fear, and finally it served a feeling of superiority.* The patient himself hit upon this explanation when, in the course of several sessions, he reconstructed the way he had found to keep at bay the misery of his childhood. Hence, the meaning was: "Nothing can harm me; I am immune to everything." It was in the latter sense that the smile had become a resistance in the analysis, a defense against the resuscitation of the old conflicts. Infantile fear seemed to be the essential motive for this defense. A dream which the patient had at about the end of the fifth month of analysis revealed the deepest layer of his fear, the fear of being deserted by his mother. The dream went as follows: "Accompanied by an unknown person, I am riding in a car through a completely deserted and dreary looking town. The houses are dilapidated, the windows smashed. No one is to be seen. It is as if death has ravaged this place. We come to a gate, and I want to turn back. I tell my companion we should have another look around. A man and a woman in mourning are kneeling on the sidewalk. I walk toward them with the intent of asking them something. As I touch their shoulders, they are startled, and I wake up in fear." The most important association was that the town was similar to the one he had lived in until he was four. Symbolically, the death of the mother and the feeling of infantile desertion were clearly intimated. The companion was the analyst. For the first time the patient took a dream completely seriously and without smiling. The character resistance had been broken through and the connection had been established to the infantile material. From this point on, apart from the usual interruptions caused by relapses into the old character resistance, the analysis proceeded without any particular difficulty. But a deep depression ensued, which disappeared only with time.

Naturally, the difficulties were far greater than may be evident from this brief summary. The resistance phase from beginning to end lasted almost six months and was marked by continuing mockery of the analysis. If it had not been for the necessary patience and confidence in the effectiveness of consistent interpretation of the character resistance, one might easily have "thrown in the sponge."

Let us now endeavor to decide whether the subsequent analytic insight into the mechanism of this case would justify the use of a different technical procedure. It is true that the manner of the patient's behavior could have been given less prominence in the analysis; instead, the scanty dreams could have been subjected to more exact analysis. It is also true that he might have produced interpretable associations. Let us pass over the fact that, until he entered analysis, this patient always forgot his dreams or didn't dream at all. And it wasn't until his behavior was consistently interpreted that he produced dreams of a definite content and of a specific relevance to the analytic situation. I am prepared for the objection that the patient would have produced the corresponding dreams spontaneously. To enter into such a discussion is to get into an argument about things that cannot be proven. There are ample experiences which show that a situation such as the one presented by this patient is not easily resolved solely through passive waiting; and if it is, then it happens only by chance, i.e., the analyst does not have the analysis under control.

Let us assume that we had interpreted his associations relating to the castration complex, that is, tried to make him conscious of the repressed content, the fear of cutting or of being cut. Eventually this approach, too, *might have* achieved success. But the very fact that we cannot say with certainty that that would have been the case, the fact that we admit the element of chance, compels us to reject as unanalytic this kind of technique which violates the essence of psychoanalytic work. Such a technique would mean a reversion to that stage of analysis where one did not bother about the resistances because one did not recognize them, and therefore interpreted the meaning of the unconscious directly. It is evident from the case history itself that this technique would also have meant a neglect of the ego defenses.

It might also be objected that, while the technical handling of the case was absolutely correct, my polemics were uncalled for. What I am saying is quite obvious and not at all new—that's the way all analysts work. I do not deny that the general principles are not new, that character analysis is merely the special application of the principle of resistance analysis. But many years of experience in the seminar have clearly and unequivocally shown that while the principles of resistance technique are generally known and acknowledged, in practice one proceeds almost exclusively according to the old technique of direct interpretation of the unconscious. This discrepancy between theoretical knowledge and actual practice was the cause of all the mistaken objections to the systematic attempts on the part of the Vienna seminar to develop the consistent application of theory to therapy. Those who said that all this was commonplace and that there was nothing new in it were basing their statements on their theoretical knowledge; those who contended that this was all wrong and not "Freudian analysis" were thinking of their own practice, which, as we have said, deviated considerably from theory.

A colleague once asked me what I would have done in the following case. For four weeks he had been treating a young man who immured himself in complete silence but who was otherwise very friendly and, before and after the analytic session, feigned a very genial disposition. The analyst had already tried everything possible, threatened to terminate the analysis, and finally, when even a dream interpretation failed to achieve any results, had set a definite termination date. The scanty dream material had contained nothing but sadistic murders; the analyst had told the patient that his dreams showed quite clearly that he conceived of himself as a murderer in fantasy. But this had not served any purpose. The analyst was not satisfied with my statement that it does not do to make a deep interpretation to a patient who has an acute resistance, even though the material appears quite manifestly in a dream. He was of the opinion that there was no alternative but to do that. To my suggestion that, to begin with, the patient's silence should have been interpreted as a resistance, he said that this was not possible: there was "no material" available for such an interpretation. Wasn't there, quite apart from the content of the dreams, sufficient "material" in the patient's behavior itself, the contradiction between his silence during the analytic session and his friendliness outside of it? Wasn't at least one thing clear from the situation, namely that through his silence the patient—to put it in very general terms—expressed a negative attitude or a defense; expressed, to judge from his dreams, sadistic impulses which he sought to counter and conceal through his obtrusively friendly behavior? Why is it that an analyst will venture to infer unconscious processes from a patient's slip—e.g., the forgetting of an object in the analyst's consultation room—but is afraid to make inferences, from the patient's behavior, which will have bearing on the meaning of the analytic situation? Does a patient's behavior offer less conclusive material than a slip? Somehow I couldn't get this across to my colleague. He stuck to his view that the resistance could not be tackled because there was "no material." There can be no doubt that the interpretation of the murderous wish was a mistake; the result of such an interpretation can only be that the patient's ego becomes even more frightened and even more inaccessible to analysis. The difficulties offered by the cases presented in the seminar were of a similar nature. There was always an underestimation of or disregard for the patient's behavior as interpretable material; the repeated attempt to eliminate the resistance from the position of the id, instead of through the analysis of the ego defense; and finally the oft-repeated idea, which served as an excuse, that the patient simply did not want to get well or was "much too narcissistic."

The technique of breaking down the narcissistic defense in other types is not fundamentally different from that described above. If, for example, a patient never becomes emotionally involved and remains indifferent, regardless of what material he produces, one is dealing with a dangerous emotional block, the analysis of which must take precedence over everything else if one does not want to run the risk of having all the material and interpretations lost. If this is the case, the patient may acquire a good knowledge of psychoanalytic theory, but he will not be cured. If, confronted with such a block, the analyst elects not to give up the analysis because of the "strong narcissism," he can make an agreement with the patient. The patient will be given the option to terminate the analysis at any time; in turn, he will allow the analyst to dwell upon his emotional lameness until it is eliminated. Eventually—it usually takes many months (in one case it took a year and a half)—the patient begins to buckle under the continual stressing of his emotional lameness and its causes. In the meantime, the analyst will gradually have obtained sufficient clues to undermine the defense against anxiety, which is what an emotional block is. Finally, the patient rebels against the threat of the analysis, rebels against the threat to his protective psychic armor, of being put at the mercy of his drives, particularly his aggressive drives. By rebelling against this "nonsense," however, his aggressiveness is aroused and it is not long before the first emotional outbreak ensues (i.e., a negative transference) in the form of a paroxysm of hate. If the analyst succeeds in getting this far, the contest has been won. When the aggressive impulses have been brought into the open, the emotional block has been penetrated and the patient is capable of analysis. From this point on, the analysis runs its usual course. The difficulty consists in drawing out the aggressiveness.

The same holds true when, because of the peculiarity of their character, narcissistic patients vent their resistance verbally. For example, they speak in a grandiloquent manner, use technical terminology, always rigidly chosen or else confused. This manner of speaking constitutes an impenetrable wall; until it is subjected to analysis, no real progress can be made. Here, too, the consistent interpretation of the patient's behavior provokes a narcissistic rebellion: the patient does not like to hear that he speaks in such a stilted, grandiloquent manner, or uses technical terminology to conceal his inferiority complex from himself and from the analyst, or that he speaks confusedly because he wants to appear especially clever—the truth of the matter being that he cannot formulate his thoughts simply. In this way the hard terrain of the neurotic character has been loosened in an essential area and an approach has been paved to the infantile foundation of the character and the neurosis. Needless to say, it is not enough to make passing allusions to the nature of the resistance. The more tenacious it proves to be, the more consistently it must be interpreted. If the negative attitudes toward the analyst which are provoked by this consistent interpretation are simultaneously analyzed, then there is little danger that the patient will terminate the treatment.

The immediate result of the analytic loosening of the character armor and the disruption of the narcissistic protective apparatus is twofold: (1) *the loosening of the affects from their reactive anchorings and concealments*; (2) *the establishment of an entry into the central area of the infantile conflict, the Oedipus complex and the castration anxiety.* There is an advantage in this procedure which should not be underestimated: it is not only the content of infantile experiences that is reached. More important, they are brought directly to analysis in the specific context in which they have been assimilated, i.e., *in the form in which they have been molded by the ego.* It is seen again and again in analysis that the dynamic value of the same element of repressed material varies depending on the degree to which the ego defenses have been loosened. In many cases the affect-cathexis of the childhood experiences has been absorbed into the character as a defensive mechanism, so that, by simply interpreting the content, one reaches the remembrances but not the affects. In such cases, to interpret the infantile material *before* the affects assimilated into the character have been loosened is a grave mistake. It is, for example, to this neglect that the long, bleak, and more or less fruitless analyses of compulsive characters are to be traced.[5] If, on the other hand, the affects pertaining to the defensive formation of the character are liberated first, then a new cathexis of the infantile instinctual expressions takes place automatically. The character-analytic interpretation of resistances all but excludes remembering without affects because of the disturbance of the neurotic balance, which always occurs at the outset in character analysis.

In still other cases, the character erects itself as a hard protective wall against the experiencing of infantile anxiety and thus maintains itself, notwithstanding the great forfeiture of *joie de vivre* which this entails. If a patient having such a character enters analytic treatment because of some symptom or other, this protective wall continues to serve in the analysis as a character resistance; and it soon becomes ap-

---

[5]Let the following case serve as an example of how decisive it is to take into consideration or neglect a patient's mode of behavior. A compulsive character who had twelve years of analysis behind him without any commensurate improvement and was well informed on his infantile motivations, e.g., on the central father-conflict, spoke in a strange monotone in the analysis, in a somewhat singsong cadence and kept wringing his hands. I asked whether this behavior had ever been analyzed. It had not. At first, I had no insight into the case. One day it struck me that he spoke as if he were praying. I informed him of my observation, whereupon he told me that as a child he had been forced by his father to attend prayer meetings, which he had done very reluctantly. He had prayed, but under protest. In the same way he had recited to the analyst for twelve years, "Fine, I'll do as you say, but under protest." The uncovering of this apparently insignificant detail in his behavior threw open the analysis and led to the most deeply buried affects.

parent that nothing can be accomplished until the character armor, which conceals and consumes the infantile anxiety, has been destroyed. This, for example, is the case in moral insanity and in manic, narcissistic-sadistic characters. Here, the analyst is often faced with the difficult question whether the existing symptom justifies a thoroughgoing character analysis. For let there be no doubt about it: when the analysis of the character destroys the character compensation, especially in cases where that defense is a relatively good one, a temporary condition is created which approximates a breakdown of the ego. In some extreme cases, it is true, such a breakdown is necessary before the new reality-oriented ego structure can develop. (However, we must admit that the breakdown would have come of itself sooner or later—the formation of a symptom was the first sign of this.) Yet one is reluctant, unless an urgent indication exists, to adopt a measure which involves such grave responsibility.

Nor can it be ignored in this connection that, in every case in which it is used, character analysis provokes violent emotions; indeed, often creates dangerous situations. Hence, the analyst must have technical mastery of the analysis at all times. Some analysts will perhaps reject the character-analytic procedure for this reason. If such is so, however, the analytic treatment of quite a number of patients can be counted upon to fail. There are neuroses which simply cannot be reached through mild means. The methods employed in character analysis, the consistent stressing of the character resistance and the persistent interpretation of its forms, means, and motives, are as powerful as they are disagreeable to the patient. This has nothing to do with preparing the patient for analysis; it is a strict analytic principle. However, it is good policy to make the patient aware, at the very outset, of all the foreseeable unpleasantness and difficulties of the treatment.

On the Optimal Conditions for the Analytic Reduction to the Infantile Situation from the Contemporary Situation

Since the consistent interpretation of a patient's behavior spontaneously provides access to the infantile sources of the neurosis, a new question arises: are there criteria for determining when the contemporary mode of behavior should be reduced to its infantile prototype? Indeed, one of the main tasks of analysis consists precisely in this reduction. In these general terms, however, the formula is not applicable in everyday practice. Should this reduction take place immediately, as soon as the first signs of the germane infantile material become apparent, or are there factors which indicated that it would be better to wait until a certain specific time? To begin with, it must be borne in mind that the purpose of reduction, namely the dissolution of the resistance and the elimination of amnesia, is not immediately encompassed in many cases. This much we know from definite experiences. Either the patient does not get beyond an intellectual understanding or the attempt at reduction is foiled by doubt. This is explained by the fact that, just as in the case of making an unconscious idea conscious, the topographical process of conversion actually culminates only when combined with the *dynamic-affective* process of becoming conscious. Two things are necessary to achieve this: (1) the main resistance must at least be loosened; (2) the cathexis of the idea which is to become conscious or (as in the case of reduction) which is to be exposed to a definite connection must have attained a minimum degree of intensity. As we know, however, the libido-charged affects of the repressed ideas are usually split off, i.e., bound in the character or in the acute transference conflicts and transference resistances. If the contemporary resistance is now reduced to its infantile source, before it has been fully developed (that is, as soon as a trace of its infantile foundation has been spotted), then the intensity of its cathexis has not been fully taken advantage of. The content of the resistance has been analytically utilized in the interpretation, but the corresponding affect has not been included. If, in other words, both the topographical and the dynamic points of view are taken into consideration in making one's interpretations, then we have the following stricture imposed upon us: the resistance must not be nipped in the bud. On the contrary, it must be allowed to reach full maturity in the heat of the transference situation. In the case of torpid character encrustations which have become chronic, the difficulties cannot be gotten at in any other way. To Freud's rule that the patient has to be led from acting out to remembering, from the contemporary to the infantile, must be added that, *before* this takes place, what has been chronically stultified has to attain a new living reality in the contemporary transference situation. This is the same process involved in the healing of chronic inflammations— i.e., they are first made acute by means of irritation—and this is always necessary in the case of character resistances. In advanced stages of the analysis, when the analyst is sure of the patient's cooperation, "irritation therapy," as Ferenczi called it, is no longer as necessary. One gets the impression that when an analyst reduces a wholly immature transference situation he does so out of fear of the stresses which are part and parcel of strong transference resistances. So, despite one's better theoretical knowledge, the resistance is often regarded as something highly unwelcome, as merely disruptive. This is also the reason for the tendency to circumvent the resistance, instead of allowing it to develop and then attacking it. It seems to be forgotten that the neurosis itself is contained in the resistance, that, in dissolving a resistance, we also dissolve a part of the neurosis.

Allowing the resistance to develop is necessary for another reason. In view of the complicated structure of each resistance, all its determinants and meaningful contents are comprehended only with time; and the more thoroughly a resistance situation has been comprehended, the more successful its interpretation will be, quite apart from the previously mentioned dynamic factor. The double nature of the resistance, its contemporary and its historical motives, requires that the forms of the ego defense which it contains must be brought to complete consciousness first. Only after the contemporary meaning of the resistance has become clear should its infantile origin be interpreted in light of the material which has been produced. This also holds true for patients who have already revealed the infantile material necessary to the understanding of the *subsequent* resistance. In other cases, probably the majority, it is necessary to allow the resistance to develop, if only to be able to obtain the infantile material in sufficient measure.

Thus, the resistance technique has two aspects: (1) *comprehending the resistance from the contemporary situation through interpretation of its contemporary meaning*; (2) *dissolving the resistance by linking the ensuing infantile material with the contemporary material*. In this way, escape into the contemporary as well as the infantile situation is easily avoided, inasmuch as both are given equal consideration in interpretation.

Thus, the resistance, once a therapeutic obstruction, becomes the most powerful vehicle of analysis.

Character Analysis in the Case of Abundantly Flowing Material

In cases in which the patient's character impedes the recall work from the very beginning, character analysis as described above is unquestionably indicated as the solely legitimate analytic method of introducing the treatment. But what about those patients whose characters admit of ample recall work in the beginning? We are faced with two questions. Is character analysis as we have described it here also necessary in these cases? If so, how should the analysis be introduced? The first question would have to be answered in the negative if there were any patients who did not exhibit character armor. However, since there are no such patients, since the narcissistic protective mechanism sooner or later becomes a character resistance, varying only in intensity and depth, no *fundamental* difference exists. There is merely a circumstantial difference: in patients whose character impedes the recall work, the mechanism of narcissistic protection and defense lies wholly on the surface and immediately appears as a resistance, whereas in the other patients the protective and defensive mechanism lies deeper in the personality, so that it is not at all obvious at first. But it is precisely these patients who are dangerous. With the former, one knows in advance where one stands. With the latter, one goes on believing for quite some time that the analysis is progressing very well because the patient seems to accept everything very readily; indeed, even shows signs of improvement, and produces prompt reactions to the interpretations. It is with such patients that one experiences the greatest disappointments. The analysis has been carried out, but there is no sign of final success. One has used up all one's interpretations, is confident that the primal scene and the infantile conflicts have been made completely conscious; yet the analysis is stuck in bleak, monotonous repetitions of the old material—the cure refusing to take effect. It is still worse when a transference success deludes the analyst into thinking that the patient is cured, only to find that he suffers a complete relapse soon after discharge.

The countless bad experiences with such cases lead me to believe—a self-evident belief, really—that something has been neglected, not with regard to content, for the thoroughness of these analyses leaves little to be desired in this area. What I have in mind is an unknown and unrecognized, a concealed resistance which causes all therapeutic efforts to fail. Closer examination shows that these concealed resistances are to be sought precisely in the patient's docility, in his manifestly weak defense against the analysis. And these analyses, on closer comparison with other cases which succeed, are shown to have followed a steady, even course, never disrupted by violent affective outbursts, and, above all—something which did not become clear until the very end—to have been conducted almost exclusively in a "positive" trans-ference. Seldom or never had there been violent negative impulses against the analyst. Although the hate impulses had been analyzed, they just had not appeared in the transference or had been remembered without affects. The narcissistic affect-lame and the passive-feminine characters are the prototypes of these cases. The former are characterized by a tepid and steady "positive" transference; the latter by an effusive "positive" transference.

So it had to be admitted that in these so-called going cases—referred to as "going" because they produce infantile material, i.e., again on the basis of a one-sided overestimation of the contents of the material—the character had operated as a resistance in a concealed form throughout the entire analysis. Very often these cases were held to be incurable, or at least difficult to master, an appraisal for which, formerly, I too thought I saw sufficient evidence in my own experiences. However, since I gained a knowledge of their concealed resistances, I can consider them among my most rewarding cases.

In terms of character analysis, the introductory phase of such cases differs from other cases in that the flow of the communications is not disturbed and the analysis of the character resistance is not taken up until the flood of material and the behavior itself have become clearly recognizable resistances. The following typical case of a passive-feminine character is intended to illustrate this and, moreover, to demonstrate how, here too, the entry into the deeply repressed infantile conflicts ensues of itself. Furthermore, by pursuing the analysis into advanced stages, we want to demonstrate the legitimate unwinding of the neurosis on the spool of the transference resistances.

A CASE OF PASSIVE-FEMININE CHARACTER

Anamnesis

A twenty-four-year-old bank employee turned to analysis because of the anxiety states which had seized him a year before while he was visiting a hygiene exhibition. And prior to that occasion, he had suffered from acute hypochondriac fears, e.g., that he had a *hereditary taint*, would become *mentally ill* and *perish in a mental institution*. He was able to offer a number of rational reasons to account for these fears: his fa-

ther had contracted syphilis and gonorrhea ten years before his marriage. His paternal grandfather was also supposed to have had syphilis.
One of his father's brothers was very nervous and suffered from insomnia. On his mother's side the hereditary taint was even worse: his maternal grandfather had committed suicide, as had one of his maternal
uncles. One of the sisters of his maternal grandmother was "mentally
abnormal" (apparently melancholic-depressive). The patient's mother
was a nervous, anxiety-ridden woman.

This double "hereditary taint" (syphilis on his father's side; suicide
and psychosis on his mother's side) made the case that much more interesting: psychoanalysis does not deny a hereditary etiology of the
neurosis but merely accords it the importance of one of many etiologies
and, for this reason, finds itself in opposition to orthodox psychiatry.
We shall see that the patient's idea about his heredity also had an irrational basis. Notwithstanding his severe handicaps, he was cured. His
subsequent freedom from relapses was followed up over a period of five
years.

This report covers only the first seven months of treatment, which
were taken up with the unfolding, objectification, and analysis of the
character resistances. The last seven months are considered only very
briefly; from the point of view of resistance and character analysis, this
part had little of interest to offer. For us it is chiefly important to describe the introductory phase of the treatment, the course pursued by
the analysis of the resistances, and the way in which it found access to
the early infantile material. In deference to the difficulties of describing
an analysis and also to make it easier to comprehend, we shall report
the analysis without any of the accessories and repetitions. We shall
concentrate solely on the resistances and how they were worked
through. We shall, as it were, reveal only the scaffolding of the analysis
and attempt to lay bare its most important stages and to relate them to
one another. In reality, the analysis was not so simple as it may appear
here in print. As the months passed, however, one manifestation was
added to another and a definite outline began to take shape regarding
certain events; it is this outline which we shall attempt to describe
here.

The patient's *attacks of anxiety* were accompanied by *palpitations* and
a paralysis of all *volition*. Even in the intervals between these attacks he
was never wholly free of a feeling of *uneasiness*. Frequently, the attacks
of anxiety occurred quite suddenly, but they were also easily provoked

when, for example, he read about mental illnesses or suicide in the newspaper. In the course of the previous year his work capacity had shown marked signs of deteriorating, and he feared that he might lose his job because of his *reduced performance*.

He had severe *sexual* disturbances. Shortly before his visit to the *hygiene exhibition*, he had attempted to have intercourse with a prostitute but had failed. This had not bothered him very much, or so he said. Nor were his conscious sexual needs very strong. Apparently, abstinence created no problem for him. Several years earlier, a sexual act had worked out, but he had had a premature and pleasureless ejaculation.

Asked whether he had ever suffered states of anxiety before this time, the patient reported that even as a *child* he had been *very timorous* and, especially during puberty, had been *afraid of world catastrophes*. He had been very much afraid in 1910 when there was talk of the end of the world through a collision with a comet, and he had been astonished that his parents spoke about it so calmly. This "fear of catastrophes" subsided gradually, but it was later replaced by the idea of having a hereditary taint. He had suffered from vivid states of anxiety ever since he was a child. In recent years, however, they had become less frequent.

Apart from the *hypochondriac idea of having a hereditary taint*, the *states of anxiety*, and the *sexual debility*, there were no other neurotic symptoms. At the beginning of the treatment, the patient had an insight into his states of anxiety, for he suffered the most from these. The hereditary idea was too well rationalized, and his libido debility (impotence) did not trouble him enough to make him sense them as an illness. In terms of the symptoms, we had here the *hypochondriac form of anxiety-hysteria* having the customary, in this case especially well developed, *actual neurotic core (stasis neurosis)*.

The diagnosis, *hysterical character with hypochondriac anxiety-hysteria*, was based on the analytic findings with respect to his fixations. Phenomenologically, he came under the type of the *passive-feminine character*: his demeanor was always excessively friendly and humble; he was forever excusing himself for the most trifling matters. Both when he arrived and when he departed, he bowed deeply several times. In addition, he was *awkward, shy*, and *ceremonious*. If he were asked, for example, whether he had any objection to rescheduling his hour, he would not simply answer "no." He would assure me that he was at my service, that everything was quite agreeable with him, etc. If he had a request to make, he stroked the arm of the analyst while making it. Once, when it was intimated that perhaps he distrusted the analyst, he returned on the same day very much upset. He could not, he said, endure the thought that his analyst regarded him as distrustful, and he repeatedly begged forgiveness in the event he had said something that might have caused me to make such an assumption.

The Development and Analysis of the Character Resistance

The analysis, marked by resistances which stemmed from his character, developed as follows:

Acquainted with the basic rule, he began, fluently and seldom at a loss for words, to tell about his family background and the hereditary taint. Gradually, he came to talk about his relationship to his parents. He maintained that he loved both of them the same; indeed, he said that he had a very high regard for his father. He depicted him as an energetic, level-headed person. *His father had repeatedly warned him against masturbation and extramarital intercourse.* The father had told him about his own bad experiences in this area, about his syphilis and gonorrhea, about his relationships with women which had ended badly. All this had been done with the best of intentions, i.e., in the hope of sparing the son similar experiences. The father had never beaten him as a means of enforcing his will. He had always used a more subtle approach: "I'm not forcing you; I'm merely advising you . . . " Needless to say, this was said with great energy. The patient described his relationship to his father as being extremely good; he was devoted to him; he had no better friend in the whole world.

He did not dwell upon this subject very long. The sessions were taken up almost exclusively with descriptions of his relationship to the mother. She had always been affectionate and extremely attentive to his welfare. He, too, behaved affectionately toward her. On the other hand, he let himself be waited on hand and foot. She laid out his clothes for him, served him breakfast in bed, sat beside his bed until he fell asleep (still at the time of the analysis), combed his hair; in a word, he led the life of a pampered child.

He progressed rapidly in the discussion of his relationship to his mother and *within six weeks was on the verge of becoming conscious of the desire for coitus.* With this exception, he had become fully conscious of his affectionate relationship to his mother—to some extent he had been aware of this even before the analysis: he was fond of throwing her on his bed; to which she submitted with "*glowing eyes* and *flushed cheeks.*" When she came in her nightgown to wish him goodnight, he would embrace her impetuously. Though he always endeavored to stress the sexual excitement of the mother—in an effort, no doubt, to betray his own intentions as little as possible—he mentioned several times, parenthetically as it were, that he himself had felt clear sexual excitation.

My extremely cautious attempt to make him aware of the real meaning of these practices met with prompt and violent resistance. He could assure me, he said, that he would have responded in the same way to other women. I had not made this attempt with the intent of interpreting the incest fantasy but merely to ascertain whether I had been right in assuming that his rigid advance in the direction of the historically important incestuous love was a clever evasion of other material having greater *contemporary* importance. The material which he produced on the relationship to his mother was not in the least ambiguous; it really appeared as if he were on the verge of grasping the true situation. In principle, therefore, there was no reason why an interpretation could not be given. Yet the striking disparity between the content of his communications and the content of his dreams and his excessively friendly demeanor cautioned me against such an interpretation.

Thus, my attention had to become more and more focused on his behavior and dream material. He did not produce any associations to his dreams. During the session itself, he was enthusiastic about the analysis and the analyst; outside of the session, he was deeply worried about his future and had sullen thoughts about his hereditary taint.

The dream material had a twofold nature: in part, it was concerned with his incestuous fantasies. What he did not express during the day, he betrayed in the manifest content of his dreams. Thus, in his dream he followed his mother with a paper knife, or he crawled through *a hole* in front of which *his mother was standing*. On the other hand, it *frequently* dealt with a *dark story of murder*, with the *hereditary idea*, a *crime* which someone had committed, jeering *remarks* made by somebody, or an expression of distrust.

In the first four to six weeks, I had the following analytic material at my disposal: his communications about his relationship to his mother;

his contemporary states of anxiety and the hereditary idea; his excessively friendly, submissive behavior; his dreams, those which clearly
followed up his incest fantasies and those which dealt with murder and
distrust; certain indications of a positive mother transference.

Faced with the choice of interpreting his completely clear incest material or of stressing the indications of his distrust, I chose the latter.
For, in fact, we were dealing here with a *latent resistance* which, over a
period of weeks, remained concealed. And it was precisely for this reason that the patient offered too much material and was not sufficiently
inhibited. As was shown later, this was also the first major *transference
resistance*, the special *nature* of which was determined by the patient's
character. *He gave a deceptive impression:* (1) through his divulgence of
therapeutically worthless material relating to his experiences;
(2) through his excessively friendly demeanor; (3) through the frequency and clarity of his dreams; (4) through the sham trust which he
showed in the analyst. *His attitude toward the analyst was "complaisant,"*
in the same way as he had been devoted to his father throughout his
life, and, in fact, for the same reason, i.e., *because he was afraid of him.* If
this had been my first case of this kind, it would have been impossible
for me to know that such behavior is a strong, dangerous resistance;
nor would I have been able to resolve it, for I could not have divined its
meaning and its structure. However, previous experiences with similar
cases had taught me that such patients are not capable of producing
any manifest resistance for months, indeed years on end, and that they
do not react at all therapeutically to the interpretations which the clear
material induces the analyst to give. Hence, it cannot be said that, in
such cases, one has to wait until the transference resistance sets in; the
truth of the matter is that it is already completely developed from the
very beginning. The resistance is concealed in a form peculiar to the
patient's character.

Let us consider also whether the heterosexual incest material which
was offered actually represents material that had broken through from
the depth of the unconscious. The answer must be in the negative. If
the contemporary function of the material currently offered is considered, it can often be ascertained that deeply repressed impulses, without any change whatever in the fact of repression, are temporarily
drawn upon by the ego to ward off *other* contents. This very peculiar
fact is not easily comprehensible in terms of depth psychology. It is a
decided error of judgment to interpret such material. Such interpreta-

tions not only do not bear fruit, they thwart the maturation of this repressed content for future use. In theory, we can say that psychic
contents can appear in the conscious system under one of two highly
diverse conditions: borne by *native*, specifically libidinal affects which
pertain to them, or by *foreign*, nonrelated interests. In the first instance, the internal pressure of dammed-up excitation forces the content into consciousness; in the second instance, the content is brought
to the surface for purposes of defense. An illustration of this is freely
flowing expressions of love as compared with those whose purpose is to
cover up repressed hate, i.e., reactive testimonies of love.

The resistance had to be tackled, a task which was of course much
more difficult in this case than if the resistance had been manifest.
Though the meaning of the resistance could not be derived from the
patient's communications, it was certainly possible to derive it from his
demeanor and from the seemingly insignificant details of some of his
dreams. From these it could be seen that, fearing to rebel against his father, he had masked his obstinacy and distrust with reactive love and
by means of his obedience had spared himself anxiety.

The first interpretation of the resistance was made as early as the
fifth day of the analysis, in connection with the following dream: "*My
handwriting is sent to a graphologist for an expert evaluation. Answer: this
man belongs in an insane asylum. Deep despair on the part of my mother. I
want to make an end of my life. I wake up.*"

He thought of Professor Freud in connection with the graphologist;
the professor had told him, the patient added, that sicknesses such as
the one from which he suffered could with "absolute certainty" be
cured by analysis. I called his attention to the contradiction: since, in
the dream, he thought of an insane asylum and was afraid, he was undoubtedly of the opinion that the analysis could not help him. He refused to admit this, insisting that he had full confidence in the efficacy
of the analysis.

Until the end of the second month, he had many dreams, though
few were capable of interpretation, and continued to talk about his
mother. I allowed him to go on speaking, without interrupting or
inciting him, and was careful not to miss any indication of distrust.
After the first resistance interpretation, however, he masked his secret
distrust even better, until finally he had the following dream:

"*A crime, possibly a murder, has been committed. I have become involuntarily implicated in this crime. Fear of being detected and punished. One of*

my co-workers, by whose courage and determined nature I am impressed, is present. I am aware of his superiority."

I singled out only his fear of detection and related it to the analytic situation by telling him point-blank that his entire demeanor indicated that he was concealing something.

On the very next night, he had a long dream confirming what I had said:

> I have learned that there is a plan to commit a crime in our apartment. It is night and I am on the dark staircase. I know that my father is in the apartment. I want to go to his aid, but I am afraid of falling into the hands of the enemy. It occurs to me to notify the police. I have a roll of paper in my possession which contains all the details of the criminal plot. A disguise is necessary, otherwise the leader of the gang, who has planted many spies, will frustrate my undertaking. Putting on a large cape and a false beard, I leave the house stooped over like an old man. The chief of the adversaries stops me. He orders one of his subordinates to search me. The roll of paper is noticed by this man. I feel that all will be lost if he reads its contents. I try to appear as innocent as possible and tell him that they are notes having no meaning whatever. He says that he has to have a look anyhow. There is a moment of agonizing suspense; then, in desperation, I look for a weapon. I find a revolver in my pocket and pull the trigger. The man has disappeared, and I suddenly feel very strong. The chief of the adversaries has changed into a woman. I am overcome by a desire for this woman; I seize her, lift her up, and carry her into the house. I am filled with a pleasurable sensation and I wake up.

The entire incest motif appears at the end of the dream, but we have also, at the beginning, unmistakable allusions to his dissimulation in the analysis. I stressed only this element, again bearing in mind that a patient who is so self-sacrificing would first have to give up his deceptive attitude in the analysis before deeper interpretations could be given. But this time I went one step further in the interpretation of the resistance. I told him that not only was he distrustful of the analysis but he feigned to be the exact opposite. The patient became terribly excited at this and produced three different hysterical actions over a period of six sessions.

1. He reared up, his arms and legs thrashing in all directions, as he screamed, "Leave me alone, do you hear, don't come near me, I'll kill

you, I'll pulverize you." This action often modulated imperceptibly into a different one:

2. He seized himself by the throat, produced a whining sound, and cried in a rattling voice, "Oh, leave me alone, please leave me alone, I won't do anything again."

3. He did not behave like one who has been violently attacked but like a girl who has been raped: "Leave me alone, leave me alone." This was spoken without sounds of strangulation and, whereas he had curled up in the earlier action, he now spread his legs wide apart.

During these six days, the flow of his communications faltered; he was definitely in a state of manifest resistance. He spoke continuously of his hereditary taint; between times he occasionally lapsed into that peculiar condition in which, as we described, he reenacted the above scenes. The strange thing was that, as soon as the action ceased, he went on speaking calmly as if nothing had happened. He merely remarked, "But this is a strange thing that is going on in me here, Doctor."

I now explained to him, without going into any details, that he was obviously enacting something for me which he must have experienced or at least fantasized sometime in his life. He was visibly delighted with this first explanation, and he enacted far more frequently from then on. It had to be admitted that my interpretation of the resistance had roused an important unconscious element, which now expressed itself in the form of these actions. But he was a long way from an analytic clarification of the actions; he was still making use of them as part of his resistance. He thought that he was being especially pleasing to me with his frequent reenactments. I learned later that, during his evening attacks of anxiety, he behaved as described in 2 and 3 above. Though the meaning of the actions was clear to me and I could have communicated it to him in connection with the murder dream, I persisted in the analysis of his character resistance, toward the understanding of which his reenactments had already contributed a great deal.

I was able to form the following picture of the *stratification of the contents of the character transference resistance.*

The *first action* represented the transference of the murderous impulses which he harbored toward the father (the deepest layer).

The *second action* portrayed the fear of the father because of the murderous impulses (intermediate layer).

The *third action* represented the concealed, crudely sexual content of his feminine attitude, the identification with the (raped) female, and at the same time the passive-feminine warding off of the murderous impulses.

Thus, *he surrendered himself to prevent the father from executing the punishment* (castration).

But even the actions which corresponded to the topmost layer could not be interpreted yet. The patient might have accepted every interpretation *pro forma* ("to be pleasing"), but none would have had therapeutic effect. For, between the unconscious material which he offered and the possibility of a deep understanding, there was the inhibiting factor of the *transferred feminine warding off of a similarly transferred fear of me*, and this fear, in turn, was related to a *hate impulse* and a distrust which were transferred from the father. In short, hate, fear, and distrust were concealed behind his submissive, confiding attitude, a wall against which every symptom interpretation would have been dashed to pieces.

So I continued to restrict myself to the interpretation of the intentions of his unconscious deceptions. I told him that he was now reenacting so frequently in an effort to win me over to his side; I added that this acting out was in fact very important. But we could not begin to understand it until he had grasped the meaning of his contemporary behavior. His opposition to the interpretation of the resistance weakened, but he still did not agree.

During the following night, he dreamed, for the first time *openly*, of his distrust of the analysis:

> Dissatisfied with the failure of the analysis thus far, I turn to Professor Freud. As a remedy for my illness, he gives me a long rod, which has the form of an ear-pick. I have a feeling of gratification.

In the analysis of this dream fragment, he admitted for the first time that he had been mildly distrustful of Freud's words, and then had been disagreeably surprised that he had been recommended to so young an analyst. I was struck by two things: first, this communication about his distrust was made to oblige me; second, he was suppressing something. I called his attention to both of these points. Sometime later I learned that he had cheated me in the matter of remuneration.

While his character resistance, his deceptive obedience and submissiveness, was being consistently worked on, more and more material continued to flow automatically from all periods of his life, material about his childhood relationship to his mother and his relationship to young men, his childhood anxiety, the pleasure he had had in being sick as a child, etc. This was interpreted only insofar as it related to his character resistance.

He began to have more and more dreams relating to his distrust and to his suppressed sarcastic attitude. Among others, he had this dream several weeks later:

> To a remark by my father that he does not have any dreams, I reply that this is definitely not the case, that he evidently forgets his dreams, which, to a large extent, are prohibited fancies. He laughs derisively. I point out in excitement that this is the theory of no less a person than Professor Freud, but I feel ill at ease in saying this.

I explained that he had his father laugh derisively because he himself was afraid to, and I substantiated my claim by referring to the uneasiness which he experienced in the dream. This I interpreted as the sign of a bad conscience.

He accepted this interpretation, and during the next ten days the question of remuneration was discussed. It turned out that, during the preliminary talk before the beginning of the analysis, he had consciously lied to me, inasmuch as, without having been asked, he quoted a smaller sum than he actually had at his disposal. He had done this, he said, "to protect himself," that is, because he doubted my honesty. As is my custom, I had quoted him my usual fee and my minimum fee, and I had accepted him as a patient at the latter rate. However, he could afford to pay more, not only because he had a larger savings and a better income than he had said he had, but also because his father was covering half of the cost of the analysis.

Linking the Analysis of the Contemporary Material to the Infantile

In the discussion of the "money matter," which was always taken up in connection with his character resistance (i.e., his concealed fear and concealed distrust), he once committed a slip of the tongue. He said, "I wanted my savings in the bank to get *bigger!*" instead of saying that he wanted his savings to increase. Thus, he betrayed the relationship of money to the phallus and the relationship of *the fear of losing money to the fear for the phallus.* I did not point any of this out to him, nor did I analyze his slip of the tongue, for I did not want to interpret the castration anxiety as such too soon. I merely made a few remarks to the effect that his thrift must be related to his fear of catastrophes, that he evidently felt more secure when he had more money. He showed a good and genuine understanding of this explanation and produced confirmatory associations from his childhood: he had begun to save pennies at a very early age, and he could never forget the fact that his father had once taken his savings and spent it, without asking his permission. *For the first time he spontaneously expressed disapproval of the father;* on a conscious level, this disapproval related to the money, but unconsciously of course it was related to the castration danger. In this connection I also explained that, while his father had evidently acted in good faith, he had been unwise to suppress his son's sexuality to such an extent. The patient admitted that he himself had often puzzled about these things in secret but had never had the courage to oppose his father, who, as the patient assumed, had only the patient's best interest in mind. I still could not tell him that a deep guilt feeling and fear of the father were the driving forces of his obedience.

From now on, the analysis of the transference resistance went hand in hand with the analysis of the concealed rebellious attitude toward the father. Every element of the transference situation was related to the father and understood by the patient, while producing a wealth of *new material on his true attitude toward his father.* To be sure, everything which he brought forward was still strictly censored, still inaccessible to deep interpretation, but the analysis of his childhood had been duly begun. He no longer divulged the material for the purpose of escaping other things; now, because of the analysis of the character resistance, he was deeply shaken and the conviction had begun to grow in him that his relationship to his father was not what he had thought it was and that it had had a detrimental influence on his development.

Every time he came close to the murder fantasy, his fear grew stronger. He dreamed less frequently and had shorter dreams, but they were more compact and had a closer connection to the analytic situation. To a large extent, the material which had been previously *pushed forward* now faded into the background. What came forth from other psychic layers had a close connection to the father complex: his fantasy of being a woman and his incest desire. In the course of the next six weeks, undisguised castration dreams appeared for the first time, notwithstanding the fact that I had given no interpretations or suggestions along these lines.

1. I am lying in my bed, suddenly I am roused and notice that my former high-school principal, Mr. L, is sitting on me. I overpower him and get him under me, but he frees one of his hands and threatens my phallus.
2. My older brother climbs through a window in our hallway and gets into our apartment. He commands that someone bring him a sword because he wants to kill me. I beat him to it and I slay him.

Thus, we see how the central father conflict emerges more and more clearly, *without* any special effort on my part, but solely as a result of correct resistance analysis.

Repeated stagnations occurred in this phase, and there were loud exclamations of distrust concerning the analysis. Now the resistance was tied up with the question of remuneration: he doubted my honesty. Doubt and distrust always cropped up when he came close to his antipathy toward the father, the castration complex, and the murder fantasy. True, the resistances sometimes masked themselves behind feminine devotedness, but it was no longer difficult to draw them out of their concealment.

After a five-week vacation, we resumed the analysis. Because his parents were away on a trip and he was afraid to stay alone, the patient, who had not taken a vacation, had lived with a friend during this time. There had been no letup in his anxiety states; on the contrary, they had become very severe after my departure. In this connection he told me that as a child he had always been afraid when his mother went away, that he had always wanted to have her with him and was angry with his father when he took her to the theater or to a concert.

Thus, it was fairly clear that, alongside the negative father transference, he had realized a strong, affectionate mother transference. Comparing the situation during the vacation with the situation in the months before my departure, the patient said he had felt quite well and secure with me. This shows that the mother transference had been present from the very beginning, alongside the reactive passive-feminine attitude. He himself deduced that he felt as sheltered with me as he felt with his mother. I did not go into this communication any further, for the affectionate mother transference was not causing any trouble then. It was still premature for an analysis of the mother relationship and, as a result of the interruption, his reactive-feminine father transference was again as strong as ever. He spoke in a meek and submissive manner, as he had done at the beginning of the analysis, and his communications were again focused upon his relationship to his mother.

On the third and fourth day after we had resumed the analysis, he had two dreams which contained *the incest desire*, his *infantile attitude toward his mother, and his womb fantasy*. In connection with these dreams, the patient remembered scenes which he had experienced with his mother in the bathroom. She had washed him until he was twelve years old, and he could never understand why his school friends teased him about this. Then he remembered his childhood fear of criminals who might force their way into the apartment and murder him. Thus, the analysis had already brought to the surface the infantile anxiety-hysteria, without any interpretations or suggestions along these lines. A deeper analysis of the dreams was avoided, because the remainder of his behavior was again marked by deceptive tendencies.

The dreams of the following night were even more distinct:

1. I am hiking through the Arnbrechtthal (the site of our summer vacations when I was five and six) with the intent of refreshing my childhood impressions. Suddenly, I come to a large place, to leave which one has to go through a castle. The doorkeeper, who is a woman, opens the gate for me and explains that I cannot visit the castle at this time. I reply that this is not my intention; I merely want to go through the castle to get into open country. The owner of the castle appears, an elderly lady who seeks to find favor with me flirtatiously. I want to withdraw, but suddenly notice that I have forgotten my key (which opens my suitcase and also appears to be of great importance to me otherwise) in the private coffer of the lady of the castle. Unpleasant feeling, which soon passes, however, for the coffer is opened and the key is given back to me.

2. I am called by my mother, who lives on the floor above mine. I seize a newspaper, form it into a penis, and go to my mother.

3. I am in a large hall in the company of my cousin and her mother. My cousin, who causes a tingle of delight in me, is clad solely in a shift. I, too. I embrace her. It strikes me that I am suddenly considerably smaller

than she, for my penis is only halfway up her thighs. I have an involuntary ejaculation and feel terribly ashamed because I fear that this will cause stains on my shift which might be easily noticed.

He himself recognizes his mother in the cousin. With respect to his nudity, he remembered that he never undressed in his attempts at sexual intercourse. He had a vague fear of doing so.

Thus, the incest fantasy (parts 2 and 3) and the castration anxiety (part 1) were revealed quite clearly. Why did he censor so little? In view of his barefaced diversions, I did not give any interpretations, nor did I make any effort to get the patient to produce further communications or associations. On the other hand, I did not interrupt the patient's associations. I wanted this subject to develop further and, most important of all, *I did not want anything to happen until the next transference resistance had emerged and had been eliminated.*

It wasn't long in making its appearance, and it was touched off by a remark, which I had made involuntarily and against my better judgment, relating to the second dream. I called his attention to the fact that once before he had had a dream about a paper penis. It was a needless observation. Notwithstanding the unambiguous manifest content of the dream, he reacted to it defensively in his usual way. He saw my point, he said, "but . . . " On the night following this incident, he had a violent attack of anxiety and had two dreams: the first related to his "money resistance" (transferred castration anxiety); the second revealed *the primal scene for the first time*, which, when all was said and done, motivated the money resistance.

1. I am standing in front of an amusement stand in the midst of a large crowd at the Prater. Suddenly, I notice that a man standing behind me is trying to purloin my wallet from my back pocket. I reach for my wallet and prevent the theft at the last moment.

2. I am riding in the rear car of a train in a part of the country south of Wörther See. At a curve I suddenly notice that another train is coming toward me on the single-line stretch of railroad. There seems to be no way of averting the catastrophe; to save myself, I jump from the platform.

This dream made it quite clear that I had been right in not interpreting his incest dreams. A latent but strong resistance was in front of it. We also see that the resistance dream was intimately related to his infantile anxiety (fear of castration, fear of the primal scene). Between the ages of three and six, he had spent his summer vacations at Wörther See.

No associations came to mind with reference to the dream. Relating the man in the first dream to myself, I once again focused the discussion upon his entire attitude, his suppressed fear of me and his concealed distrust in the matter of remuneration, without, for the time being, touching upon the connection with the fear of catastrophes. In the second dream, I singled out only the "unavoidable catastrophe." We of course already knew, I told him, that for him money meant protection against catastrophes, and he feared I could deprive him of this protection.

He did not admit this immediately (indeed, he appeared to be shocked at the idea that he might conceive of me as a thief), but he did not reject it either. During the next three days, he produced dreams in which he assured me of his devotion and trust. I also appeared as his mother. There was also a new element: *his mother as a man*; she appeared in the dream as a Japanese. We didn't understand this element until many months later, when the meaning of his childhood fantasies about the Russo-Japanese War became clear. The Russian represented the father; the Japanese, because of his slight stature represented the mother. His mother, moreover, had worn Japanese pajamas at that time: *the mother in pants*. He made repeated slips, referring, e.g., to "mother's penis." Even his "school friend" who appeared in some dreams represented his cousin, who resembled his mother.

However, the clear incest dreams were resistance dreams, the intent of which was to conceal his fear of woman (having a penis).

From this point on — for about six weeks — the analysis followed a strange zigzag course: dreams and communications relating to his money resistance alternating with dreams which revealed his longing for the mother, the mother as a man, the dangerous father, and the most diverse variations of the castration anxiety. In my interpretations, I always proceeded from his money resistance (= castration anxiety) and, using this as a base, continued to deepen the analysis of the infantile situation. This was quite easy since *the infantile material was always intimately connected with the transference situation*. Of course all the childhood fears and desires which now emerged did not appear in the transference, which was brought to a head more and more every day. (At this time, the salient feature of the transference was the castration anxiety.) Only the core of the infantile situation had appeared in the transference resistance. Since I had a secure feeling that the analysis was proceeding correctly, I had no misgivings about reserving the deep content interpretations for the proper time. Instead, I consistently worked on his fear of me by always relating it to his fear of his father.

It was my intention, by working through and eliminating as thoroughly as possible the transferred father resistance, to penetrate to his childhood incest fantasies. In this way I would receive them relatively free of resistance and be able to interpret them. Thus, I hoped to prevent the wasting of my main interpretations. For the time being, therefore, I made no effort to interpet the incest material which flowed ever more clearly and compactly from the unconscious.

At the beginning of this phase, the topographical stratification of the resistance and of the material was as follows:

1. The castration anxiety, in the form of his money resistance, occupied the top layer.

2. He continually sought to ward this off by means of his feminine behavior toward me; but this was no longer so easy for him as it had been in the beginning.

3. The feminine behavior concealed a sadistic-aggressive attitude toward me (toward his father) and was accompanied by a deep affectionate attachment to the mother, which was also transferred to me.

4. Connected with this ambivalent behavior, which was concentrated in the transference resistance, were the incest desires, the fear of masturbation, his longing for the womb, and the great fear stemming from the primal scene, all of which appeared in his dreams but were not interpreted. Only his intent to deceive and its motives, the fear of an antipathy toward the father, were interpreted.

This situation, which of course had been latently present from the very beginning but had not become concentrated in all points until now (above all, in the transference of the castration anxiety), developed in the following way.

In the fifth month of the analysis he had his first incestuous masturbation anxiety dream:

> I am in a room. A young woman with a round face is sitting at a piano. I see only the upper part of her body, for the piano conceals the rest

of her body. I hear the voice of my analyst beside me: "You see, this is the cause of your neurosis." I feel myself being drawn closer to the woman, am suddenly overwhelmed by fear and scream loudly.

On the previous day, in reference to a dream, I had told him, "You see, this is one of the causes of your neurosis," by which I meant his childish behavior, his demand to be loved and cared for. As if the patient had known the true cause of his neurosis, he connected this "statement of the preceding day" with his repressed *masturbation anxiety*. The masturbation idea was again associated with the incest idea. He woke up in a state of fear. There was a good reason for the fact that the lower part of the woman's body was concealed. (Representation of the aversion to the female genital.)

However, since his resistance was still at its height and nothing occurred to him with respect to the dream, I did not pursue the subject.

The patient subsequently had a dream in which a "naked family," father, mother, and child, were clasped by an enormous snake.

Another dream ran as follows:

1. I am lying in bed; my analyst is sitting beside me. He says to me: 'Now I will show you the cause of your neurosis.' I cry out in fear (not only fear, perhaps with a trace of voluptuousness) and almost lose consciousness. He repeats that he will analyze me in our bathroom. I am pleasantly taken with this idea. It is dark as we open the door to the bathroom.

2. I am walking with my mother through a woods. I notice that we are being pursued by a robber. I notice a revolver in my mother's dress and I take it into my possession to shoot down the robber when he gets closer. Walking at a rapid pace, we reach an inn. The robber is hard on our heels as we climb up the steps. I fire a shot at him. However, the bullet is transformed into a banknote. We are safe for the time being, but I am not sure whether the robber, who is sitting in the lobby, still has evil intentions. To put him in a good humor, I give him another banknote.

That I made the right move in not going into these clear dreams was confirmed by the fact that the patient, who already had sufficient analytic knowledge, made no reference whatever to the figure of the robber. Nor was he able to come up with any associations. Either he said nothing or he spoke excitedly about the "large sums of money" which he had to pay and about his doubts as to whether the analysis would help him, etc.

There could be no doubt, of course, that this resistance was also directed against the discussion of the incest material, but an interpretation to this effect would not have served any purpose. I had to wait for a suitable opportunity to interpret his money anxiety as phallus anxiety.

In the first part of the robber dream it is said that I am going to analyze him in the bathroom. It came out later that he felt safest in the bathroom when he masturbated. In the second part of the dream, I (the father) appeared as a robber (= castrator). Thus, *his contemporary resistance* (distrust due to money) *was intimately related to the older masturbation anxiety* (castration anxiety).

With respect to the second part of the dream, I told him that he was afraid I might hurt him, that I might endanger his life. Unconsciously, however, it was his father he was afraid of. After some opposition, he accepted this interpretation and, in this connection, he himself began to discuss his exaggerated friendliness. He required very little help in this. He recognized the meaning of his obsequious attitude toward his boss as an expression of a vague fear of being blamed for something. Nor were other people to notice that he sneered at them in secret. The more he succeeded in objectifying and unmasking his character, the more free and more open he became, both in and outside the analysis. Already he ventured to offer criticism and began to be ashamed of his former mode of behavior. *For the first time he began to sense the neurotic character trait as something alien.* This, however, also marked the first success of the character analysis: *the character had been analyzed.*

The money resistance continued. *Without the least bit of help from me,* the deepest layer of material, the *fear for his penis,* began to appear in his dreams more and more clearly in connection with *the primal scene.*

This fact has to be especially emphasized: when the analysis of the character resistance is carried out in a systematic and consistent manner, it is not necessary to make a special effort to obtain the infantile material pertaining to it. It emerges of its own accord, always more clearly and always more closely connected with the contemporary resistance, provided, naturally, that this process has not been disturbed by premature interpretations of the childhood material. The less effort that is made to penetrate to the childhood sphere and the more accurately the contemporary resistance material is worked through, the more rapidly the infantile material is reached.

This was again proven when he dreamed, after the interpretation, that he was afraid of being hurt. He dreamed that he was walking past a chicken farm and saw how a chicken was killed. A woman also lay stretched out on the ground, and another woman stuck a large fork into her a number of times. Then he embraced one of his female co-workers; his *phallus was halfway up her thighs* and he had an involuntary ejaculation.

Since his money resistance had grown somewhat weaker, an attempt was made to analyze this dream. With respect to the chicken farm, he was now able to remember that as a child he had often witnessed animals in the act of copulation during his summer vacations in the country. We had no way of knowing at this time what meaning the detail "summer in the country" had. He identified the first woman as his mother, but had no way of explaining her position in the dream.

However, he was able to tell us more about the involuntary ejaculation. He was convinced that he appeared as a child in the dream. He remembered that he liked to and was in the habit of pressing himself against women until he ejaculated involuntarily.

It appeared to me to be a good sign that this intelligent patient did not offer an interpretation, despite the fact that everything lay before him in a rather transparent state. If, *prior* to the analysis of his resistances, I had interpreted symbols or essential contents of the unconscious, he would have immediately accepted these interpretations for reasons of resistance, and we would have leaped from one chaotic situation into another.

Through my interpretation of his fear of being injured, the analysis of his character had been brought into full swing. For days on end there was no trace of his money resistance; he discussed his infantile behavior at great length, and produced one example after another of his "cowardly" and "furtive" way of doing things, which now he wholeheartedly condemned. I made an effort to persuade him that his father's influence had been chiefly responsible for this. Here, however, I encountereed the most passionate opposition. *He still lacked the courage to speak critically of his father.*

Sometime after this, he again dreamed about that subject behind which I surmised the primal scene:

I am standing along the shore of the ocean. A number of large polar bears are romping about in the water. Suddenly they become restless. I see the back of a gigantic fish emerging. The fish pursues one of the polar bears, upon which he inflicts injuries by terrible bites. Finally, the fish turns away from the mortally wounded bear. However, the fish itself has been severely wounded; a stream of blood shoots out of its gills as it struggles to breathe.

I call his attention to the fact that his dreams always have a cruel character. He responded to this and went on for several sessions to tell about the sexual fantasies he had while masturbating and the cruel acts he had indulged in until the age of puberty. I had him write them down after they had been analyzed. Almost all of them were determined by the "sadistic conception of the sexual act."

(Three to five years old). At the *summer resort* I accidentally witness how pigs are slaughtered. I hear the squealing of the animals and see the blood spurting from their bodies, which have a white gleam in the darkness. I feel a deep sensation of pleasure.

(Four to six years old). The idea of slaughtering animals, especially horses, evokes a sensation of deep pleasure in me.

(Five to eleven years old). I very much like to play with tin soldiers. I stage battles which always end up in hand-to-hand fighting. In this, I press the bodies of the soldiers against one another. The soldiers which I favor overpower the enemy.

(Six to twelve years old). I press two ants together in such a way that they fasten upon one another with their nippers. Thus locked into one another, these two insects are forced to fight to the death. I also engineer battles between two different colonies of ants by sprinkling sugar in the area between their hills. This lures the insects from their hostile camps and causes them to engage in regular battles. It also affords me pleasure to imprison a wasp and a fly in a water glass. After a while, the wasp pounces upon the fly and bites off its wings, legs, and head, in that order.

(Twelve to fourteen years old). I keep a terrarium and like to observe how the males and females engage in the sexual act. I like to observe the same thing in the chicken yard; it also gives me pleasure to see the stronger cocks drive away the weaker ones.

(Eight to sixteen years old). I like to scuffle with the housemaid. In later years, I usually lifted the girls up, carried them to a bed, and threw them down on it.

(Five to twelve years old). I like to play with trains. I run my little trains throughout the apartment, whereby tunnels improvised out of boxes, stools, etc., are gone through. In this, I also attempt to imitate the sound of the locomotive as it builds up steam and picks up speed.

(*Fifteen years old: masturbation fantasies*). *I am always an onlooker.* The woman defends herself against the *man,* who, in many instances, *is considerably smaller than she is.* After a struggle of some duration, *the woman is overpowered.* Brutally, the man clutches at her breasts, thighs, or hips. *Neither the male nor female genital nor the sexual act itself is ever part of the fantasy.* At the moment that the woman ceases to offer resistance, I have an orgasm.

The two major aspects of the situation at this time were: (1) he was ashamed of his cowardice; (2) he remembered his past sadism. The analysis of the fantasies and acts which are summarized above lasted until the end of the treatment. He became much freer in the analysis, bolder and more aggressive; but his behavior was still characterized by fear. His states of anxiety were not as frequent, but they always reappeared with the money resistance.

Here again we can be assured that the chief object in producing the genital-incest material was to conceal the infantile sadism, even though, at the same time, it represented an attempt to move toward a genital-object cathexis. But his genital strivings were imbued with sadism and, economically, it was important to extract them from their entanglement with the sadistic impulses.

At the beginning of the sixth month of the analysis, the first opportunity presented itself to interpret his *fear for the penis.* It was in connection with the following dream:

1. I am lying on a sofa in an open field (at the summer resort!). One of the girls whom I know comes toward me and lies on top of me. I get her under me and attempt to have intercourse. I get an erection, but I notice that my phallus is too short to complete the sexual act. I am very sad about this.

2. I am reading a drama. The characters: three Japanese—father, mother, and a four-year-old child. I sense that this play will have a tragic ending. I am deeply moved by the role of the child.

For the first time, an attempt to have intercourse appeared as a manifest part of a dream. The second part, which alludes to the primal scene (four years old), was not analyzed. In continuously discussing his cowardice and timidity, he himself began to speak about his penis. I took this opportunity to point out that his fear of being injured and cheated, etc., referred in actual fact to his genital. Why and of whom he was afraid were not yet discussed. Nor was any effort made to interpret the real meaning of the fear. The explanation seemed plausible to him, but now he fell into the clutches of a resistance which lasted for six weeks and *was based on a passive-feminine homosexual defense against the castration anxiety.*

It was the following which told me that he was in a fresh state of resistance: he did not rebel openly, expressed no doubt, but again became excessively polite, docile, and obedient. His dreams, which had become shorter, clearer, and less frequent during the analysis of the previous resistance, were again as they had been at the beginning — long and confused. His states of anxiety were again very prevalent and intense. But he did not voice any doubts about the analysis. The hereditary idea also cropped up again, and in this connection his doubts about the analysis were expressed in a veiled manner. As he had done at the beginning of the analysis, he again enacted a raped woman. The passive-homosexual attitude was also dominant in his dreams. He no longer had any dreams involving coitus or an involuntary ejaculation. Hence, we see that, notwithstanding the advanced stage of the analysis of his character, the old character resistance immediately assumed its full force when a new layer of his unconscious — this time the most crucial layer for his character, i.e., the castration anxiety — moved into the forefront of the analysis.

Accordingly, the analysis of the new resistance did not go into the phallus anxiety, the point at which the resistance had been aroused. Indeed, I again referred to his attitude as a whole. Throughout six full weeks the analysis was taken up almost exclusively with the consistent interpretation of his behavior as a defense against danger. Every detail of his conduct was examined from this perspective and impressed upon him again and again, gradually moving forward to the central motive of his behavior, the phallus anxiety.

The patient made repeated efforts to slip away from me through "analytic sacrifices" of infantile material, but I consistently interpreted the meaning of this procedure also. Gradually, the situation came to a head. He felt like a woman toward me, told me so, and added that he also sensed sexual excitations in the region of the perineum. I explained the nature of this transference phenomenon. He construed my attempt to explain his behavior to him as a reproach, *felt guilty, and wanted to expiate his guilt through feminine devotion.* For the time being, I did not enter into the deeper meaning of this behavior, namely that he identified with the mother because he was afraid to be the man (i.e., the father).

Among other things, he now produced the following confirmatory dream:

> I meet a young chap at the Prater and get into a conversation with him. He appears to misconstrue one of my statements and remarks that he is willing to give himself to me. In the meantime, we have reached my apartment; the young man lies down in my father's bed. I find his underwear very distasteful.

In the analysis of this dream, I could again trace the feminine transference back to the father. In association with this dream, he remembered that there had been a time in his masturbation fantasies when he had had the desire to be a woman and also had had fantasies in which he was a woman. The "dirty underwear" led to the analysis of the anal activities and habits (toilet ceremonies) which related to his behavior. Another character trait, his punctiliousness, was also clarified.

Finally, the resistance had been resolved; in the process, both its old form and its erogenous, anal basis had been discussed. Now I went a step further in the interpretation of his character: I explained the connection between his submissive attitude and his "female fantasy," telling him that he behaved in a feminine, i.e., exaggeratedly faithful and devoted, manner because he was afraid to be a man. And I added that the analysis would have to go into the reasons for his fear to be a man (in his sense of the word: brave, open, honest, proud).

Almost as an answer to this, he produced a short dream in which the castration anxiety and the primal scene were again conspicuous:

> I am at my cousin's, an attractive young woman [*the mother, W.R.*]. Suddenly, I have the sensation that I am my own grandfather. I am gripped by an oppressive despondency. At the same time I somehow have the feeling that I am the center of a stellar system and that planets are revolving around me. At the same time (still in the dream) I suppress my fear and am annoyed at my weakness.

The most important detail of this incest dream is his appearance in it as *his own grandfather*. We were immediately agreed that his fear of having a hereditary taint played an important role here. It was clear that, identifying himself with the father, he fantasized being his own procreator, i.e., having intercourse with his mother; but this was not discussed until later.

He was of the opinion that the planetary system was an allusion to his egotism, i.e., "everything revolves around me." I surmised that there was something deeper at the bottom of this idea, namely the primal scene, but I made no mention of it.

After the Christmas vacation, he went on for several days speaking almost exclusively about his egotism, about his desire to be a child who is loved by everyone — at the same time realizing that he himself neither wanted to love nor was able to love.

I showed him the connection between his egotism and his fear for his adored ego and his penis[6] whereupon he had the following dream, giving me, as it were, a glimpse of the infantile groundwork:

1. I am completely nude and regard my penis, which is bleeding at the tip. Two girls are walking away; I am sad because I assume that they will hold me in contempt due to the smallness of my penis.

2. I am smoking a cigarette with a holder. I remove the holder and notice with astonishment that it is a cigar holder. As I put the cigarette back into my mouth, the mouthpiece breaks off. I feel disturbed.

Thus, without my having done anything, the castration idea began to assume definite forms. Now he interpreted the dreams without my assistance, and he produced an abundance of material on his aversion to the female genital and on his fear of touching his penis with his hand and of having someone else touch it. The second dream is clearly a matter of an oral fantasy (cigar holder). It occurred to him that he desired everything about a woman (*most of all the breast*) except the genital, and in this way he came to speak of his oral fixation on the mother.

I explained to him that mere awareness of the genital anxiety was

---

[6]In view of the total picture at this point, perhaps some psychologists will understand why we analysts cannot acknowledge the inferiority complex as an absolute agent, because the real problem and the real work begin precisely at the point at which it ceases for Alfred Adler.

not much help. He had to find out why he had this anxiety. After this explanation, he again dreamed about the primal scene, not realizing that he had entered into my question:

> I am behind the last car of a standing train right at a fork in the tracks. A second train travels past and I am sandwiched between the two trains.

Before continuing the description of the analysis itself, I must mention here that, in the seventh month of the treatment, after the dissolution of his passive-homosexual resistance, the patient made a courageous effort to involve himself with women. I had no knowledge of this whatever—he told me about it later, in passing. He followed a girl and carried out his intentions in this way: in the park he pressed himself against her, had a strong erection, and an involuntary ejaculation. The anxiety states gradually ceased. It did not occur to him to engage in sexual intercourse. I called his attention to this and told him that he was evidently afraid to have coitus. He declined to admit this, using the lack of opportunity as an excuse. Finally, however, he too was struck by the infantile nature of his sexual activity. Naturally, he had dreams in which this kind of sexual activity was depicted. Now he remembered that as a child he had pressed himself against his mother in this same way.

The incest theme with which, in the hope of diverting me, he had begun the analysis, reappeared, but this time it was fairly free of resistance—at any rate, free of secondary motives. Thus, there was a parallel between the analysis of his demeanor during the analytic session and the analysis of his outside experiences.

Again and again he refused to accept the interpretation that he had really desired his mother. In the course of seven months, the material which he had produced in confirmation of this desire was so clear, the connections—as he himself admitted—were so evident, that I made no effort to persuade him, but began, instead, to analyze why he was afraid to avow this desire.

These questions had been simultaneously discussed in connection with his penis anxiety, and now we had two problems to solve:

1. What was the etiology of the castration anxiety?
2. Why, notwithstanding conscious agreement, did he refuse to accept the sensuous incest love?

From now on, the analysis advanced rapidly in the direction of the primal scene. This phase began with the following dream:

> I am in the hall of a royal palace where the king and his retinue are gathered. I ridicule the king. His attendants pounce upon me. I am thrown down and feel that mortal cuts are inflicted upon me. My corpse is carried away. Suddenly, it seems as if I were still alive, but I keep still so as not to undeceive the two gravediggers, who take me for dead. A thin layer of earth lies on top of me, and breathing becomes difficult. I make a movement which catches the eyes of the gravediggers. I keep myself from being detected by not moving. Somewhat later I am liberated. Once again I force my way into the royal palace, a terrible weapon in each hand, perhaps thunderbolts. I kill everyone who gets in my way.

It seemed to him that the idea of the gravediggers must have something to do with his fear of catastrophes, and now I was able to show him that these two fears, the hereditary idea and the penis anxiety, related to one and the same thing. It was very likely, I added, that the dream reproduced the childhood scene from which the penis anxiety originated.

With respect to the dream, it struck him that he pretended to be "dead," that he remained still in order not to be detected. Then, he recalled that, in his masturbation fantasies, he was usually the onlooker. And he himself posed the question whether he might have witnessed "such a thing" between his parents. He immediately rejected this possibility, however, arguing that he had never slept in his parents' bedroom. Naturally, this greatly disappointed me, for, on the basis of his dream material, I was convinced that he had actually witnessed the primal scene.

I, too, pointed out the inconsistency and asserted that one must not allow oneself to be put off so easily—the analysis would clarify the situation in due course. In the very same session, the patient felt fairly sure that he must have seen a certain maid together with her friend. Then it occurred to him that there were two other occasions when he might have eavesdropped on his parents. He remembered that, when guests were visiting, his bed was pushed into his parents' bedroom. *On summer holidays in the country*, moreover, he had slept in the same room with his parents until he was of school age. There was also the representation of the primal scene through the killing of chickens (rural scene), and the many dreams about Ossiacher See and Wörther See, where he had often spent his summer vacations.

In this connection, he again spoke about his acting out at the beginning of the analysis and about the states of nocturnal anxiety which he had experienced in childhood. One of the details of this anxiety was clarified here. He was afraid of a white female figure emerging from between the curtains. Now he remembered that, when he screamed at nights, his mother used to come to his bed in her nightgown. Unfortunately, the element, "someone behind the curtains," was never clarified.

Evidently, however, we had ventured too far into forbidden territory in this session. That night, he had a resistance dream whose content was clearly derisive:

> I am standing on a pier and am on the verge of boarding a steamship, as the companion, it turns out, of a mental patient. Suddenly the whole operation appears to me to be a spectacle in which I have been assigned a definite role. On the narrow plank which leads from the pier to the steamer, I have to repeat the same thing three times – which I do.

He himself interpreted the boarding of the steamer as a desire for coitus, but I directed his attention to an element of the dream which had greater contemporary importance, namely the "play acting." His having to repeat the same thing three times was a mocking allusion to my consistent interpretations. He admitted that he had often been quietly amused at my efforts. It also occurred to him that he had a mind to call on a woman and to engage in the sexual act three times – "to please me," I told him. But I also explained to him that this resistance had a deeper content, namely the warding off of his coital intentions out of fear of the sexual act.

On the following night, he again had the two complementary dreams: homosexual surrender and coital anxiety:

> 1. I meet a young chap on the street who belongs to the lower classes, but who has a healthy, vigorous appearance. I have the feeling that he is physically stronger than I, and I endeavor to gain his favor.
> 2. I go on a ski trip with the husband of one of my cousins. We are in a narrow pass which drops down precipitately. I examine the snow and

find it sticky. I remark that the terrain is not very suitable for skiing—one would often have to take a spill on going down. As we continue our trip, we come to a road which runs along the declivity of a mountain. On a sharp curve, I lose a ski, which falls over the precipice.

He did not, however, go into this dream. Instead he took up the question of "remuneration"; he had to pay so much and had no idea whether it would do him any good. He was very dissatisfied, was again afraid—and more of the same.

It was no difficult matter now to show him the connection between the money resistance and the nonresolved coitus anxiety and genital anxiety—and to overcome this resistance. He could also be shown the deeper intentions of his feminine surrender: *when he approached a woman, he became afraid of the consequences and became a woman himself, i.e., became homosexual and passive in character.* As a matter of fact, he understood very well that he had made himself into a woman, but he was at a loss to explain why and what he was afraid of. It was clear to him that he was afraid of sexual intercourse. But, then, what could possibly happen to him?

Now he devoted his full attention to this question. Instead of discussing his fear of the father, however, he talked about his fear of women. In the anxiety-hysteria of his childhood, the woman was also an object to be feared. From first to last, instead of a woman's genital, he spoke of a "woman's penis." Until the age of puberty he had believed that the woman was made in the same way as the man. He himself was able to see a connection between this idea and the primal scene, the reality of which he was now firmly convinced.

At the end of the seventh month of the analysis, he had a dream in which he saw how a girl lifted her skirt so that her underwear was visible. He turned away as someone "who sees something which he isn't supposed to see." Now I felt that the time had come to tell him that he was afraid of the female genitalia because it looked like an incision, a wound. On seeing it for the first time, he must have been terribly shocked. He found my explanation plausible, for his feelings toward the female genitalia were a mixture of disgust and antipathy; fear was aroused in him. He had no recollection of a real incident.

Now the situation was this: whereas the central element of his symptoms, the castration anxiety, had been worked through, it was still unresolved in its ultimate and deepest meaning because the more intimate, individual connections to the primal scene were missing; these connections had been disclosed but not analytically assimilated.

Another time, in a resistance-free period, as we were discussing these relationships and not achieving any tangible results, the patient mumbled to himself, "I must have been caught once." Upon closer questioning, he said that he had a feeling that he had once done something wrong in a sneaky way and had been caught in the act.

Now the patient remembered that, even as a small boy, he had secretly rebelled against his father. He had ridiculed and made faces behind his father's back, while feigning obedience to his face. But this rebellion against the father had ceased completely in puberty. (Complete repression of the hatred of the father out of fear of the father.)

Even the hereditary-taint idea turned out to be a severe reproach against the father. The complaint, "*I have a hereditary taint,*" meant: "*My father handicapped me in giving me birth.*" The analysis of the fantasies about the primal scene revealed that the patient fancied himself in the womb while his father was having intercourse with his mother. The idea of being injured in the genitalia combined with the womb fantasy to form the notion that *he had been castrated by the father in the womb.*

We can be brief in our description of the remainder of the analysis. It was relatively free of resistance and was clearly divided into two parts.

The first part was taken up with the working through of his childhood masturbation fantasies and the masturbation anxiety. For some time, his castration anxiety was anchored in the fear of (or aversion to) the female genitalia. The "incision," the "wound," was not an easily refutable proof of the feasibility of castration. Finally, the patient plucked up enough courage to masturbate, whereupon the anxiety states disappeared completely, a proof that the attacks of anxiety originated from the libido stasis and not from the castration anxiety, for this anxiety continued. By working through additional infantile material, we finally succeeded in subduing the castration anxiety to such an extent as to enable him to attempt intercourse, which, as far as his erection was concerned, succeeded well. Further sexual experiences with women brought out two disturbances: he was orgastically impotent, i.e., he derived less sensual pleasure from coitus than he did from masturbation; and he had an indifferent, contemptuous attitude toward the woman. There was still a cleavage in the sexual impulse between tenderness and sensuality.

The second phase was taken up with the analysis of his orgastic impotence and his infantile narcissism. As had always been his habit, he wanted everything from the woman, from the mother, without having to give anything in return. With great understanding and even greater eagerness, the patient himself took the initiative in dealing with his disturbances. He objectified his narcissism, realized that it was a burden, and finally overcame it when the final remnant of his castration anxiety, which was anchored in his impotence, had been resolved analytically. He was *afraid of the orgasm*; he thought the excitement it produced was harmful.

The following dream was the projection of this fear:

> I am visiting an art gallery. One picture catches my eye — it is entitled "Inebriated Tom." It is a painting of a young handsome English soldier in the mountains. There is a storm. It appears that he has lost his way; a skeleton hand has taken hold of his arm and appears to be leading him away, evidently a symbol that he is going to his doom. A painting "Difficult Profession": also in the mountains, a man and a small boy plunge down an incline; at the same time, a rucksack empties its contents. The boy is surrounded by a whitish pap.

The plunge represents the orgasm,[7] the whitish pap the sperm. The patient discussed the anxiety which, in puberty, he experienced when he ejaculated and when he had an orgasm. His sadistic fantasies with regard to women were also thoroughly worked through. A few months later — it was then summer — he began a liaison with a young girl; the disturbances were considerably milder.

The resolution of the transference did not offer any difficulties, because it had been systematically dealt with from the very beginning, both in its negative and in its positive aspects. He was happy to leave the analysis and was full of hope for the future.

I saw the patient five times in the course of the next five years, full of health in both mind and body. His timidity and attacks of anxiety had wholly disappeared. He described himself as completely cured and ex-

---

[7]Cf. my discussion of the symbolism of the orgasm in *The Function of the Orgasm*.

pressed his satisfaction that his personality had been cleansed of its servile and underhanded traits. Now he was able to face all difficulties courageously. His potency had increased since the termination of the analysis.

SUMMARY

Having arrived at the conclusion of our report, we become keenly aware of the inadequacies of language to depict analytic processes. Notwithstanding these linguistic difficulties, we want to outline at least the most salient features of character analysis in the hope of improving our understanding of it. Hence, let us summarize:

1. Our patient is the prototype of the passive-feminine character who, regardless of what symptoms cause him to seek analytic help, always confronts us with the same kind of character resistance. He also offers us a typical example of the mechanism of the latent negative transference.

2. In terms of technique, the analysis of the passive-feminine character resistance (i.e., deception through excessive friendliness and submissive demeanor) was given priority. The result was that the infantile material became manifest in the transference neurosis according to its own inner logic. This prevented the patient from delving into his unconscious in a solely intellectual way, that is, to satisfy his feminine devotion ("to be obliging"), which would have had no therapeutic effect.

3. It becomes clear from this report that, if the character resistance is systematically and consistently stressed and if premature interpretations are avoided, the germane infantile material emerges *of itself* even more clearly and distinctly. This ensures that the content and symptom interpretations which follow will be irrefutable and therapeutically effective.

4. The case history showed that the character resistance can be taken up as soon as its contemporary meaning and purpose have been grasped. It was not necessary to have a knowledge of the infantile material pertaining to it. By *stressing* and interpeting its contemporary meaning, we were able to draw out the corresponding infantile material, without having to interpret symptoms or have preconceptions. *The dissolution of the character resistance* began with the establishment of

contact with the infantile material. The subsequent symptom interpretations took place free of resistance, with the patient turning his full attention to the analysis. Typically, therefore, the analysis of the resistance fell into two parts: (a) *stressing* of the resistance's form and of its contemporary meaning; (b) its *dissolution* with the help of the infantile material drawn to the surface by that emphasis. The difference between a character resistance and an ordinary resistance was shown here in that the former was manifested in his politeness and submissiveness, whereas the latter was manifested in simple doubting and distrusting of the analysis. Only the former attitudes were a part of his character and constituted the *form* in which his distrust was expressed.

5. Through consistent interpretation of the latent negative transference, the repressed and masked aggressiveness against the analyst, superiors, and father was liberated from repression, whereby the passive-feminine attitude, which of course was merely a reaction formation against the repressed aggressiveness, disappeared.

6. Since the repression of the aggressiveness toward the father also entailed the repression of the phallic libido toward women, the active-masculine genital strivings returned with the aggressiveness in the process of analytic dissolution (*cure of impotence*).

7. As the aggressiveness became conscious, the timidity which was a part of his character vanished, along with the castration anxiety. And the attacks of anxiety left off when he ceased to live in abstinence. Through the orgastic elimination of the actual anxiety, the "core of the neurosis" was also finally eliminated.

Finally, it is my hope that by describing a number of cases, I have shattered the opinion held by my opponents, namely that I approach each and every case with a "fixed scheme." Hopefully, the point of view which I have advocated for years, that there is only *one* technique for each case and that this technique has to be deduced from the structure of the case and applied to it, will have become clear from the foregoing representation.

CHAPTER 4

Technique and Resistance

Anna Freud

Anna Freud's classic book on defensive functions, The Ego and the Mechanisms of Defense (1936), *covers much more than the title indicates. A far-reaching work, it deals with structural elements, technique of treatment (and inherent problems in this area), and both very specific and very broad areas of personality dynamics. Because it covers the defense mechanisms and the functions of the ego, it is a work that always, either implicitly or explicitly, has some relevance to resistance analysis.*

We will begin with a brief section that deals with two aspects of technique, free association and dream analysis, and see how clearly she relates technique to ego psychology theory and to resistance.

FREE ASSOCIATION

Even in free association—the method which has since replaced hypnosis as an aid to research—the role of the ego is at first still a negative one. It is true that the patient's ego is no longer forcibly eliminated. Instead, it is required to eliminate itself, to refrain from criticizing the associations and to disregard the claims of logical connection, which are at other times held to be legitimate. The ego is, in fact, requested to be silent and the id is invited to speak and promised that its derivatives shall not encounter the usual difficulties if they emerge into consciousness. Of course, it is never promised that, when they make their ap-

117

pearance in the ego, they will attain their instinctual aim, whatever that may be. The warrant is valid only for their translation into ideas of words: it does not entitle them to take control of the motor apparatus, which is their real purpose in emerging. Indeed, this apparatus is put out of action in advance by the strict rules of analytic technique. Thus we have to play a double game with the patient's instinctual impulses, on the one hand encouraging them to express themselves and, on the other, steadily refusing them gratification – a procedure which incidentally gives rise to one of the numerous difficulties in the handling of analytic technique.

Even to-day many beginners in analysis have an idea that it is essential to succeed in inducing their patients really and invariably to give all their associations without modification or inhibition, i.e. to obey implicitly the fundamental rule of analysis. But, even if this ideal were realized, it would not represent an advance, for after all it would simply mean the conjuring-up again of the now obsolete situation of hypnosis, with its one-sided concentration on the part of the physician upon the id. Fortunately for analysis such docility in the patient is in practice impossible. The fundamental rule can never be followed beyond a certain point. The ego keeps silence for a time and the id-derivatives make use of this pause to force their way into consciousness. The analyst hastens to catch their utterances. Then the ego bestirs itself again, repudiates an attitude of passive tolerance which it has been compelled to assume and by means of one or other of its customary defence-mechanisms intervenes in the flow of associations. The patient transgresses the fundamental rule of analysis, or, as we say, he puts up 'resistances.' This means that the inroad of the id into the ego has given place to a counter-attack by the ego upon the id. The observer's attention is now diverted from the associations to the resistance, i.e. from the content of the id to the activity of the ego. The analyst has an opportunity of witnessing, then and there, the putting into operation by the latter of one of those defensive measures against the id, which I have already described and which are so obscure, and it now behooves him to make it the object of his investigation. He then notes that with this change of object the situation in the analysis has suddenly changed. In analysing the id he is assisted by the spontaneous tendency of the id-derivatives to rise to the surface: his exertions and the strivings of the material which he is trying to analyse are similarly directed. In the analysis of the ego's defensive operations there is, of course, no such community of aim. The unconscious elements in the ego have no inclination to become conscious and derive no advantage from so doing. Hence any piece of ego-analysis is much less satisfactory than the analysis of the id. It has to proceed by circuitous paths, it cannot follow out the ego-activity directly, the only possibility is to reconstruct it from its influence on the patient's associations. From the nature of the effect produced — whether it be omission, reversal, displacement of meaning, etc. — we hope to discover what kind of defence the ego has employed in its intervention. So it is the analyst's business first of all to recognize the defence-mechanism. When he has done this, he has accomplished a piece of ego-analysis. His next task is to undo what has been done by the defence, i.e., to find out and restore to its place that which has been omitted through repression, to rectify displacements and to bring that which has been isolated back into its true context. When he has re-established the severed connections, he turns his attention once more from the analysis of the ego to that of the id.

We see then that what concerns us is not simply the enforcement of the fundamental rule of analysis for its own sake but the conflict to which this gives rise. It is only when observation is focussed now on the id and now on the ego and the direction of interest is twofold, extending to both sides of the human being whom we have before us, that we can speak of *psycho-analysis*, as distinct from the one-sided method of hypnosis.

The various other means employed in analytic technique can now be classified without difficulty, according as the attention of the observer is directed to one side or the other.

INTERPRETATION OF DREAMS

The situation when we are interpreting our patient's dreams and when we are listening to his free associations is the same. The dreamer's psychic state differs little from that of the patient during the analytic hour. When he obeys the fundamental rule of analysis he voluntarily suspends the function of the ego; in the dreamer this suspension takes place automatically under the influence of sleep. The patient is made to lie at rest on the analyst's couch, in order that he may have no opportunity to gratify his instinctual wishes in action; similarly, in sleep, the motor system is brought to a standstill. And the effect of the censorship, the translation of latent dream-thoughts into manifest dream-content, with the distortions, condensations, displacements, reversals and omissions which this involves, corresponds to the distortions which take place in the associations under the pressure of some resistance. Dream-interpretation, then, assists us in our investigation of the id, in so far as it is successful in bringing to light latent dream-thoughts (id-content), and in our investigation of the ego-institutions and their defensive operations, in so far as it enables us to reconstruct the measures adopted by the censor from their effect upon the dream-thoughts.

> *Another technical issue central to the analytic process, transference, is succinctly addressed by Anna Freud. In the section that follows we have included general material on the subject because it cogently presents the multifaceted nature of the transference, something that is essential in understanding transference resistance.*

The same theoretical distinction between observation of the id on the one hand and observation of the ego on the other may be drawn in the case of that which is perhaps the most powerful instrument in the analyst's hand: the interpretation of the transference. By transference we mean all those impulses experienced by the patient in his relation with the analyst which are not newly created by the objective analytic situation but have their source in early—indeed, the very earliest—object-relations and are now merely revived under the influence of the repetition-compulsion. Because these impulses are repetitions and not new creations they are of incomparable value as a means of information about the patient's past affective experiences. We shall see that we can distinguish different types of transference-phenomena according to the degree of their complexity.

TRANSFERENCE OF LIBIDINAL IMPULSES

The first type of transference is extremely simple. The patient finds himself disturbed in his relation to the analyst by passionate emotions, e.g. love, hate, jealousy and anxiety, which do not seem to be justified by the facts of the actual situation. The patient himself resists these emotions and feels ashamed, humiliated and so forth, when they manifest themselves against his will. Often it is only by insisting on the fundamental rule of analysis that we succeed in forcing a passage for them to conscious expression. Further investigation reveals the true character of these affects—they are irruptions of the id. They have their source in old affective constellations, such as the Oedipus and the castration-complex, and they become comprehensible and indeed are justified if we disengage them from the analytic situation and insert them into some infantile affective situation. When thus put back into their proper place, they help us to fill up an amnestic gap in the patient's past and provide us with fresh information about his infantile instinctual and affective life. Generally he is quite willing to co-operate with us in our interpretation, for he himself feels that the transferred affective impulse is an intrusive foreign body. By putting it back into its place in the past we release him from an impulse in the present which is alien to his ego, thus enabling him to carry on the work of analysis. It should be noted that the interpretation of this first type of transference assists in the observation of the id only.

TRANSFERENCE OF DEFENCE

The case alters when we come to the second type of transference. The repetition-compulsion, which dominates the patient in the analytic situation, extends not only to former id-impulses but equally to former defensive measures against the instincts. Thus he not only transfers undistorted infantile id-impulses, which become subject to a censorship on the part of the adult ego secondarily and not until they force their way to conscious expression; he transfers also id-impulses in all those forms of distortion which took shape while he was still in infancy. It may happen in extreme cases that the instinctual impulse itself never enters into the transference at all but only the specific defense adopted by the ego against some positive or negative attitude of the libido, as, for instance, the reaction of flight from a positive love-fixation in latent female homosexuality or the submissive, feminine-masochistic attitude, to which Wilhelm Reich has called attention in male patients whose relations to their fathers were once characterized by aggression. In my opinion we do our patients a great injustice if we describe these transferred defence-reactions as 'camouflage' or say that the patients are 'pulling the analyst's leg' or purposely deceiving him in some other way. And indeed we shall find it hard to induce them by an iron insistence on the fundamental rule, that is to say, by putting pressure upon them to be candid, to expose the id-impulse which lies hidden under the defence as manifested in the transference. The patient *is* in fact candid when he gives expression to the impulse or affect in the only way still open to him, namely, in the distorted defensive measure. I think that in such a case the analyst ought not to omit all the intermediate stages in the transformation which the instinct has undergone and endeavour at all costs to arrive directly at the primitive instinctual impulse against which the ego has set up its defence and to introduce it into the patient's consciousness. The more correct method is to change the focus of attention in the analysis, shifting it in the first place from the instinct to the specific mechanism of defence, i.e. from the id to the ego. If we succeed in retracing the path followed by the instinct in its various transformations, the gain in the analysis is twofold. The transference-phenomenon which we have interpreted falls into two parts, both of which have their origin in the past: a libidinal or aggressive element, which belongs to the id, and a defence-mechanism, which we must attribute to the ego—in the most instructive cases to the ego of the same infantile period in which the id-impulse first arose. Not only do we fill in a gap in the patient's memory of his instinctual life, as we may also do when interpreting the first, simple type of transference, but we acquire information which completes and fills in the gaps in the history of his ego-development or, to put it another way, the history of the transformations through which his instincts have passed.

The interpretation of the second type of transference is more fruitful than that of the first type but it is responsible for most of the technical difficulties which arise between analyst and patient. The latter does not feel the second kind of transference-reaction to be a foreign body, and this is not surprising when we reflect how great a part the ego plays—even though it be the ego of earlier years—in its production. It is not easy to convince him of the repetitive nature of these phenomena. The form in which they emerge in his consciousness is ego-syntonic. The distortions demanded by the censorship were accomplished long ago and the adult ego sees no reason for being on its guard against their making their appearance in his free associations. By means of rationalization he easily shuts his eyes to the discrepancies between cause and effect which are so noticeable to the observer and make it evident that the transference has no objective justification. When the transference-reactions take this form, we cannot count on the patient's willing co-operation, as we can when they are of the type first described. Whenever the interpretation touches on the unknown elements of the ego, its activities in the past, that ego is wholly opposed to the work of analysis. Here evidently we have the situation which we commonly describe by the not very felicitous term, 'character-analysis.'

From the theoretical standpoint, the phenomena revealed by interpretation of the transference fall into two groups: that of id-contents and that of ego-activities, which in each case have been brought into consciousness. The results of interpretation during the patient's free association may be similarly classified: the uninterrupted flow of associations throws light on the contents of the id, the occurrence of a resistance on the defence-mechanisms employed by the ego. The only difference is that interpretations of the transference relate exclusively to the past and may light up in a moment whole periods of the patient's past life, while the id-contents revealed in free association are not connected with any particular period and the ego's defensive operations, manifested during the analytic hour in the form of resistance to free association, may belong to his present life also.

ACTING IN THE TRANSFERENCE

Yet another important contribution to our knowledge of the patient is made by a third form of transference. In dream-interpretation, free association, the interpretation of resistance and in the forms of transference hitherto described, the patient as we see him is always inside the analytic situation, i.e. in an unnatural endopsychical state. The relation of the two institutions in respect of strength has been upset: the balance is weighted in favour of the id, in the one case through the influence of sleep and, in the other, through the observance of the fundamental rule of analysis. The strength of the ego-factors when we encounter them—whether in the form of the dream-censorship or in that of resistance to free associations—has always been impaired and their influence diminished, and often it is extremely difficult for us to picture them in their natural magnitude and vigour. We are all familiar with the accusation not infrequently made against analysts—that they may have a good knowledge of a patient's unconscious but are bad judges of his ego. There is probably a certain amount of justification in this criticism, for the analyst lacks opportunities of observing the patient's whole ego in action.

Now an intensification of the transference may occur, during which for the time being the patient ceases to observe the strict rules of analytic treatment and begins to act out in the behaviour of his daily life both the instinctual impulses and the defensive reactions which are embodied in his transferred affects. This is what is known as *acting* in the transference—a process in which, strictly speaking, the bounds of analysis have already been overstepped. It is instructive from the analyst's standpoint, in that the patient's psychic structure is thus automatically revealed in its natural proportions. Whenever we succeed in interpreting this 'acting,' we can divide the transference-activities into their component parts and so discover the actual quantity of energy supplied at that particular moment by the different institutions. In contrast to the observations that we made during the patient's free associations this situation shows us the absolute and the relative amount naturally contributed by each institution.

Although in this respect the interpetation of 'acting' in the transference affords us some valuable insight, the therapeutic gain is generally small. The bringing of the unconscious into consciousness and the exercise of therapeutic influence upon the relations between id, ego and super-ego clearly depend upon the analytic situation, which is artificially produced and still resembles hypnosis in that the activity of the ego-institutions is curtailed. As long as the ego continues to function freely or if it makes common cause with the id and simply carries out its behests, there is but little opportunity for endopsychical displacements and the bringing to bear of influence from without. Hence this third form of transference, which we call *acting*, is even more difficult for the analyst to deal with than the transference to the various modes of defence. It is natural that he should try to restrict it as far as possible by means of the analytical interpretations which he gives and the non-analytical prohibitions which he imposes.

It is clear that Anna Freud can bring theoretical and technical material into focus very concisely. It is also apparent that she clearly perceives the intricate and complex process that ensues in structure rebuilding. Indeed, both her clarity and brevity are epitomized in the more extended excerpt that follows. Within this section, she brilliantly intertwines and explicates the notions of defense and resistance in regard to instinct, character, and symptom. She concludes by concretizing these theoretical constructs with illustrative case material from a child analysis.

DEFENCE AGAINST INSTINCT, MANIFESTING ITSELF AS RESISTANCE

[Elsewhere] I tried for the purposes of this study to draw a theoretical distinction between the analysis of the id and that of the ego, which in our practical work are inseparably bound up with one another. The result of this attempt is simply to corroborate afresh the conclusion to which experience has led us, that in analysis all the material which assists us to analyse the ego makes its appearance in the form of resistance to the analysis of the id. The facts are so self-evident that explanation seems almost superfluous. The ego becomes active in the analysis whenever it desires by means of a counter-action to prevent an inroad by the id. Since it is the aim of the analytic method to enable ideational representatives of repressed instincts to enter consciousness, i.e. to encourage these inroads by the id, the ego's defensive operations against such representatives automatically assume the character of active resistance to analysis. And since, further, the analyst uses his personal influence to secure the observance of the fundamental rule which enables such ideas to emerge in the patient's free associations, the defence set up by the ego against the instincts takes the form of direct opposition to the analyst himself. Hostility to the analyst and a strengthening of the measures designed to prevent the id-impulses from emerging coincide automatically. When, at certain moments in the analysis, the defence is withdrawn and instinctual representatives can make their appearance unhindered in the form of free associations, the relation of the ego to the analyst is relieved of disturbance from this quarter.

There are, of course, many possible forms of resistance in analysis besides this particular type. As well as the so-called ego-resistances there are, as we know, the transference-resistances, which are differently constituted, and also those opposing forces, so hard to overcome in analysis, which have their source in the repetition-compulsion. Thus we cannot say that every resistance is the result of a defensive measure on the part of the ego. But every such defence against the id, if set up during analysis, can be detected only in the form of resistance to the analyst's work. Analysis of ego-resistances gives us a good opportunity of observing and bringing into consciousness the ego's unconscious defensive operations in full swing.

DEFENCE AGAINST AFFECTS

We have other opportunities besides those provided by the clashes between ego and instinct for a close observation of the activities of the former. The ego is in conflict not only with those id-derivatives which try to make their way into its territory in order to gain access to consciousness and to obtain gratification. It defends itself no less energetically and actively against the affects associated with these instinctual impulses. When repudiating the claims of instinct, its first task must always be to come to terms with these affects. Love, longing, jealousy, mortification, pain and mourning accompany sexual wishes, hatred, anger and rage the impulses of aggression; if the instinctual demands with which they are associated are to be warded off, these affects must submit to all the various measures to which the ego resorts in its efforts to master them, i.e. they must undergo metamorphosis. Whenever transformation of an affect occurs, whether in analysis or outside it, the ego has been at work and we have an opportunity of studying its operations. We know that the fate of the affect associated with an instinctual demand is not simply identical with that of its ideational representative. Obviously, however, one and the same ego can have at its disposal only a limited number of possible means of defence. At particular periods in life and according to its own specific structure the individual ego selects now one defensive method, now another—it may be repression, displacement, reversal, etc.—and these it can employ both in its conflict with the instincts and in its defence against the liberation of affect. If we know how a particular patient seeks to defend himself against the emergence of his instinctual impulses, i.e. what is the nature of his habitual ego-resistances, we can form an idea of his probable attitude towards his own unwelcome affects. If, in another patient, particular forms of affect-transformation are strongly in evidence, such as complete suppression of emotion, denial, etc., we shall not be surprised if he adopts the same methods of defence against his instinctual impulses and his free associations. It is the same ego, and in all its conflicts it is more or less consistent in using every means which it has at its command.

PERMANENT DEFENCE-PHENOMENA

Another field in which the ego's defensive operations may be studied is that of the phenomena to which Wilhelm Reich refers in his remarks on 'the consistent analysis of resistance.' Bodily attitudes such as stiffness and rigidity, personal peculiarities such as a fixed smile, contemptuous, ironical and arrogant behaviour – all these are residues of very vigorous defensive processes in the past, which have become dissociated from their original situations (conflicts with instincts or affects) and have developed into permanent character-traits, the 'armour-plating of character' (*Charakterpanzerung*, as Reich calls it). When in analysis we succeed in tracing these residues to their historical source, they recover their mobility and cease to block by their fixation our access to the defensive operations upon which the ego is at the moment actively engaged. Since these modes of defence have become permanent, we cannot now bring their emergence and disappearance into relation with the emergence and disappearance of instinctual demands and affects from within or with the occurrence and cessation of situations of temptation and affective stimuli from without. Hence their analysis is a peculiarly laborious process. I am sure that we are justified in placing them in the foreground only when we can detect no trace at all of a present conflict between ego, instinct and affect. And I am equally sure that there is no justification for restricting the term 'analysis of resistance' to the analysis of these particular phenomena, for it should apply to that of all resistances.

SYMPTOM-FORMATION

Analysis of the resistances of the ego, of its defensive measures against the instincts and of the transformations undergone by the affects reveals and brings into consciousness in a living flow the same methods of defence as meet our eyes in a state of petrification when we analyse the permanent 'armour-plating of character.' We come across them, on a larger scale and again in a state of fixation, when we study the forma-

tion of neurotic symptoms. For the part played by the ego in the formation of those compromises which we call symptoms consists in the
unvarying use of a special method of defence, when confronted with a
particular instinctual demand, and the repetition of exactly the same
procedure every time that demand recurs in its stereotyped form. We
know that there is a regular connection between particular neuroses
and special modes of defence, as, for instance, between hysteria and repression or between obsessional neurosis and the processes of isolation
and undoing. We find the same constant connection between neurosis
and defence-mechanism when we study the modes of defence which a
patient employs against his affects and the form of resistance adopted
by his ego. The attitude of a particular individual towards his free associations in analysis and the manner in which, when left to himself, he
masters the demands of his instincts and wards off unwelcome affects
enable us to deduce *a priori* the nature of his symptom-formation. On
the other hand, the study of the latter enables us to infer *a posteriori*
what is the structure of his resistances and of his defence against his affects and instincts. We are most familiar with this parallelism in the
case of hysteria and obsessional neurosis, where it is specially apparent
between the formation of the patient's symptoms and the form assumed by his resistances. The symptom-formation of hysterical patients in their conflict with their instincts is based primarily on
repression: they exclude from consciousness the ideational representatives of their sexual impulses. The form of their resistance to free association is analogous. Associations which put the ego on its defence are
simply dismissed. All that the patient feels is a blank in consciousness.
He becomes silent; that is to say, the same interruption occurs in the
flow of his associations as took place in his instinctual processes during
the formation of his symptoms. On the other hand, we learn that the
mode of defence adopted in symptom-formation by the ego of the
obsessional neurotic is that of isolation. It simply removes the instinctual impulses from their context, while retaining them in consciousness. Accordingly, the resistance of such patients takes a different
form. The obsessional patient does not fall silent; he speaks, even
when in a state of resistance. But he severs the links between his associations and isolates ideas from affects when he is speaking, so that his associations seem as meaningless on a small scale as his obsessional
symptoms on a large scale.

ANALYTIC TECHNIQUE AND THE DEFENCE AGAINST INSTINCTS AND AFFECTS

A young girl came to me to be analysed on account of states of acute anxiety, which were interfering with her daily life and preventing her regular attendance at school. Although she came because her mother urged her to do so, she showed no unwillingness to tell me about her life both in the past and in the present. Her attitude towards me was friendly and frank, but I noticed that in all her communications she carefully avoided making any allusion to her symptom. She never mentioned anxiety-attacks which took place between the analytic sessions. If I myself insisted on bringing her symptom into the analysis or gave interpretations of her anxiety which were based on unmistakable indications in her associations, her friendly attitude changed. On every such occasion the result was a volley of contemptuous and mocking remarks. The attempt to find a connection between the patient's attitude and her relation to her mother was completely unsuccessful. Both in consciousness and in the unconscious that relation was entirely different. In these repeated outbursts of contempt and ridicule the analyst found herself at a loss and the patient was, for the time being, inaccessible to further analysis. As the analysis went deeper, however, we found that these affects did not represent a transference-reaction in the true sense of the term and were not connected with the analytic situation at all. They indicated the patient's customary attitude towards herself whenever emotions of tenderness, longing or anxiety were about to emerge in her affective life. The more powerfully the affect forced itself upon her, the more vehemently and scathingly did she ridicule herself. The analyst drew down these defensive reactions upon herself only secondarily, because she was encouraging the demands of the patient's anxiety to be worked over in consciousness. The interpretation of the content of the anxiety, even when this could be correctly inferred from other communications, could have no result so long as every approach to the affect only intensified her defensive reaction. It was impossible to make that content conscious until we had brought into consciousness and so rendered inoperative the patient's method of defending herself against her affects by contemptuous disparagement — a process which had become automatic in every department of her life. Historically this mode of defence by means of ridicule and scorn was explained by her identification of herself with her dead father, who used to try to train the little girl in self-control by making mocking remarks when she gave way to some emotional outburst. The method had become stereotyped through her memory of her father, whom she had loved dearly. The technique necessary in order to understand this case was to begin with the analysis of the patient's defence against her affects and to go on to the elucidation of her resistance in the transference. Then, and then only, was it possible to proceed to the analysis of her anxiety itself and of its antecedents.

From the technical standpoint this parallelism between a patient's defence against his instincts and against his affects, his symptom-formation and his resistance, is of great importance, especially in child-analysis. The most obvious defect in our technique when analysing children is the absence of free association. To do without this is very difficult and that not only because it is through the ideational representatives of a patient's instincts, emerging in his free associations, that we leant most about his id. After all, there are other means of obtaining information about the id-impulses. The dreams and day-dreams of children, the activity of their phantasy in play, their drawings and so forth reveal their id-tendencies in a more undisguised and accessible form than is usual in adults, and in analysis they can almost take the place of the emergence of id-derivatives in free association. But, when we dispense with the fundamental rule of analysis, the conflict over its observance also disappears, and it is from that conflict that we derive our knowledge of the ego-resistances when we are analysing adults—our knowledge, that is to say, of the ego's defensive operations against the id-derivatives. There is therefore a risk that child-analysis may yield a wealth of information about the id but a meagre knowledge of the infantile ego.

In the play-technique advocated by the English school for the analysis of little children the lack of free association is made good in the most direct way. These analysts hold that a child's play is equivalent to the associations of adults and they make use of his games for purposes of interpretation in just the same way. The free flow of associations corresponds to the undisturbed progress of the games; interruptions and inhibitions in play are equated with the breaks in free association. It follows that, if we analyse the interruption to play, we discover that it represents a defensive measure on the part of the ego, comparable to resistance in free association.

If for theoretical reasons, as, for instance, because we feel some hesitation in pressing the interpretation of symbols to its extreme limits, we cannot accept this complete equation between free association and play, we must try to substitute some new technical methods in child-analysis to assist us in our investigation of the ego. I believe that analysis of the transformations undergone by the child's affects may fill the gap. The affective life of children is less complicated and more transparent than that of adults; we can observe what it is which evokes the affects of the former, whether inside or outside the analytic situation. A child sees more attention paid to another than to himself; now, we say, he will inevitably feel jealousy and mortification. A long-cherished wish is fulfilled: the fulfilment must certainly give him joy. He expects to be punished: he experiences anxiety. Some anticipated and promised pleasure is suddenly deferred or refused: the result is sure to be a sense of disappointment, etc. We expect children normally to react to these particular occurrences with these specific affects. But, contrary to expectation, observation may show us a very different picture. For instance, a child may exhibit indifference when we should have looked for disappointment, exuberant high spirits instead of mortification, excessive tenderness instead of jealousy. In all these cases something has happened to disturb the normal process; the ego has intervened and has caused the affect to be transformed. The analysis and bringing into consciousness of the specific form of this defence against affect—whether it be reversal, displacement or complete repression— teaches us something of the particular technique adopted by the ego of the child in question and, just like the analysis of resistance, enables us to infer his attitude to his instincts and the nature of his symptom-formation. It is therefore a fact of peculiar importance in child-analysis that, in observing the affective processes, we are largely independent of the child's voluntary co-operation and his truthfulness or untruthfulness in what he tells us. His affects betray themselves against his will.

The following is an illustration of what I have just said. A certain little boy used to have fits of military enthusiasm whenever there was any occasion for castration-anxiety: he would put on a uniform and equip himself with a toy sword and other weapons. After observing him on several such occasions I guessed that he was turning his anxiety into its opposite, namely, into aggressiveness. From that time I had no difficulty in deducing that castration-anxiety lay behind all his fits of aggressive behaviour. Moreover I was not surprised to discover that he was an obsessional neurotic, i.e. that there was in his instinctual life a tendency to turn unwelcome impulses into their opposite. One little girl appeared to have no reaction at all to situations of disappointment. All that could be observed was a quivering of one corner of her mouth. She betrayed thereby the capacity of her ego to get rid of unwelcome psychic processes and to replace them by physical ones. In this case we should not be surprised to find that the patient tended to react hysterically in the conflict with her instinctual life. Another girl, still in the latency-period, had succeeded in so completely repressing her envy of her little brother's penis — an affect by which her life was entirely dominated — that even in analysis it was exceptionally difficult to detect any traces of it. All that the analyst could observe was that, whenever she had occasion to envy or be jealous of her brother, she began to play a curious imaginary game, in which she herself enacted the part of a magician, who had the power of transforming and otherwise influencing the whole world by his gestures. This child was converting envy into its opposite, into an over-insistence on her own magical powers, by means of which she avoided the painful insight into what she supposed to be her physical inferiority. Her ego made use of the defence-mechanism of reversal, a kind of reaction-formation against the affect, at the same time betraying its obsessional attitude towards the instinct. Once this was realized, it was easy for the analyst to deduce the presence of penis-envy whenever the game of magic recurred. We see, then, that what we acquire by applying this principle is simply a kind of technique for the translation of the defensive utterances of the ego, and this method corresponds almost exactly to the resolution of the ego-resistances as they occur in free association. Our purpose is the same as in the analysis of resistance. The more completely we succeed in bringing both the resistance and the defence against affects into consciousness and so rendering them inoperative, the more rapidly shall we advance to an understanding of the id.

CHAPTER 5

Resistance Analysis

Ralph Greenson

Greenson is one of the outstanding contributors to both the theory and technique of psychoanalysis. At the risk of some redundancy, we will start the excerpts from his major work, The Technique and Practice of Psychoanalysis (1967), *with his exceptionally clear general review of resistance.*

Resistance refers to all the forces within the patient which oppose the procedures and processes of psychoanalytic work. To a greater or lesser degree it is present from the beginning to the end of treatment (Freud, 1912). The resistances defend the *status quo* of the patient's neurosis. The resistances oppose the analyst, the analytic work, and the patient's reasonable ego. Resistance is an operational concept, it is not newly created by the analysis. The analytic situation becomes the arena where the resistances reveal themselves.

The resistances are repetitions of all the defensive operations that the patient has used in his past life. All varieties of psychic phenomena may be used for the purpose of resistance, but no matter what its source, the resistance operates through the patient's ego. Although some aspects of a resistance may be conscious, an essential part is carried out by the unconscious ego.

Psychoanalytic therapy is characterized by the thorough and systematic analysis of resistances. It is the task of the psychoanalyst to uncover how the patient resists, what he is resisting, and why he does so. The immediate cause of a resistance is always the avoidance of some painful affect like anxiety, guilt or shame. Behind this motive will be found an instinctual impulse which has triggered the painful affect. Ultimately one will find that it is the fear of a traumatic state which the resistance is attempting to ward off (A. Freud, 1936, pp. 45–70; Fenichel, 1945a, pp. 128–167).

There are many ways of classifying resistances. The most important practical distinction is to differentiate the *ego-syntonic* resistances from the *ego-alien* ones. If a patient feels a resistance is alien to him, he is ready to work on it analytically. If it is ego syntonic, he may deny its existence, belittle its importance, or rationalize it away. One of the crucial early steps in analyzing a resistance is to convert it into an ego-alien resistance for the patient. Once this has been accomplished, the patient will form a working alliance with the analyst. He will have temporarily and partially identified himself with the analyst in his willingness to work analytically on his resistances.

Other forms of psychotherapy attempt to evade or overcome resistances by means of suggestions or by using drugs or exploiting the transference relationship. In the covering-up or supportive therapies the therapist attempts to strengthen the resistances. This may well be necessary in patients who may be slipping into a psychotic state. It is only in psychoanalysis that the therapist seeks to uncover the cause, purpose, mode, and history of the resistances (Knight, 1952).

Greenson pursues an understanding of resistance from many different perspectives. However, because the concepts of resistance and defense have been intimately connected since the inception of these terms, his exploration of this area provides a broad view of the interrelationship of the two constructs.

The concept of resistance is of basic significance for psychoanalytic technique and because of its central position, its ramifications touch upon every important technical issue. Resistance has to be approached from multiple points of view in order to be properly comprehended. The present theoretical discussion will touch only on a few fundamental considerations which are of general importance for understanding the clinical and technical problems. More specific theoretical questions will be dealt with in relation to particular problems. For a more comprehensive metapsychological approach, the reader is referred to the classical psychoanalytic literature (Freud, 1912, 1914,

1926, 1937; A. Freud, 1936; Fenichel, 1945a, Chapt. VIII, IX; Gill, 1963, Chapt. 5, 6).

Resistance opposes the analytic procedure, the analyst, and the patient's reasonable ego. Resistance defends the neurosis, the old, the familiar, and the infantile from exposure and change. It may be adaptive. The term resistance refers to all the *defensive operations* of the mental apparatus as they are evoked in the analytic situation.

Defense refers to processes which safeguard against danger and pain and is to be contrasted to instinctual activities which seek pleasure and discharge. In the psychoanalytic situation, the defenses manifest themselves as resistances. Freud used the terms synonymously throughout most of his writings. The function of defense is originally and basically an ego function, although every kind of psychic phenomenon may be used for defensive purposes. This touches upon the question raised by Anna Freud when she stated that the many strange modes of representation which occur in the dream work are instigated at the behest of the ego, but are not carried out completely by it. Analogously, the various measures of defense are not entirely the work of the ego; the properties of instinct may also be made use of (A. Freud, 1936, p. 192). This idea seems related to the notions of the prestages of defense and the special problem of defenses in the psychotic patient as contrasted to the psychoneurotic (Freeman, 1959, pp. 208, 211).

I believe it is safe to state that no matter what its origin may be, for a psychic phenomenon to be used for defensive purposes, it must oper- ate through the ego. This is the rationale for the technical rule that the analysis of resistance should begin with the ego. Resistance is an operational concept; it is nothing new that is created by the analysis; the analytic situation only becomes the arena for these forces of resist- ance to show themselves.

It is to be remembered that during the course of analysis the forces of resistance will utilize all the mechanisms, modes, measures, methods, and constellations of defense which the ego has used in the patient's outside life. They may consist of the elementary psychodynamisms which the unconscious ego uses to preserve it synthetic function, such as the mechanisms of repression, projection, introjection, isolation, etc. Or the resistances may consist of more recent complicated acquisi- tions, such as rationalization or intellectualization which are used for defensive purposes (Sperling, 1958, pp. 36–37).

The resistances operate within the patient, essentially in his unconscious ego, although certain aspects of his resistance may be accessible to his observing, judging ego. We have to distinguish between the fact *that* the patient is resisting, *how* he does it, *what* he is warding off, and *why* he does so (Fenichel, 1941, p. 18; Gill, 1963, p. 96). The defense mechanism itself is by definition always unconscious, but the patient may be aware of one or another secondary manifestation of the defensive process. The resistances come to light during the process of analysis as some form of opposition to the procedures or processes of being analyzed. In the beginning of the analysis the patient will usually feel this as some contrariety in regard to the analyst's requests or interventions rather than as an intrapsychic phenomenon. As the working alliance develops, as the patient identifies with the analyst's working attitudes, the resistance will be perceived as an ego-alien defensive operation within the patient's experiencing ego. This shifts during the course of the analysis in accordance with the fluctuations of the working alliance. It should be stressed, however, that throughout the course of the analysis, along every step of the way, there will be some contention with resistances. It may be felt intrapsychically or in terms of the relationship to the analyst; it may be conscious, preconscious, or unconscious; it may be negligible or monumental in its effects, but resistance is omnipresent.

The concept of defense entails two constituents: a danger and a protecting agency. The concept of resistance consists of three agencies: a danger, a force impelling to protect the (irrational) ego, and a force pushing toward taking a risk, the preadaptive ego.

Another parallel in the relation between defense and resistance is the recognition of the existence of hierarchies of resistance just as we postulate hierarchies of defense. The conception of defense refers to a variety of unconscious activities of the ego, but we can distinguish between the deep, unconscious, automatic defense mechanisms and those closer to the conscious ego. The more primitive the place in this hierarchy occupied by a particular defense, the more closely it is connected to repressed material, the less likely it is to become conscious. Those defenses higher up on the scale operate more in accordance with the secondary process and regulate more neutralized discharges (see Gero, 1951, p. 578; Gill, 1963, p. 115). This reasoning can be carried over to our understanding of resistances. The resistances too include a wide range of processes both in terms of whether they make use of primary or secondary process in their functioning and also in regard to whether they are attempting to regulate an instinctual or neutralized discharge. I believe I can illustrate this point by a description of the goings-on in a patient who stated that he was afraid to "let me enter into him" because then he would be devoured, he would be destroyed, gone. How different is this resistance from that of a patient who revealed to me that he always quietly hummed a tune when I began to speak in order to lessen the impact of what I might say.

Defense and resistance are relative terms; the defense and what is defended against form a unit. Defensive behavior will provide some discharge for that which is defended against. All behavior has impulse and defense aspects (Fenichel, 1941, p. 57). The cruel self-reproach of the obsessional clearly betrays the underlying sadistic impulses he is attempting to ward off. All defense is "relative defense" (p. 62). A given fragment of behavior may be a defense in regard to a drive more primitive than itself, and this same behavior may be reacted to as a drive in relation to a defense more advanced than itself (Gill, 1963, p. 122).

> I can illustrate this in terms of resistance-impulse units as they emerge in the course of an analysis. A middle-aged man, a psychiatrist, tells me that he thoroughly enjoys sex with his wife, "even her moist, smelly vagina." Then he adds that "strangely enough" after intercourse he usually awakens from a deep sleep to find himself washing his genitals in the bathroom. In light of the previous discussion I will try to explain his resistance activities as follows: the patient's telling me he thoroughly enjoys sex is clearly instinctual in content; but on the other hand it is an attempt to please me, to show me how healthy he is, and to obscure any doubts I might have about his potency. One can readily observe impulse manifestation and then resistance in this. All of this, however, is defensive in regard to the next phrase, "even her moist, smelly vagina." The defensive aspect is betrayed by the word "even." But this description too obviously contains an impulse-gratifying exhibitionistic element. It is also a resistance against facing the meaning of the next piece of behavior, the washing in the bathroom. This last activity was reacted to like an ego-alien resistance in view of the previous statement of how he enjoyed her vagina and by the fact that he found the washing strange. But it was also a defensive action against a feeling of dirtiness that had awakened him and that he felt impelled to overcome by washing.

I believe this brief analysis exemplifies and confirms the concept of the relativity of resistance or defense. The concepts of "resistance to resistance" and "defenses against defense" are analogous approaches to this theme (see Freud, 1937, p. 239; Fenichel, 1941, p. 61).

The hierarchy and layering of resistances and impulses should not lead one to expect to find an orderly stratification of these components in the minds of people undergoing psychoanalysis. This was carried to an extreme by Wilhelm Reich (1928, 1929), who advocated analyzing resistance-impulse units in reverse chronological order. Fenichel (1941, pp. 47–48) and Hartmann (1951, p. 147) stressed the many factors which may disrupt this historical stratification and which cause "faulting" and other more chaotic conditions.

I would like to summarize this part of the theoretical discussion about resistances and defense by quoting a paragraph from Merton Gill (1963, p. 123): "We cannot draw a hard-and-fast line between the various levels of defense. If the defenses exist in a hierarchy, the lower levels must be unconscious and automatic, and may be pathogenic. The defenses high in the hierarchy must be conscious and voluntary, and may be adaptive. And, of course, specific defensive behaviors may include both kinds of characteristics. The idea that defenses can disappear after an analysis could be held only by someone who maintained a very restricted view of defense, since in a hierarchical conception the defenses are as much the woof of personality functioning as the drives and drive derivatives are its warp."

Let us now turn to the question of relating the motives and mechanisms of defense to the motives and mechanisms of resistance (A. Freud, 1936, pp. 45–70; Fenichel, 1945a, pp. 128–167). By motive of defense we are referring to what *caused* a defense to be brought into action. The immediate cause is always the avoidance of some painful affect like anxiety, guilt, or shame. The more distal cause is the underlying instinctual impulse which stirred up the anxiety, guilt, or shame. The ultimate cause is the traumatic situation, a state in which the ego is overwhelmed and helpless because it is flooded with anxiety it cannot control, master, or bind—a state of panic. It is this state which the patient tries to avoid by instituting the defenses upon any sign of danger. (For a compact, lucid discussion of the ego in anxiety, see Schur, 1953).

Let me illustrate with a simple clinical example. An ordinarily good-natured male patient begins to talk evasively in an analytic hour when he describes seeing me at a concert the night before. It is clear that he is embarrassed and anxious. After this point is acknowledged by the patient, we explore the underlying reasons and we discover that he felt jealous and resentful that I seemed to be enjoying the company of a young man. In subsequent hours we uncover the fact that this rivalry situation mobilized in him a tendency to a terrible rage outburst. He had suffered from frightening temper tantrums as a child when his younger brother seemed to be favored over him. Part of his later neurotic character deformation was an unreasonably rigid good-naturedness. I believe this example demonstrates the immediate, distal, and ultimate causes of resistance. The embarrassment was the immediate motive. The jealous resentment was the distal cause of resistance. The ultimate basis for the resistance was the fear of the violent rage.

The danger situations, which may evoke a traumatic state, go through a sequence of development and change with the different phases of maturation (Freud, 1926, pp. 134–143). They can be characterized roughly as the fear of abandonment, the fear of bodily annihilation, feeling unloved, the fear of castration, and the fear of loss of self-esteem. In the course of analysis every thought, feeling, or fantasy which stirs up a painful emotion, be it from free association, a dream or from the analyst's intervention, will evoke some degree of resistance. If one probes what lies behind the painful affect, one will discover some dangerous instinctual impulse and eventually some link to a relatively traumatic event in the patient's history.

The problem of working through has a particular relevance to the theory of resistance since it was in his discussion of this matter that Freud introduced the terms "compulsion to repeat," "adhesiveness of the libido," and "psychical inertia" (1914, p. 150; 1937, pp. 241–242). These phenomena were linked together by what Freud designated "perhaps not quite correctly" as "resistance from the id," a manifestation of the death instinct (1937, p. 242). Without intending to dismiss these ideas summarily, I must say that the concept of a resistance stemming from the id seems either imprecise or a contradiction. According to our working definition of resistance: all resistances operate through the ego, no matter where the danger or mode originates. The clinging to old gratifications as implied in the terms adhesiveness of the libido and psychical inertia may have some special instinctual basis, but my clinical experiences indicate that in such instances it is an underlying fear of the new or mature satisfactions which makes the old gratification intractable.

In my opinion, the role of the death instinct in regard to resistances seems too complex and too remote to warrant a thorough discussion in a book on technique. I am referring to the concept of a death instinct as distinct from the concept of aggressive instinctual drives. Interpreting clinical material to a patient in terms of a death instinct tends too readily to be facile and mechanistic.

From a technical point of view, the compulsion to repeat can best be handled therapeutically by recognizing it as an attempt at belated mastery of an old traumatic situation. Or the repetition may represent the hope for a happier end to a past frustration. Masochism, self-destructiveness, and the need for suffering can be best approached clinically as manifestations of aggression turned upon the self. In my experience, the interpretation of resistances as an expression of a death instinct leads only to intellectualization, passivity, and resignation. It has seemed clinically valid to me that in the final analysis we find the same basic motive true for resistance as well as for defense: the main motive for resistance and for defense is to avoid pain.

Resistance and transference are the basic theoretical cornerstones of psychoanalytic technique. As previously indicated, defenses have been closely associated with the concept of resistance; resistance, in turn, is closely associated with the notion of transference resistance. We turn to Greenson's concise yet full description of the basic tenet.

Transference and resistance are related to each other in many ways. The phrase "transference resistance" is commonly used in the psychoanalytic literature as a shorthand expression for the close and complex relationship between transference phenomena and resistance functions. However, transference resistance can mean different things, and I believe it would be wise to clarify this term before going on to the clinical material.

I have already discussed Freud's (1905a, 1912, 1914) basic formulation that transference phenomena are the source of the greatest resistances as well as the most powerful instrument for psychoanalytic therapy. Transference reactions are a repetition of the past, a reliving without memory. In this sense, all transference phenomena have a resistance value. On the other hand, the reactions to the analyst provide the most important bridges to the patient's inaccessible past. Transference is a detour on the road to memory and to insight, but it is a pathway where hardly any other exists. Not only does the transference offer clues to what is warded off, it also may supply the motive and incentive for work in the analysis. This is an unreliable ally because it is capricious and also produces superficial "transference improvements" which are deceptive (Fenichel, 1945a; Nunberg, 1951).

Certain varieties of transference reactions *cause* resistances because they contain painful and frightening libidinal and aggressive impulses. Sexual and hostile transference responses are particularly prone to be the source of important resistances. Very often the erotic and aggressive components appear together. For example, a patient develops sexual feelings for her analyst and then becomes furious at his lack of reciprocity, which she perceives as a rejection. Or the patient is unable to work in the analytic situation because of the fear of humiliation in exposing infantile or primitive fantasies.

It may occur that the transference reaction itself makes the patient unable to work. For example, a patient may regress to an extremely passive, dependent stage of object relationship. The patient may not be aware of this but will act it out in the analytic hours. It may appear as a pseudostupidity or a blissful inertia. The patient may be re-experiencing some early aspect of the mother-child relationship. In such a state the patient cannot perform the analytic work unless the analyst succeeds in re-establishing a reasonable ego and a working alliance.

The situation becomes more complicated when certain transference reactions are clung to tenaciously in order to hide other types of transference feelings. There are patients who stubbornly maintain a façade of realistic cooperation with the analyst for the purpose of concealing their irrational fantasies. Sometimes a patient will split off certain feelings and displace them onto others in order to remain unaware of his ambivalence toward the analyst. It often happens that my patients will express great hostility toward other psychoanalysts while they profess great admiration for me. Analysis will reveal that both sets of feelings actually pertain to me.

The most difficult resistances to overcome are the so-called "character transference" reactions. In such situations, general traits of character and attitudes which have a defensive function are manifested toward the analyst as well as toward people in everyday life. These are so deeply rooted in the patient's character structure and so well rationalized that they are difficult to make the subject of analysis. These problems [are] described in greater detail [later in this excerpt].

To summarize: Transference and resistance are related to each other in many ways. The term transference resistance condenses this clinical fact. Transference phenomena in general are a resistance to memory despite the fact that they indirectly lead in this direction. Transference reactions may cause a patient to become unable to work analytically because of the nature of the reaction. Some transference reactions may be used as a resistance against revealing other transference reactions. The analysis of transference resistances is the "daily bread," the regular work of psychoanalytic therapy. More time is spent in analyzing the transference resistances than in any other apsect of therapeutic work.

> In greater detail, Greenson elaborates on the different types and forms of transference resistance that are part and parcel of the psychoanalytic work.

From a clinical and technical point of view, it is worthwhile to distinguish various types of transference resistance because they differ greatly in their dynamics and structure and in the difficulty of the technical task. The form and structure of the transference resistance change in the patient during the course of psychoanalysis and every patient is unique in the sequence of the different types of resistance. There is also considerable variation in what forms of transference resistance predominate in a particular patient. It should further be borne in mind that a variety of transference resistances may be operating simultaneously, and one of our technical problems is to ascertain what constellation of transference resistance we shall choose for our therapeutic work at a given time. I have selected for special elaboration those types of transference resistance which occur with the greatest frequency and which can be isolated with the greatest clarity.

THE SEARCH FOR TRANSFERENCE GRATIFICATION

One of the simplest and most frequent sources of transference resistance occurs when the patient develops strong emotional and instinctual urges toward the analyst and strives to satisfy them rather than do the analytic work. This may be derived from libidinal and aggressive instinctual drives or from the emotions of love or hatred. Further, any and all of the developmental phases of the instincts and emotions may be involved. For example, the patient may have sexual desires toward the analyst on a phallic-oedipal level and have incestuous wishes and castration anxiety. Or a patient may have passive-anal impulses toward the analyst or oral wishes to be fed and taken care of, etc. Any of these libidinal elements may impel the patient to try to obtain some form of gratification and to renounce the analytic work.

As an illustration, let me cite the case of a patient who at different times was driven by each of the libidinal components just mentioned. In the beginning of her analysis (she was a depressed patient with a problem of overeating), she was frequently sadly silent because she wanted me to talk to her. At that time, my speaking to her meant that I was willing to feed her. If I would talk, then it meant I was truly concerned about her, would take care of her, feed her, and not abandon her. Then, if these wishes were gratified she would be able to work, to produce, otherwise she felt empty and forlorn and unable to communicate. Later on in the analysis she felt strong sexual impulses toward me which were unmistakably of an incestuous nature. She came to her hour in a flirtatious, frivolous mood, determined to provoke me into some kind of sexual play, even if it were only verbal. For a period of time she refused to work with this material, she demanded that I first had to indicate some reciprocity in my feelings. Still later on in her analysis, she went through a phase in which she refused to produce analytic material unless I prodded her. She insisted that I insert even a small comment into her silence and then she would be able to let out all her stored-up communications. All these different urges became a source of resistance, until she was able to relinquish her desire for satisfaction. Only then was she willing to establish a working alliance and attempt to work analytically on her different instinctual impulses toward me.

Allied to the above examples, and extremely frequent as a source of resistance, is the patient's wish or need to be loved. All patients, to a greater or lesser degree and in a variety of ways, go through periods in which their wish to be loved by their analyst supersedes and blocks their desire to accede to the analytic procedures. The fear of loss of love or respect from the therapist is an ever-present and underlying source of resistance. It may operate alone or it may be found to be on the surface or underlying the different forms of transference resistance. The family romance may also be repeated in the transference (Freud, 1905b; Frosch, 1959).

Let me illustrate this problem from the analysis of Mrs. K. I was alerted to the patient's enormous need to be loved by her history of having been brought up by an irresponsible mother and having been deserted by her father at age two. Her first dream exposed this need. I had seen Mrs. K. in the preliminary interviews and we agreed she would begin analysis in about two months, when I would have an opening. She came to the first analytic hour and we talked briefly about the interim events and about the use of the couch. She was eager to begin. As soon as she lay down she reported the following dream: "I come to my first analytic hour, but you seem different, you look like Dr. M. You lead me into a small room and tell me to undress. I am surprised and ask you whether you're supposed to do that as a classical Freudian. You assure me it is alright. I get undressed and you begin to kiss me all over. Then you finally 'went down' on me. I was pleased, but I kept wondering if it was right."

The patient acknowledged her embarrassment about the dream, and began to talk. Dr. M. is the doctor who referred her to me, and she had a crush on him for a while. He seemed to be very competent, but then she saw he had his shortcomings. He seemed to enjoy her flirtatiousness, which proved to her there was something wrong in his home life. She knows I am married and that reassures her. She is so excited to be lying on the couch doing psychoanalysis. She was so afraid I would not accept her as a patient, she heard I have few private patients. Maybe I will throw her out when I find out how "nothing" she is. She felt I was a bit brusque the last time I saw her, not as warm as in the first few hours. But she was determined to get into analysis with me. She would have waited as long as necessary. She was tired of taking rejects and castoffs. "I want the best [pause]. I want the best, but can I hold on to it? What makes me think I deserve it? [Pause.] Everything worthwhile I ever got I got because I was attractive. Maybe that's why you accepted me as a patient. But why should I dream of you 'going down' on me. I don't even know how to say it politely. Maybe you will teach me how to speak proper English. Or are you already fed up with my drivel? [Pause.] I have trouble with sex. I like the idea of it, but I can't have an orgasm with intercourse. The only way I sometimes do is when my husband uses his mouth on me. I suppose that means something—something bad."

This dream posed several difficult problems because it had overt sexual activity in it as well as resistances, and it is the patient's first analytic hour. The manifest dream seemed to be saying that I reminded her of someone she was infatuated with and that I, not she, want to do sexual things with my mouth to her. Further, she was concerned about doing the correct thing and I was primarily interested in giving her sexual pleasure. One could see how our roles had been interchanged. Her associations kept going back to the question of will I accept her, keep her as a patient. They also indicated her feeling of being unworthy, empty, and uneducated, whereas I am looked upon as worthy and the "best." There was also the statement that she can have an orgasm only from cunnilingus.

The special technical problem was how to handle the overt sexual element in the dream in this, the fearful patient's first hour? I decided I would point out her need to be loved, her fear of being rejected by me, and somehow tie this in with the sexual element. To ignore the sexual would be to make it seem "bad," to talk about it might obscure the resistance elements and perhaps get us too deep too early in the analysis. However, since the patient was able to dream it and remember it, I decided I had to comment upon the sexual activity. I said to her approximately as follows: "You must have been very worried after the last hour when I seemed brusque and you wondered if I would really take you as a patient. Then you dream that I use my mouth on you sexually as proof that I really do accept you." I had made a reconstruction upward as described by Berta Bornstein (1949) and Loewenstein (1951, p. 10).

The patient listened attentively and replied: "It's funny that you recognized that I always felt that if a man loved you, he should be able to use his mouth on you sexually. Lots of men are great at making speeches about love, but they back down when it comes to 'that.' I am always embarrassed when they do it at first because I wonder how can they stand it, but I guess it does prove a person loves you, at least in a sexual way."

The need to be loved and the terror of being rejected were major factors in Mrs. K.'s transference resistances. She equated being rejected with being abandoned. Abandonment stirred up great rage, which she turned inward, and consequently she felt like a "nothing." In part this was done to preserve, to hold on to, the idealized analyst because she dreaded that her hostility would destroy him and then she would really be alone, i.e., "nothing."

I can give illustrations from the aggressive side of the ledger as well. There are patients who become full of hostile, destructive impulses, who are bent unconsciously upon destroying their analyst and their analysis instead of analyzing their impulses.

A neurotic depressive male patient of mine with ulcerative colitis had a quarrel with his wife who he claimed neglects to prepare the proper food for him. He stormed out of the house to his analytic hour. It seemed clear to me he had displaced his hostility from his mother onto his wife. When he seemed relatively reasonable, I pointed this out to him. All he heard in this interpretation was that I was on his wife's side. That evening, despite following a strict diet for years, he went to a restaurant alone and ate all the forbidden foods he was able to swallow. He topped it off with a great deal of brandy and black coffee. That night he was in acute pain with severe vomiting and diarrhea. The fury he felt toward his wife, his mother, and me he vented on himself as a means of revenge according to the formula: "I will kill myself and then you will all be sorry." In addition to all its other meanings, this behavior was an attempt to wreck the analysis and hurt the analyst.

Patients who suffer from what is called an "eroticized" transference are prone to very destructive acting out (Rappaport, 1956). This is also seen in impulse-ridden characters, perversions, borderline cases, etc. All these patients have transference resistances that stem from underlying impulses of hatred. They seek only to discharge these feelings and oppose the analytic work. The technical task is to find the moment when one can mobilize the reasonable ego. Usually, once the intensity of the feelings has worn off, once the instinctual demands are less urgent, a reasonable ego does become accessible.

The less intense, subtle, and chronic demands for gratification are harder to detect and to demonstrate to the patient. Once they become recognizable by the patient, then they too become accessible to analytic work.

DEFENSIVE TRANSFERENCE REACTIONS

Another typical form of transference resistance occurs when the patient repeats and relives, in regard to his analyst, his defenses against instinctual and emotional involvement (A. Freud, 1936, pp. 19–25). This may become the outstanding quality and function of the transference reaction. This form of transference may be designed as defensive transference reactions. Such reactions are always transference resistances and serve the purpose of warding off other aspects and forms of transference phenomena. Several typical clinical varieties occur with great frequency and deserve to be singled out for discussion (see Fenichel, 1941, pp. 68–69).

One of the most frequently seen forms of defensive transference re-actions is the persistence of reasonable and rational behavior toward the analyst. Such prolonged absence of irrational reactions appears on the surface to be an absence of transference, but it is actually a transfer-ence reaction, albeit a defensive transference reaction. The persistent reasonable and rational behavior is the defensive side of a set of reac-tions, underneath which is hidden the instinctual, the emotional, and the irrational. This kind of defensive transference reaction is often seen at the beginning of an analysis in patients who want to be "good" patients (Gitelson, 1948, 1954).

> Let me illustrate this situation by briefly describing a patient of mine, a man in his late thirties who came to analysis because of sexual impo-tence of some eight years' duration. The impotence was limited to his wife, he was potent with other women, but he felt guilty both for his in-fidelity and for his impotence. However, he was unable to give up his extramarital affairs despite loving his wife.
>
> He was extremely competent and successful in his professional work, in a field of cut-throat competition and where success required a high degree of aggressivity and even combativeness.
>
> In his analysis he was very conscientious and cooperative. He tried hard to free-associate, he brought in dreams, he tried to follow my inter-pretations, he spoke with a moderate amount of feeling, he was not cold or overly intellectualized. At times he would fall silent and would wish that I would say something, but he knew analysts were supposed to be silent. He often felt he was making little progress, but he blamed himself since he was satisfied I was a competent analyst. When he had embar-rassing material to talk about, he reproached himself for being so child-ish since he knew that I would not be critical of him; analysts were accustomed to such material. When I made interpretations he could not agree with or follow, he supposed I must be right and he was just a bit thick or slow-witted.
>
> I then began to point out the persistent reasonableness of his reac-tions to me and wondered whether he ever had any other feelings or fantasies about me. He was unaware of anything but the feeling that I was a competent analyst doing his best. I pointed out that in some of his dreams there were situations where I was depicted as dead, or mutilated, and such pictures must come from within him. He agreed it seemed plausible, but he could not find such feelings within himself. When I

tried to find the figure in the past to whom he had similar reactions, it turned out to be his father. For the patient, the father was a decent, conscientious, hardworking man toward whom he also had persistent reasonable, rational, and warmhearted feelings. He was always tolerant and good-natured about any of his father's shortcomings. This was in marked contrast to his hostile and pugnacious behavior toward other men of authority or toward his competitors. He seemd to protect me and his father from his unconscious instinctual impulses — but why?

A dream supplied the key material. He is on a sailboat. The sail is suspended from a totem pole which had three figures on it, two men and a baby. The top figure looks like me, then comes the baby and at the bottom is his father. His associations lead to the following: When he was seven years old, his father had suffered a heart attack and the patient was given to believe that it was his (the patient's) emotional outbursts that had almost killed the father. This material was not new, but it seemed to have new import for the patient. He hesitates for several moments and then quietly tells me he had heard that I had once had a heart attack. He goes on by saying heartily that he is sure I must take very good care of myself, after all I am a physician. I detect a thinness in his attempt to talk reassuringly. I interrupt him and ask: "Something is worrying you, what else are you thinking?" The patient sighs, pretends to laugh, and then says he heard that I was over fifty years old and that came as a shock to him. He thought I was in my forties. I seem to look young and act young.

I intervene: "My being over fifty shocked you. What occurs to you to that idea — over fifty years old?" The patient says quickly: "My father died at fifty-three and I can't bear the possibility of you dying. I have enough on my conscience. I don't think I ever told you this, but the baby on the totem pole made me think back to the death of our first baby. I told you my wife had placenta previa, but I didn't realize until just now that I felt guilty for having caused it by having intercourse with her shortly before she hemorrhaged."

I interpret to him: "And you became impotent with your wife to make sure you would never hurt another baby." He replies: "Yes, I didn't deserve intercourse with a good woman. Only destructive things seem to come out of me when I let go. You ought to be grateful I am so well controlled here." Pause. Silence.

It has now become clear that behind this patient's chronic reasonableness, behind his defensive transference lay tumultuous feelings and impulses. His reasonableness with me was his way of protecting and preserving me from his destructive hostility. Analyzing the history of his defensive reasonableness eventually made it possible for the patient to experience the stormy impulses which lay behind this protective barrier.

The apparent lack of transference reactions turned out to be a defensive transference. The patient repeated with his analyst a set of defensive reactions he had found it necessary to use in relationship to his father and then in regard to his wife. These defensive reactions were a resistance and opposed the uncovering of the instinctual and affective components which lay hidden underneath.

In the above example, the patient transferred an entire set of defenses onto the analyst, but one sees cases where only a single defensive attitude may be transferred. There are patients who always react to an interpretation by seeming to accept it. They may be repeating a submissive attitude from the past in order to ward off aggressive feelings. One of my patients never made an interpretation on his own initiative, no matter how obvious the material was. He always waited for me to give the interpretation. This defensive behavior was derived from the fact that his older brother was fiercely competitive with him and would attack him severely if the patient in any way threatened his supremacy. Thus the patient acted with me the naîve, unknowing one—the same defensive role he had adopted toward his older brother.

Thus far, the examples of defensive transference reactions described are those in which certain defenses are in the foreground of the transference phenomena. However, there are other defensive transference reactions in which certain instinctual and affective reactions are used as a defense against other instinctual and affective phenomena. For example, a woman patient maintains for long periods of time a strong sexual and erotic transference in order to ward off a deeper underlying hostile, aggressive transference. In patients of the same sex as the analyst, a persistent hostile transference may be used to defend against homosexual feelings. A similiar situation exists with attitudes. Persistent submissiveness can be a defense against rebelliousness, or rebelliousness may be a defense against submissiveness which may mean passive homosexuality to the patient, etc. The above illustrations are examples of reaction formations occurring in the transference.

Defensive transference reactions always indicate there is a fear of some underlying instinctual and affective component. Defensive transference is usually ego syntonic and therefore presents an additional technical hurdle. It is first necessary to make the defensive transference ego alien and only then can one proceed to analyze it effectively. Defensive transference reactions are frequently found in pseudonormal characters, in candidates undergoing training analysis, in clinic cases treated without fee, and also in neurotic character disorders who need to maintain a normal façade. The additional technical problem such patients present is the need to expose the defensive transference as a resistance, to make it ego dystonic, to make it appear to the patient as a symptom (Reider, 1950; Gitelson, 1954). Only then can one go on to the analysis of the underlying impulses and affects.

GENERALIZED TRANSFERENCE REACTIONS

Thus far in our discussion of the different types of transference phenomena and transference resistances, we have described reactions to the analyst which are derived from experience with specific significant persons in the patient's past. The patient loves or hates or dreads the analyst as he once dreaded or loved his father or mother or brother, etc. The patient's transference behavior toward his analyst is usually quite distinct and different from his behavior toward most of the people in his outside life except for those few who are similar transference figures. Transference reactions are ordinarily specific and circumscribed.

However, under the heading of Generalized Transference Reactions, I should like to describe a form of transference phenomenon which differs from all other previous forms precisely in being unspecific and uncircumscribed. Here the patient reacts to the analyst as he reacts to many or most of the people in his life. The transference behavior is not distinctive, it is typical and habitual. This behavior has been designated as "character transference" by Wilhelm Reich (1928, 1929), but others have considered this term misleading and ambiguous (A. Freud, 1936; Sterba, 1951).

What distingushes this form of transference from others is that the reactions to the analyst are the patient's habitual, representative, and typical responses to people at large; the transference is characteristic of the patient's object relations in general. It is this quality of nonspecificality, of characteristicness, which led to the use of the term "character transference." However, the term "character" has other meanings and I find the term "generalized transference reaction" more precise.

Patients who react to their analyst with generalized transference will have feelings, attitudes, impulses, expectations, desires, fears, and defenses which had been molded into their character and which have become their presenting surface to the world at large. These traits are the relatively fixed results, the residuals, the compromises of various conflicts between instincts and defenses. This aspect of the personality contains both defensive and instinctual components, often condensed. During the course of psychoanalytic therapy, such transference reactions always serve an important resistance function. The student is referred to the standard works on the subject of character formation for a more thorough description of the dynamics (W. Reich, 1928, 1929; Fenichel, 1945a).

Let me give a typical example of a generalized transference reaction. A man in his middle fifties came for analysis because of a sleep disturbance and a fear of becoming addicted to sleeping pills. He was exceptionally successful in his profession and apparently so also in his family and social life. A vital factor in his various successes was his propensity for enthusiasm. He was a hail-fellow-well-met, witty, hearty, joyous, emotionally generous, outspoken, gregarious, the life of the party, etc. In short, he was an enthusiast.

He began his analysis just as he undertook any other project, eagerly, vigorously, and optimistically. He began each hour with a booming hello, interspersed his associations with jokes; his life's experiences were woven into fascinating stories; he found my interpretations brilliant, remarkable, or delightful. If my remarks pained him, he was awed and eager to confirm my findings. He admired me, flattered me, proclaimed my virtues to one and all, and recruited new patients for me. Although he knew the standard procedure of psychoanalysis, he repeatedly invited me to parties, even arranged parties with special celebrities he thought would interest me, and although I constantly declined, he was sure that sooner or later I would give in. He was convinced he was my favorite patient, although he knew I was bound by psychoanalytic convention to withhold this information. This manner of reacting to me was typical and characteristic of the way in which he reacted to most people, with whom it was highly successful. He was considered lovable and charming by people in all walks of life, by his family, his employees, his many mistresses, important executives, and famous artists.

This generalized transference reaction was difficult to handle. First of all, it was necessary for me to constrain my real and countertransference responses. Then I consistently had to point out to him the indiscriminateness of his behavior, the promiscuity of his loves, the constant restlessness which indicated a hidden discontent. Slowly I was able to demonstrate that this chronic enthusiasm, this feeling of being the favorite was a myth, a screen he tried to perpetuate. It failed him only in his sleep and in his dreams, when he had to relinquish his conscious controls. After many months of work, his enthusiasm became ego alien, he no longer approved of it, he realized it was fraudulent, and he dared let himself feel the underlying depression. Then his transference reaction changed, and I became at various times the hateful, hypocritical mother who seduced him and rejected him, the angry father, etc. Outside of the analysis his behavior changed too. Although he could still become enthusiastic and charming, it was controllable. He was eventually able to develop some worthy enemies and even at times to be boring. Then he was also able to sleep and to dream (Greenson, 1962).

The technical problems in generalized transference reactions are similar to those in defensive transference, since the generalized transference always serves an important defensive purpose and is ego syntonic. The first task is to convert the transference into an ego-dystonic, painful one so that the patient will actively work on the transference instead of trying to perpetuate it. Character resistances have to be changed into transference resistances (Fenichel, 1941, p. 68). Then the transference neurosis will evolve and fruitful analytic work can be accomplished.

Generalized transference reactions occur in patients who suffer predominantly from character disorders. Each special type will produce a typical generalized transference; for example, an obsessive character will develop a generalized transference to the analyst which will be a replica of his isolated, obsessive object relations in general.

ACTING OUT OF TRANSFERENCE REACTIONS

Since the case of Dora, whom he treated in 1900, Freud was aware of the great importance of recognizing and analyzing transference, transference resistances, and, in particular, the acting out of transference reactions. Dora broke off her treatment with Freud because he failed to recognize that a particular transference reaction of hers was derived from her lover and not from her father. Furthermore, the patient acted out this aspect of her transference. She acted toward Freud as she had wanted to do toward her lover, Herr K.; she deserted him. In reviewing the history and outcome of this case Freud (1901–1905) came to recognize the special importance of transference and the acting out of transference phenomena. He returned to the problem of acting out on several later occasions, particularly in reference to his work on the compulsion to repeat (1914, 1920, 1937). In recent years several other authors have made significant contributions to our understanding of the acting out of transference reactions (Fenichel, 1945a, 1945b; Greenacre, 1950; Spiegel, 1954; Bird, 1957). . . .

Acting out occurs under a great variety of circumstances and not only as a transference reaction. . . . In the present section acting out will be discussed as a transference phenomenon occurring during the course of analysis and as a special variety of transference reaction.

Acting out refers to a well-organized, cohesive set of actions which appear to be purposeful, consciously willed, and ego syntonic, and which turn out to be a re-enactment of a past memory. The action is a slightly disguised repetition of the past, but the patient is not able to recall the past memory or memories. The patient seems intent upon acting instead of remembering; it is a defense against memory. During the course of analysis, patients will act out their transference reactions instead of reporting them in words and feelings. This may be acted out toward the analyst himself or outside the analysis toward others.

Some amount of acting out is inevitable in every analysis. This is due partly to the fact that the analyst attacks the neurotic defenses and thus encourages the discharge of affects and impulses in less distorted ways. This facilitates the breakthrough into actions. Secondly, transference itself is a reliving, a repetition of the past, and so mobilizes impulses from the past which may be expressed in behavior and actions. However, acting out will also be caused by the mishandling of the transference, particularly by the insufficient analysis of the negative transference. Errors in dosage, timing, and tact of interpretation often lead to acting out. Transference reactions of the analyst toward the patient can also set off acting out. However, the tendency to re-enact instead of remember will arise when nonverbal or preverbal material is attempting to gain expression during analysis or when traumatic material is approached.

Acting out is always a resistance even though it may serve some useful function temporarily. It is a defense against remembering, it is a defense against thinking, and it opposes the integration of thinking, memory, and behavior and thus opposes structural changes in the ego. However, some forms of acting out may serve a constructive purpose. I refer here to the transient, sporadic acting out which may occur in the breaking down of rigid, inhibiting defenses. This type should be differentiated from the habitual acting out of the chronic re-enactor. Then, too, acting out may be a form of trial recollection, a first testing out of a daring to remember (Ekstein and Friedman, 1957). In this sense it is a detour on the road to memory. My clinical experience seems to indicate that the memory which is re-enacted is a screen memory (Greenson, 1958). The distortion inherent in the acting out is always in the direction of wish fulfillment. The overt actions are like the manifest content of a dream, an attempted fulfillment of a wish (Lewin, 1955). Finally, acting out is a form of nonverbal communication; despite its resistance functions, it is also a reaching out toward an object (Bird, 1957; Greenson, 1959). It may be a cry for help (Winnicott, 1956).

Acting out is only one specific form of neurotic re-enactment which may occur in and outside of analysis. It should be differentiated from reliving and symptomatic action, although this is not always clinically possible. In reliving there is a simple repetition and duplication of a past event. There is no distortion and it readily leads to memory. Usually this occurs in altered ego states, under the influence of intense emotions or drugs, fugue states, etc. Symptomatic actions are not well organized and coherent; they are felt as bizarre, ego alien, and represent a failure of ego functioning. The past event has been greatly distorted and only a fragment of the event may be reported in the symptomatic action. Let me illustrate simple examples of acting out, reliving, and symptomatic action.

> Mrs. K. ended each hour by standing up and picking up the Kleenex upon which her head had been resting upon the pillow. As she would walk to the door she would crumple the Kleenex in her hand, taking care to keep it from my view. She would then throw it into the wastebasket beneath my desk as she passed or place it in her purse. This was done as deftly as possible and I had the impression the patient hoped these actions would escape my notice. When I pointed out this behavior to Mrs. K., she readily acknowledged this but seemed surprised that I questioned it. Her attitude was: doesn't everybody? She felt her reactions were self-explanatory and indicated ordinary decorum. She continued

to act in this way despite my attempts to understand the underlying meaning.

In one hour I was able to make some headway when I asked her to associate to the "soiled napkin" she tried to hide from me. This led to painful memories about her shame concerning menstruation. The behavior with the Kleenex continued. Finally, we began to analyze her terrible shame about her anus, the part of her she had to hide at all costs. She could not move her bowels when strangers were in her home for fear of being overheard or for fear the odors might betray her. After a bowel movement she spent considerable time in the bathroom to make it seem as if nothing had transpired. I pointed out she acted with the Kleenex as though it indicated a toilet activity she had to hide. Then she recalled many memories of her mother's fanaticism about toilet matters and cleanliness in the bathroom. Only then could she leave the Kleenex upon the pillow at the end of the hour.

Mrs. K. acted out at the end of each analytic hour: I am a clean girl who makes sure her toilet activities are not seen by others. Nobody must know I engage in such actions. It is not true that I do such dirty things; there is no evidence of it left behind. It was a cohesive, well-organized, purposeful set of actions, consciously willed and ego syntonic, serving to deny her past pleasurable toilet activities which she could not remember. In short, it was a form of acting out.

During World War II I gave a tail-gunner on a B-17 bomber, just returned from combat, an intravenous injection of sodium pentothal. He had been suffering from insomnia, nightmares, tremor, profuse sweating, and pronounced startle reaction. He had completed fifty combat missions, but was not aware of any troublesome anxiety and was reluctant to talk about combat. He agreed to take the pentothal because he had been told it felt like being drunk, and besides it meant he didn't have to talk to any other officer. As soon as he had about 5 cc. in his vein, he jumped on top of the bed, tearing the needle out of his arm and began to scream at the top of his voice: "They're coming in at four o'clock, they're coming in at four o'clock, get 'em, get 'em, get 'em or they'll get us, those sons of bitches, get 'em. Oh Lord, get 'em, get 'em. Here they come again at one o'clock, at one o'clock, get 'em, get 'em, you bastards, get 'em, oh God, I'm hurt, I can't move, get 'em, get 'em, someone help me, I'm hit, I'm hit, I can't move, help me. Oh you bastards, help me, get 'em, get 'em."

The patient shouted and screamed like this for twenty minutes with his eyes full of terror and sweat pouring down his face. His left hand clutched his right arm which dangled limply. He was quivering and taut. I finally said, "Okay, Joe, I got 'em. I got 'em." With that he collapsed on the bed and fell into a deep sleep.

The next morning I saw him and asked if he recalled the pentothal interview. He smiled sheepishly and said he recalled yelling, but it's all hazy. I told him he talked about a mission when his right hand was hurt and he kept yelling "get 'em, get 'em." He interrupted me: "Oh, yes, I remember we were coming back from Schweinfurt and they jumped us and they started coming in at four o'clock and then at one o'clock and we got hit by flak, etc., etc."

The patient could easily recall the past event he had relived under the sodium pentothal. It was undistorted and accessible, which is typical of reliving.

I would now like to cite the following as a symptomatic action. One of my patients, a middle-aged man, cannot sit down in my waiting room. He stands embarrassedly in the corner until I open the door to my treatment room, and then instantly walks toward me. This behavior distresses him, he knows it is strange, yet he is overpowered by a strong fear when he tries to sit down. He has had similar reactions in other waiting rooms which he would conceal by coming late or leaving and re-entering on one pretext or another. It became more transparent when he began coming regularly for his analytic hour and I began to analyze his tendency to come late.

Over a period of about a year we uncovered the following determinants of his fear of sitting down in the waiting room. To be found sitting down signified to be "caught" sitting down, which meant to be discovered masturbating. He had masturbated sitting on the toilet as a boy and would jump up as soon as he heard someone approaching out of fear they would enter. There were no locks on the bathroom door in his home. To be sitting down when I was standing meant he was little and I was big, and he felt I could assault him physically. Furthermore, his father had insisted he jump to his feet when grownups entered a room, and now he was belatedly complying. He had rebelled against his father when he entered adolescence, and he felt guilty when his father died of a stroke. He had discovered his father sitting in a chair as though he were dozing, only to discover to his horror that he was in a coma. Thus standing up meant he was alive and to be found sitting meant to be like father — dead. Finally, to sit meant to take the feminine position while urinating, and he had to stand in my presence to indicate: see, I am a man.

Here we have an example of how an ego-alien, bizarre activity is carried out against the patient's will; he is compelled to enact it, it is a symptomatic act. Analysis reveals the many historical events which are condensed, distorted, and symbolized in this activity. In clear-cut cases, acting out, reliving, and symptomatic actions are easily distinguishable from each other. In clinical practice one does not often see the pure form, and one is often dealing with some admixture of the three varieties of neurotic re-enactments. Let us now return to our study of the acting out of transference reactions.

ACTING OUT WITHIN THE ANALYTIC SETTING

The simplest form of acting out of transference reactions occurs when the patient acts out something within the analytic setting. Freud gave the example of the patient who behaves defiantly and critically toward his analyst and cannot remember this kind of behavior in his past. He not only feels these emotions toward the analyst, but he acts upon them, refusing to talk, forgetting his dreams, etc. He is acting upon his feelings instead of reporting them; he is re-enacting a piece of the past instead of remembering it (Freud, 1914, p. 150). Furthermore, he is not only unaware of the incongruity of his reactions, but he usually feels justified in his behavior. Acting out, as we have said, is ego syntonic.

Let me illustrate with the following example. A forty-year-old musician came for analysis because he suffered from chronic insomnia, colitis, and a work inhibition. When I was able to give him my first hour in the morning, at eight o'clock, he developed a remarkable pattern of beginning the hour. First of all, I could hear him coming down the hall because he would announce his arrival by loudly blowing his nose like a trumpet, each nostril separately and repeatedly. When he entered the treatment room, he would cheerfully and musically call out a good morning. Then, humming quietly, he would remove his jacket and drape it around one of the office chairs. He would walk over to the couch, sit down, and still humming quietly, he would begin to empty his pockets. First, the wallet and handkerchief from the back pockets would be placed on the side table; then the keys and change from his other pockets, and the ring from his finger. Then, with an audible groan, he would bend over and take off his shoes, placing them neatly side by side. He then would open the top button of his shirt, loosen his tie, and with an audible sigh of relief, he would lie down on the couch, turn over on his side, place his clasped hands between the pillow and his cheek, close his eyes and remain silent. Then, after a few moments he would begin to speak very softly.

At first I watched this performance silently; it seemed incredible that my patient was doing this seriously. Then, when I realized he was unaware of the inappropriateness of his behavior, I decided to try to fathom its meaning as precisely as possible before I confronted him. It was obvious that his acting out was in some way connected with going to sleep. Slowly I began to realize he was re-enacting the going to sleep of his father and mother, in which I was one parent and he was either the other parent or himself as a child. His history was full of memories of the terrible battles between his mother and father in their bedroom, which awakened him from sleep and terrified him. These fights occurred about four hours after he went to sleep as a child, and his present insomnia was characterized by his awakening after some four hours of sleep. He was acting out with me (a) how he wished his parents would have slept peacefully together, and (b) how he fantasied, as a child, he would have slept with either parent.

When I tried to draw his attention to his peculiar way of starting the hour, he was indignant. There was nothing peculiar about it, or strange, or noteworthy. He was only trying to relax and associate freely; after all, I had told him in the beginning of the analysis that all he had to do was relax and try to say whatever came to his mind. So now he was relaxing. It was true that he felt somewhat sleepy, but that was due to the earliness of the hour. Then he reluctantly admitted that when I spoke to him toward the end of the hour, he did feel it as a jarring note, an intrusion. He also realized that although for some strange reason he liked this early hour, he could hardly remember either what he had said or I had said. I then told him to continue his sleep with me. He undressed as though he was going to bed and he lay on the couch with closed eyes and blissful expression because he felt that we were sleeping together and this is the peaceful sleep he must have wished for between his father and mother or between himself and one of his parents. Up until this point in the analysis, the patient had been able to recall only his hatred toward his parents for their constant battling at night or his jealous rivalry and sexual wishes to replace either his father or his mother in their double bed. My interpretation about the peaceful sleep wishes were the first step in reconstructing the patient's preoedipal wishes toward his father and mother (Lewin, 1955).

In the instances cited, a patient has feelings toward his analyst which he does not describe or report, but acts upon. One surreptitiously disposes of the tissue, one acts defiantly, and one goes to sleep. In all three a piece of the past is being re-enacted, but the patient cannot remember it and is reluctant to analyze the activity.

Finally, it turns out that the activity is a distortion of a past event, the action is an attempt at wish fulfillment. The patient acts out with the analyst what he wishes he had done in his past. It is my clinical experience that acting out is always a re-enactment of a past wish that originally could not be acted upon. The acting out then is the belated attempt at wish fulfillment.

Acting out within the framework of the analytic hour may not be limited to a certain episode or singular event, but may occur throughout long periods of the analysis. I have seen patients, particularly candidates in training, who act out the role of the "good" patient and who try to cast me in the role of the "perfect" analyst. This may go on for months and even years until one realizes there is a certain sterility and restrictedness in the analysis. Then the task is to expose this behavior as resistance and defense and uncover the underlying hostility. I have seen a parallel situation in patients who maintain an attitude and feeling that they are my favorite patient. My eight o'clock sleepy patient was this way. He consciously believed he was my favorite patient and when I interpreted this as his wish and need, he replied that he knew that I was bound by my Freudian oath to keep my true feelings quiet. When I made interpretations which any other patient would have experienced as painful, he would react by admiring my astuteness and enjoying vicariously my supposed triumph. He loved the analysis and, above all, being analyzed by me. He felt we were a wonderful combination, he and I, me with my brains and he with his imagination. Even though his symptoms did not improve and he retained little insight, he was delighted with the analysis. I had to point out to him energetically, again and again, that he did not seem to be coming for analysis, he was coming to re-enact the delightful feeling of being the favorite. Slowly he began to recall and recount being mother's favorite and father's, too, and then these memories were found to be screens against bitter disappointments from both parents.

ACTING OUT OUTSIDE OF THE ANALYSIS

A young married woman patient began a sexual affair unexpectedly during her analysis. I became convinced, by the following clinical findings, that it was an acting out of her transference feelings: the patient had hardly known this man, and he was quite different from the men she was ordinarily attracted to. He was artistic, acted like a professor, and looked like an ancient Roman—these qualities attracted her. The affair occurred when I had to miss a few hours to attend a meeting. She had begun the analysis with a positive transference which blossomed into an erotic, sexual one. This had been interpreted and seemed to have been temporarily resolved. I recalled that during the phase of her strong love for me she had described me as a professor and an artist. Also she had once dreamed of me in a Roman toga and in association to that dream claimed I combed my hair like a Roman, and had heard my nickname was "Romi." It seemed clear that the young lady was acting out her sexual and romantic feelings with the young man. She enacted with him what she had wanted to and was unable to enact with me. These wishes were a repetition of deeply repressed feelings she had had to her stepfather.

A male patient in analysis suddenly develops a close relationship to his internist, a man he had never known socially. Now the patient invites him frequently for dinner and engages in intimate conversations with this doctor. Obviously, his wishes for intimacy with me are being acted upon outside of his analysis. When this occurs, the wish for intimacy with me is not being expressed in the analytic hour. It was my interpretation of the acting out which brought these unconscious wishes (unconscious as far as they refer to me) back into the analysis.

It is characteristic, when transference feelings are being acted out outside the analysis, that the impulses and affects which are being acted out do not appear in the analytic situation proper. A student in analysis with me is constantly critical of the stupidity of his teachers, their laziness and ineptness. At the same time, his transference feelings toward me are consistently positive. It was the lack of any hostile transference to me and the constant hostility toward the teachers that made me realize he was acting out his negative transference.

The splitting off of the ambivalent or preambivalent transference, with one aspect being acted out outside of the analysis, is a frequent form of acting out. It is often to be observed in candidates in training. Usually the ego-alien transference is vented upon some outside analyst and only the ego-syntonic feelings are expressed toward the personal analyst. Thus hostile and homosexual feelings will be discharged onto other analysts and the less disturbing emotions and impulses will be reserved for one's own analyst. Or the split will take place on a "good" and "bad" analyst basis, with some outside analyst serving in the auxiliary role.

It should be remembered that the acting out which occurs during analysis is not only connected to the transference situation. Very often it will be found that such acting out has been going on prior to the analysis. The co-actors in such situations will themselves turn out to be transference figures (Bird, 1957). . . .

> I would now like to give an illustration of a combination of acting out and symptomatic action involving the transference. For several hours a male patient finds fault with whatever I do in the analysis. He finds my silence oppressive and my interventions irritating and hostile. Actually, he admits that he likes the analytic hour until I begin to talk or until he expects me to talk. He can tell when I am about to intervene because he can hear my chair squeak or my breathing change. A short dream and the associations to it provided some important clues for the understanding of his reactions. In the dream somebody was listening to a radio commentator, Gabriel Heater, who had the voice of doom. The patient associates to this the fact that this broadcaster was his father's favorite and the entire family was forced to listen to this man whenever his father came home for dinner. This brings up the memory how father's homecoming changed the atmosphere; he was a wet blanket. He spoiled the fun for the family, at least for the patient. He could always tell when his father was coming home because he always came home twenty minutes before seven and he always whistled as he approached the house. Whenever the patient noticed the approach of seven o'clock or heard the whistle, he would become irritable and hostile.
>
> I was struck by the many parallels between how the patient behaved toward me in the hour and how he reacted to his father's homecoming. I made the following formulations to him: As long as I kept silent in the hour and let the patient talk and as long as it was early in the hour, the patient enjoyed the analytic situation just as he enjoyed being at home with his doting mother and his sisters. This was peaceful and pleasurable. About twenty minutes before the end of the hour the patient began to anticipate my interrupting his secret fun at home. The squeaking of my chair or the change in my breathing rate reminded him of his father's whistle. My interpretations were like the "voice of doom," the father's return home, the end of the patient's pleasure with his mother and his sisters. The patient confirmed these formulations by adding that "in all honesty" he had to admit that his father's homecoming was painful only to him; the mother and sisters looked forward to it. This example illustrates how in the analytic hour the patient re-enacted with

me a piece of his past history with his family. In the beginning of the hour he was the big talker and I represented the quiet and admiring mother and sisters. Toward the end of the hour, when it was my turn to speak, I became the overbearing and disturbing father. Since the situation was ego dystonic and very painful to the patient, he worked very diligently in attempting to reconstruct and remember the past events which lay behind this neurotic re-enactment.

As was stated earlier, all forms of neurotic re-enactments may occur in pure form, but usually one finds admixtures of reliving, symptomatic action, and acting out. The crux of the matter is determined by whether the neurotic re-enactment is ego syntonic or ego alien. It is always an additional resistance when the re-enactment is ego syntonic. It is then always more difficult to enlist the patient's reasonable ego, to establish a working alliance, and to uncover or reconstruct the underlying memories.

Since Greenson's book is on technique, it is a compendium of how-to approaches supported by a thorough theoretical structure of why. The positive characteristics of his approach should be evident in the preceding sections. We bring these excerpts from Greenson to a close with his pithy summary of the rules of resistance analysis and some general principles that also apply.

If we now recapitulate the general procedures in the analysis of resistance, they can be outlined as follows:

(1) Recognize the resistance.
(2) Demonstrate the resistance to the patient.
    (a) Allow the resistance to become demonstrable by waiting for several instances.
    (b) Intervene in such a way so as to increase the resistance; help it become demonstrable.
(3) Clarify the motives and modes of resistance.
    (a) What specific painful affect is making this patient resistant?
    (b) What particular instinctual impulse is causing the painful affect at this moment?
    (c) What precise mode and method does the patient use to express his resistance?

(4) Interpret the resistance.
  (a) What fantasies or memories are causing the affects and impulses behind the resistance?
  (b) Pursue the history and unconscious purposes of these affects, impulses, or events in and outside the analysis, and in the past.
(5) Interpret the mode of resistance.
  (a) Pursue this and similar modes of activity in and outside of the analysis.
  (b) Trace the history and unconscious purposes of this activity in the patient's present and past.
(6) Working through.
  Repetitions and elaborations of steps (4) (a) (b) and (5) (a) (b).

It is important to realize that only a small fragment of the work can be accomplished in a given hour. Many hours end up with only the dim awareness that there is some resistance at work, and all one can do toward the end of such an hour is to point out to the patient that he seems to be avoiding something. Sometimes one can clarify only the affect, and even that incompletely; sometimes only the historical antecedent, sometimes only the mode. Whenever possible and as much as possible one tries to explore avoidances with the patient, assaying how much of this probing the patient can meaningfully and usefully do in a given hour. The analyst's own zeal for exploration and uncovering of unconscious phenomena must play a secondary role to how much the patient is able to endure and to utilize. The patient should be neither traumatized nor allowed to enter into some playful, gamelike exploration of resistance.

It is important not to make interpretations of resistance prematurely, since that only leads the patient to rationalize or intellectualize, or it makes an intellectual contest of the interpretation of resistance. In either case it deprives the experience of emotional impact. Thus it adds to the resistances instead of diminishing them. The patient must be given the opportunity to feel his resistances, to become aware of their strength and tenacity. It is important to know when to be passive and when to be active in the analytic work. Too much patience can permit the patient to waste valuable time when he might be working effectively. Too much activity may either interfere with the patient's ability for being active and gratify his passive wishes; or it may remobilize events for which the patient is not ready and thereby stir up a traumatic situation. Above all, too much activity can serve to evade the emotional impact and turn the analysis of resistance into a guessing game (see Freud, 1914, p. 155; Fenichel, 1941, pp. 36–43).

It is important, furthermore, not to play into the resistance of the patient by using the same kind of resistance he does. If he is silent, you must be alert that your silence is not a counterresistance. Or if he uses stilted language, obscenities, or clichés, you must avoid going along with this resistance or doing the opposite. It is important to be direct and to the point without being crude, playfully provocative, or reproachful.

The steps and the order of the various steps vary from hour to hour and from patient to patient. One can pursue only what seems to be the most promising avenue of exploration at a given time. One has to keep an open and alert mind and be willing to alter one's approach or be willing to stick to it if it seems correct.

The analyst's indispensable ally in this work is the patient's reasonable ego. It must be present or it must be evoked by the analyst's interventions; otherwise one has to wait for the emotional storms to subside and for the reasonable ego to return. This can be expressed in terms of the relationship to the analyst. A working alliance must be present or evocable before one embarks on the deep analysis of resistance. It is a prerequisite for interpretation (Greenson, 1965). . . .

Finally, it is important to realize that no matter how skillfully and how correctly one works with resistances, the resistances will return. One should remember Freud's remark that resistance will be present at every step, in every aspect, in every hour of the analysis, until the analysis has been completed. Working through is necessary for a given resistance to lose its pathogenesis. Resistance analysis is not a detour of the analysis but a necessary and vital part of every analysis.

REFERENCES

Bird, B. (1957). A specific peculiarity of acting out. *Journal of the American Psychoanalytic Association* 5:630–647.

Bornstein, B. (1949). The analysis of a phobic child: some problems of theory and technique in child analysis. *The Psychoanalytic Study of the Child* 3/4:181–226.

Ekstein, R., and Friedman, S.W. (1957). The function of acting out, play action and play acting in the psychotherapeutic process. *Journal of the American Psychoanalytic Association* 5:581–629.

Fenichel, O. (1941). *Problems of Psychoanalytic Technique*, pp. 18, 36–43, 47–48, 57, 61–62, 68–69. Albany, NY: The Psychoanalytic Quarterly.

———— (1945a). *The Psychoanalytic Theory of Neurosis*, pp. 128–167; also chapters 8, 9. New York: Norton.

———— (1945b). Neurotic acting out. *Collected Papers of Otto Fenichel* 2:296–304. New York: Norton, 1954.

Freeman, T. (1959). Aspects of defence in neurosis and psychosis. *International Journal of Psycho-Analysis* 40:199–212.

Freud, A. (1936). *The Ego and the Mechanisms of Defense*, pp. 19–25, 45–70. New York: International Universities Press, 1946.

Freud, S. (1901–1905). Fragment of an analysis of a case of hysteria. *Standard Edition* 7:3–122.

———— (1905a). Psychical (or mental) treatment. *Standard Edition* 7:283–302.

———— (1905b). Three essays on the theory of sexuality. *Standard Edition* 7:125–245.

———— (1912). The dynamics of transference. *Standard Edition* 12:97–108.

———— (1914). Remembering, repeating and working-through. *Standard Edition* 12:145–156.

———— (1920). Beyond the pleasure principle. *Standard Edition* 18:3–64.

———— (1925–1926). Inhibitions, symptoms and anxiety. *Standard Edition* 20:77–175.

———— (1937). Analysis terminable and interminable. *Standard Edition* 23:209–253.

Frosch, J. (1959). Transference derivatives of the family romance. *Journal of the American Psychoanalytic Association* 7:503–522.

Gero, G. (1951). The concept of defense. *Psychoanalytic Quarterly* 20:565–578.

Gill, M.M. (1963). *Topography and Systems in Psychoanalytic Theory*, pp. 96, 115, 122–123. (Psychological Issues, Monograph 10). New York: International Universities Press.

Gitelson, M. (1948). Problems of psychoanalytic training. *Psychoanalytic Quarterly* 17:198–211.

———— (1954). Therapeutic problems in the analysis of the 'normal' candidate. *International Journal of Psycho-Analysis* 35:174–183.

Greenacre, P. (1950). General problems of acting out. *Trauma, Growth and Personality*, pp. 224–236. New York: Norton, 1952.

Greenson, R.R. (1958a). On screen defenses, screen hunger and screen identity. *Journal of the American Psychoanalytic Association* 6:242–262.

———— (1959). Phobia, anxiety and depression. *Journal of the American Psychoanalytic Association* 7:663–674.

_____ (1962). On enthusiasm. *Journal of the American Psychoanalytic Association* 10:3–21.

_____ (1965). The working alliance and the transference neurosis. *Psychoanalytic Quarterly* 34:155–181.

_____ (1972). *The Technique and Practice of Psychoanalysis.* Vol. 1. New York: International Universities Press.

Hartmann, H. (1951). Technical implications of ego psychology. *Essays on Ego Psychology,* pp. 142–154. New York: International Universities Press, 1964.

Knight, R.P. (1952). An evaluation of psychotherapeutic techniques. *Psychoanalytic Psychiatry and Psychology,* ed. R.P. Knight and C.R. Friedman, pp. 65–76. New York: International Universities Press, 1954.

Lewin, B.D. (1955). Dream psychology and the analytic situation. *Psychoanalytic Quarterly* 24:169–199.

Loewenstein, R.M. (1951). The problem of interpretation. *Psychoanalytic Quarterly* 20:1–14.

Nunberg, H. (1951). Transference and reality. *International Journal of Psycho-Analysis* 32:1–9.

Rappaport, E.A. (1956). The management of an eroticized transference. *Psychoanalytic Quarterly* 25:515–529. New York: International Universities Press.

Reich, W. (1928). On character analysis. In *The Psychoanalytic Reader,* ed. R. Fliess, Vol. 1, pp. 129–147. New York: International Universities Press, 1948.

_____ (1929). The genital character and the neurotic character. In *The Psychoanalytic Reader,* ed. R. Fliess, Vol. 1, pp. 148–169. New York: International Universities Press, 1948.

Reider, N. (1950). The concept of normality. *Psychoanalytic Quarterly* 19:43–51.

Schur, M. (1953). The Ego in Anxiety. In *Drives, Affects, Behavior,* ed. R.M. Loewenstein, Vol. 1, pp. 67–103. New York: International Universities Press.

Sperling, S.J. (1958). On denial and the essential nature of defence. *International Journal of Psycho-Analysis* 39:25–38.

Spiegel, L.A. (1954). Acting out and defensive instinctual gratification. *Journal of the American Psychoanalytic Association* 2:107–119.

Sterba, R.F. (1951). Character and resistance. *Psychoanalytic Quarterly* 20:72–76.

Winnicott, D.W. (1956). The antisocial tendency. *Collected Papers: Through Paediatrics to Psycho-Analysis,* pp. 306–315. New York: Basic Books, 1958.

CHAPTER 6

Narcissism as a Resistance and as a Driving Force in Psychoanalysis

Heinz Kohut

NARCISSISM AS A RESISTANCE IN PSYCHOANALYSIS

The existence of narcissism as resistance — and let me state immediately that I am writing here about narcissism as a *nonspecific resistance* against analysis — is fully acknowledged by all psychoanalysts; it is the only aspect of narcissism for which all analysts make allowance in their clinical work. This, at least, is the classical attitude.

Freud, in his "A Difficulty in the Path of Psycho-Analysis" (1917), compares his discovery of an unconscious mental life to the discoveries of Copernicus and Darwin. He says the findings of psychoanalysis are experienced as a narcissistic injury to mankind, especially the theory of unconscious mental life. Freud, then, speaks here about nonspecific resistance against the total edifice of psychoanalysis as a science.

This same attitude was gradually recognized also as nonspecific resistance of the individual patient against analytic treatment. The individual patient, in other words, believes that he wants to recognize his unconscious thoughts and wishes with the aid of analytic treatment. Yet, simultaneously, he fights against the treatment. He does not want to accept the fact that he is dominated by motivations of which he knows nothing.

The shift in emphasis of the concept of nonspecific narcissistic resistance—a shift from the general to the specific—reached a kind of climax and turning point with Wilhelm Reich. Reich formulated narcissistic resistance as character armor (1933–1934) and he maintained it was the task of the analyst to penetrate this narcissistic armor. The influence of Reich's teachings and writings on psychoanalytic theory and practice has now waned. His plastic descriptions of narcissistic resistance, however, and of the manner in which the analyst is to respond to it, have left their mark on analytic practice, even today.

The change which the idea of resistance during analysis underwent from Freud to Reich can be regarded as an example of the progressive concretization and intensification of a concept. What for Freud had been abstract and moderate—resistance motivated by fear—became for Reich something concrete, something hardened: an armor. Reich created an aggressive image implying hostility, fight, quarrel between patient and physician. The physician who wants to overcome the resistance turns into an attacker who undertakes breaking to pieces the armor of the analysand.

From Freud to Reich and beyond Reich, we see repetition-compulsion in successive generations. What has hurt the younger generation of analysts, what was suffered passively by them, was later repeated by them actively, rationalized as a moral stance. (What one has passively experienced as training analysand is then actively inflicted upon one's own patients, including one's training analysands.) After Reich's disappearance from the analytic scene, the narcissistic "armor" changed into a narcissistic "crust." This image still has not completely faded, and it still influences the technical attitude of many analysts. In spite of the moderation of the concept, from "armor" to "crust," traces of Reich's ideas are still present: the crust must be pierced.

This narcissistic resistance is nonspecific. The pathology whose revelation it opposes can be the outgrowth of unresolved conflicts in the area of object-instinctual drives: for instance, conflicts concerning the patient's love and hate for the objects of the oedipal period. But the pathology whose reactivations in analysis the narcissistic resistance opposes can also lie in the area of narcissistic disorders.

The intensity of this nonspecific narcissistic resistance, the hardness of the analysand's narcissistic "crust," is not proportionate to the dynamic forces of the underlying pathologic conflicts or needs. The resistance is a function of the general narcissistic vulnerability of the patient. Analytic treatment as a whole offends the pride of the analysand, contradicts his fantasy of his independence, and that is why he now resists treatment—without reference to the specific details of his psychic illness.

I submit below three typical examples of nonspecific narcissistic resistance and discuss them briefly: first two examples of narcissistic reactions to parapraxes, then an example of the narcissistic defense posture toward the analytic process (or, to express it more exactly: toward the analyst as representative of the analytic process).

First, though, some remarks about the behavior of the analyst toward parapraxes of the analysand in the early stages of analysis. In my view, it is an error if the analyst in such cases focuses on what was repressed and emerged through parapraxis. This opinion is based on many years of clinical observation; experience also taught me that nothing useful is elicited by focusing on the content of parapraxes. In the early stages of analysis—and in the analyses of some narcissistically vulnerable patients this early stage lasts a long time, often even years— the analyst should not look primarily for what was unconscious and repressed but should focus on the narcissistic injury of the analysand, i.e., he should explain to the patient that the mere fact that he has committed a parapraxis constituted a narcissistic injury. The patient feels shame, and he reacts with rage simply over the fact that a parapraxis unexpectedly got the better of him. The content of what was repressed and emerged through the parapraxis is not the most important aspect of the event. It may be mentioned, but, so to speak, only as a footnote to the interpretation proper. The proper aim of the interpretation should be the emotions caused in the patient through the feeling of relative helplessness. The temporal element—the suddenness of the loss of conscious control over one's words or actions—sometimes plays a specific (and also a specific genetic) role in this narcissistic injury through parapraxis, for instance, if a specific childhood experience concerning sudden loss of childhood self-esteem, of childhood pride, was repeated through this event.

Let us go on now to the other example of nonspecific narcissistic resistance caused through parapraxis. This example concerns not the analysand but the analyst. All of us probably have had the opportunity, for instance at a psychoanalytic meeting, to observe an analyst's public slip of the tongue. This, especially if it happens to oneself, is a very instructive event, and I advise close self-observation on the next occasion. How does the analyst behave when he makes a mistake in speaking, during a lecture perhaps, or during public scientific debate when one speaks extemporaneously? Under such circumstances one often readily admits *what* was revealed through parapraxis, often even something that was *really* hidden. But what one wants to cover up is that one lost control. "Of course I know what this means," one says; one even quickly reveals the secret. What one is ashamed of is that suddenly something broke through without one's having anything to do with this revelation. One acts as if one had almost done it intentionally; one laughs, which means that one demonstrates that one has overcome the *narcissistic* injury. (Freud explained humor [1927] as a higher form of narcissism emerging victoriously over the inevitable injuries to one's own illusory omnipotence. My own hypothesis [1966] is that humor represents a transformation of archaic narcissism.) It is very difficult not to react if one has publicly committed a parapraxis. In other words, making a parapraxis and then letting the others laugh without saying anything further oneself is most difficult.

And now the third example of nonspecific narcissistic resistance: the behavior in analysis of a young man, a successful journalist, who treated me and my attempts at explanations and interpretations at the beginning of the analysis with inimitable condescension. Instead of coming to terms with the content of what I interpreted (dynamically) and constructed (genetically), he criticized with disarming friendliness or superior irony the formal aspects of my endeavors: the grammar of my sentences, my choice of words, or similar matters. One simply cannot describe it, one has to have heard it to savor fully the expertise with which he tried to destroy my self-confidence, to degrade me.

When an inexperienced analyst feels exposed to such treatment on the part of a patient, he tends, of course, to react with anger, and he will be inclined to interpret the behavior of the patient as an offshoot of a "negative transference," for instance, as a reactivation of childhood hatred toward the rival of the Oedipus complex. But in the present case—and in my experience also in most similar cases—the behavior of the analysand is to be explained differently. The patient demonstrates through his behavior how *he* experiences the analysis, how my interpretations are received by *him*—how vulnerable and helpless *he* feels. One could say that he turns his passivity into activity, that he attacks *me* when *he* feels attacked. (That, however, is a comparatively unimportant explanation of his behavior. It is essentially based—at least in the case of this young man—on lessened differentiation between selfobject [analyst] and self [analysand].)

All this must be interpreted carefully and with true empathy. The analyst must not deny that the patient has indeed partially succeeded in hurting him, in inflicting real pain. And the analyst may admit—though probably only *sotto voce*—that he experienced an inclination to reactive anger. In other words: a tone of condescending kindness from the pedestal of the analyst's position must be avoided; what is needed is the analyst's expression of his sincere understanding for the position of the patient, including genetic reconstructions which explain the patient's sensitivity when he is confronted by pedagogic, didactic approaches toward him. (In connection with this patient, one might here recall Abraham's fine clinical contribution of 1919.)

In this case, and I could adduce many other clinical examples, we are dealing with a narcissistic defense. In all these cases, the analyst will try to reconstruct the specific history of the development of the patient's nonspecific narcissistic defensive posture (the analysand's nonspecific defensive narcissism). And he will try to illuminate more and more, especially in the later stages of analysis, the dynamic relationship between temporarily increased defensive narcissism and activation of specific aspects of the analysand's central pathology (e.g., especially strong shame and rage over the revelation of specific wishes and needs). Still, the narcissistic "crust" is not, by and large, specifically related to the nucleus of the neurosis; it is a general resistance against the analytic process which on the whole is not mobilized in order to obstruct the emergence of this or that specific pathogenic instinctual wish or this or that specific pathogenic infantile narcissistic need—it is directed against the analytic process as a whole.

One could discuss further the various possible reactions of analysts toward these narcissistic defense mechanisms of their patients. The central issue, however, is that it makes little difference what the analyst *does* so long as he *understands* what is going on in his patient. He can openly express his anger (as Freud did with patients who, it seemed to him, expressed their contempt for his empty waiting room by leaving the door open; he would send such patients to the door of the consulting room with the firmly expressed instruction to close it); or, as is my preference, he can suppress his anger and react with friendly understanding. Whatever we may do initially, it is ultimately our aim to help

the patient understand the significance of his narcissistic reactions —
the way that leads to the expansion of the patient's awareness is relatively unimportant.

A particularly instructive kind of chronic narcissistic resistance is
the complex psychic formation called schizoid personality (see Kohut,
1971). This can be explained dynamically. Such individuals are
vaguely aware of the fact that the cohesiveness of their self is maintained only very precariously. Because any injury of their self can lead
to a catastrophic fragmentation of the self, they protect themselves by
maintaining an emotional distance between themselves and others.
(Cf. the case of Mr. H [in Kohut, 1957].)

NARCISSISM AS A DRIVING FORCE IN
PSYCHOANALYSIS

I am writing here about that large number of patients whose psychopathology I have defined as narcissistic personality disorders. In the center of the illness in classical transference neuroses are structural
conflicts which relate to infantile drive demands concerning the great
objects of childhood. These objects form the nucleus of the spontaneously developing transference. In the center of the illness in narcissistic
personality disorders is the disordered self. The central content of the
spontaneously developing transference is formed not by loved or hated
autonomous and independent objects but by archaic selfobjects.
These are experienced either as a part of the self or as merged with the
self or as standing in the service of the self, i.e., as utilized for the maintenance of the stability and cohesion of the self.

How can one clinically differentiate a narcissistic personality disorder from a structural neurosis? On the basis of the following empirically ascertainable fact: that, in the psycho-analytic situation, with
patients with narcissistic personality disorders a pathognomonic transference evolves spontaneously which is directly connected with the
nucleus of the psychopathology. This transference is based on a therapeutic regression to precisely that point where the normal development of the psychic structures of the self was interrupted or where the
consolidation of those structures of the self which so far had only been
precariously established was not carried further toward completion.

The analytic situation, then, brings about a reactivation of that developmental point in time at which the basic disorder began. Thus, the interrupted psychological growth process is given the opportunity to continue beyond the point of its arrest.

To describe this in greater detail: at the point where the psychic development is traumatically interrupted, the infantile wish or the infantile need is first intensified. In the classical transference neuroses, it is an infantile instinctual wish which, after traumatic failure, is first greatly strengthened and probably also distorted and then, in this strengthened and distorted form, is repressed. In narcissistic personality disorders, it is the need for mirroring or for merging with the idealized selfobject which, after a traumatically mortifying rejection is first greatly intensified and probably also distorted and is then, in this intensified and distorted form, either repressed or split off and disavowed. [See the remarks about "vertical splits" of the personality in 1971, pp. 183–185.] In the transference we therefore see the mobilization not of a normal but of a frustrated and therefore intensified and distorted wish or need that had been repressed or split off and disavowed. Through analysis, the connection between these wishes and needs and the central sector of the personality is re-established. But then, with the help of friendly, nontraumatic, empathic interpretations and constructions – *optimal frustration* – analysis denies direct satisfaction of the infantile wish or need and prevents retreat toward its renewed repression or splitting off. Therefore, only *one* possibility remains: further psychic development through structure building. This applies to both classical transference neuroses and to narcissistic personality disorders [cf. 1971, pp. 196–199].

In classical transference neurosis, a cohesive self cannot cope with drive demands and their frustration. The sequence of: instinctual wish, anxiety, repression of the instinctual wish, and inhibition and symptom is well known to every analyst, and therefore I need not go into this any further here. Narcissistic injuries accompany these experiences, but are here secondary. It is a cohesive self that experiences the frustrations of oedipal wishes as narcissistic trauma. It may react, to be sure, with depression and rage, but its structural cohesion is not seriously threatened. The transference leads to the activation of repressed drive demands, which now, in the working-through process of analysis, are gradually integrated into the total structure of the mature personality.

At what point in psychic development does the decisive disturbance occur that leads to narcissistic personality disorder?

As you know, I maintain that the proper appreciation of the role played by narcissism in human life demands that we posit a separate line of development for it, leading from archaic to mature forms. Specifically: we postulate two lines of development (one from archaic narcissism to mature narcissism, the other, side by side with it, from archaic to mature object love), not a single line of development (from narcissism to object love).

The symptoms of narcissistic personality disorders are the result of the defective condition of the narcissistic structures: they are manifestations of a disease of the self. The disease affects either the grandiose self or the archaic omnipotent selfobject (the idealized parent imago). Specifically, these components of the self are either fragmented or enfeebled. The development of the other parts of the personality, for instance, intelligence or drives, may have progressed comparatively undisturbed. But the narcissistic structures remained fixated in their development. In their archaic form they were either repressed or split off from the other parts of the psyche. In the latter case they can strongly dominate the patients' behavior from time to time, for example, in the form of addictionlike praise-seeking or addictionlike search for idealized selfobjects. Both these strivings can also be sexualized: we then have the different forms of sexual perversion.

Conflicts over drive aims (classical structural conflicts) are secondary in narcissistic personality disorders. In some cases the patient is involved in innumerable object relations, which can create the impression that drive-related conflicts caused his psychic illness — conflicts, in other words, which concern the patient's intense love or intense hate. However, these love or hate relationships are either defensive — attempts to ward off, through an exaggerated experience of love or hate relations, the loss of the archaic selfobject, which would lead to fragmentation of the self — or they are not expressions of object-love or object-hate at all, but of the need for selfobjects in lieu of self-structure.

The spontaneously arising transference in these cases concerns the activation of the developmental stage at which the cohesive self begins to form, aided by mirroring from the side of the selfobjects of childhood and by merger with idealized aspects of these selfobjects. The structures thus formed are at first only precariously established and in constant danger of fragmentation. The formation and strengthening of the self during childhood is, in other words, the result of a long process of development. Analogously, the slowly proceeding working-through of the needs for mirroring and for idealized selfobjects which are reactivated in the form of a narcissistic transference brings about the gradual healing of the defects in the self of the analysand.

Up to this point we discussed the narcissistic transference as a driving force toward developmental progress of the damaged self in analysis in general terms. Let us now proceed to specifics.

The genesis of the disorder can, for instance, be the insufficient mirroring of the child's self by the mother (her lack of empathy for her child's need for mirroring through the gleam in the mother's eye). The child's self can therefore not establish itself securely (the child does not build up an inner sense of self-confidence; it continues to need external affirmation). But, as was mentioned above, we do not see merely fixation on a small child's normal need for mirroring—the traumatic frustration of the normal need intensifies and distorts the need: the child becomes insatiably hungry for mirroring, affirmation, and praise. It is this intensified, distorted need which the child cannot tolerate and which it therefore either represses (and may hide behind pseudoindependence and emotional coldness) or disavows and splits off. Figure 1 is a diagram of the latter case.

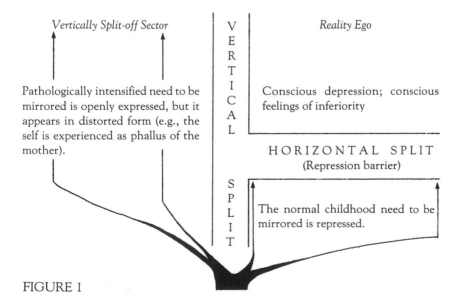

FIGURE 1

In the narcissistic transference, the infantile need for the selfobject is remobilized. (In the case shown in the diagram: the need for the mirroring selfobject.) The analyst aims at psychic reintegration of the need by reconstructing the period when, as he knows, the need was phase-appropriate and growth-promoting. Nongratification of the intensified and distorted need while yet acknowledging appropriateness of its precursor in childhood constitutes *optimal frustration* for the analysand. The analyst's acceptance of the fact that transference means reactivation of more or less normal childhood needs counteracts their renewed repression or their splitting off in distorted form. To repeat: there is only one road open to the reactivated infantile strivings for mirroring and merger with ideals: the road toward maturity. Higher forms of narcissism take shape; more precisely: the psyche acquires structures that transform the narcissistic needs.

This working-through process is kept in motion by the pressure of narcissistic needs. Again and again, in spite of strong resistance, the vulnerable, needy grandiose self offers itself to the selfobject analyst for praise, mirroring, and affirmation; or it seeks—again in spite of strong resistances—in the selfobject analyst an idealized self with which it can merge. Again and again—analogous to the conditions encountered in the classical transference neuroses where the analysand reacts to the frustration of his object-libidinal strivings—the patient reacts with regression to the frustration of his narcissistic needs as mobilized in the transference. Careful exploration of the oscillations is of great significance; knowledge of these processes contributes to their control. [See Kohut, 1971, p. 97, for a diagrammatic presentation of the usually brief but therapeutically important regressions during the working-through process of the narcissistic transferences.]

The thorough investigation of the various resistances mobilized by the analysand against the reactivation of the old narcissistic needs is, in my view, of greatest importance and will, I hope, soon be undertaken on the basis of meticulous clinical observations. In contrast to the nonspecific narcissistic resistances of which I spoke in the first part of this lecture, we are dealing here with *specific narcissistic resistances*, that is to say, in each case, with resistances against the revelation of specific narcissistic transferences in the analytic process. In the analyses of classical transference neuroses, resistances are motivated by the anxieties of a firmly cohesive self which fears either the loss of an object that is experienced as separate from the self or castration by such a separate object. By contrast, the specific resistances in the analyses of narcissistic personality disturbances are motivated by the anxieties of an insecurely established self which fears the rejection of the narcissistic needs that are reactivated in analysis, i.e., the need to be mirrored and to merge with an ideal. In other words, the specific narcissistic resistances are motivated by anxieties—I will (broadly speaking) refer to them as disintegration anxieties—which focus on the self and on an object experienced as (part of) the self. Although the analysand suffering from a narcissistic personality disorder consciously tries to express his needs openly, he nevertheless shies away from doing so because of the danger of the self's disintegration to which a possibly impending traumatic rejection of his needs exposes him. In other words, he fears the reactivation of the unempathic rejection by his childhood selfobjects, who did not respond to the need of his growing self for supportive and strengthening sustenance through mirroring and merger with the ideal.

The details of these resistances deserve, as I said, the most careful exploration. Here I can only say that they are of greatest importance during the process of psychoanalysis. They are transference resistances and, as long as they are in the ascendancy, stand in the way of the central working-through process of the analysis. They have to be dealt with time and again in the course of the treatment until they are ultimately overcome. Only then can the narcissistic transference be fully experienced and worked through. This working-through process of narcissistic personality disorders aims at integrating the repressed or split-off narcissistic structures that are mobilized in the transference into the realistic segments of the total personality. In order to achieve this end, the reactivation of these structures has to be a sustained one. With every nontraumatic frustration of the wishes of the grandiose self that are mobilized in the transference, with every nontraumatic disappointment in the omnipotent transference object, a small piece of psychic structure is laid down which increases the firmness of the self. Formerly there were gross oscillations between (1) depression and dejection on the basis of the repression of the analysand's grandiosity—to be exact: on the basis of the repression of his need for the mirroring of his grandiosity—and (2) open arrogance with self-righteous demands for an admiring audience (either on the basis of a temporary breakthrough of the archaic grandiosity across the repression barrier or, most frequently, on the basis of the displacement of the archaic narcissistic demands onto a split-off part of the personality). But gradually, as a result of the working through of the mirror transference, the analysand acquires a normal, dependable feeling of self-esteem which allows him to strive for external, self-enhancing success through realistic activities. In the area of the idealizing transference (the reactivation of the need for merger with the omnipotent selfobject), a similar development takes place. Formerly there was a quest for total merger with an omnipotent, idealized selfobject. Increasingly now, internal goal-structures are idealized instead. Previously, the patient's highly unstable self-esteem was dependent on merger with the idealized selfobject. Now the feeling of self-esteem (reacting to the vicissitudes of life with limited oscillations) can rely increasingly on the achievement of a merger between the self and its idealized goals.

REFERENCES

Abraham, K. (1919). A particular form of neurotic resistance against the psycho-analytic method. In *Selected Papers*, ed. D. Bryan and A. Strachey, pp. 303–311. New York: Basic Books, 1953.

Freud, S. (1917). A difficulty in the path of psycho-analysis. *Standard Edition* 17: 137–144.

———— (1927). Humour. *Standard Edition* 21: 161–166.

Kohut, H. (1957). Observations on the psychological function of music. In *The Search for the Self*, ed. P. Ornstein, pp. 233–253. New York: International Universities Press, 1978.

———— (1966). Forms and transformations of narcissism. In *The Search for the Self*, ed. P. Ornstein, pp. 427–460. New York: International Universities Press, 1978.

———— (1971). *The Analysis of the Self*. New York: International Universities Press.

Reich, W. (1933–34). *Character-Analysis*. New York: Touchtone Books, 1974.

PART II

Specific Techniques

CHAPTER 7

Resistances and the Basic Dimensions of Psychotherapy

Robert Langs

This chapter outlines the contributions of the communicative approach to the psychoanalytic understanding of resistances; studies the interplay between resistances and the other major dimensions of the psychotherapeutic situation and experience; and clarifies the nature of human defensive tendencies.

THE COMMUNICATIVE APPROACH

The communicative approach to psychoanalytic psychotherapy is an extension of the classical psychoanalytic position. It is based in the finding that the material from patients, as it illuminates their neuroses, contains encoded expressions that reflect the activated unconscious meanings of their emotional disturbances. Clinical studies have found that the major stimuli for these responses are virtually always contained in the conscious and especially unconscious implications of the therapist's interventions.

Since a neurosis can be illuminated only in terms of *derivative* expressions and not through manifest contents, it has proven essential to decode the material from patients in light of adaptive or adaptation-evoking contexts constituted by the therapist's interventions. The communicative approach stresses the spiraling conscious and unconscious communicative interaction between patient and therapist, and has refuted the proposition that material from patients exists as isolated intrapsychic products.

While Freud (1900, 1908) recognized the importance of derivative communications in understanding and interpreting neurotic manifestations, he nonetheless wrote of resistances mainly in terms of the manifest implications of the material from his patients (Freud 1914). Similarly, while Freud (1912) recognized that transferences are based on the *unconscious* fantasies and memories of his patients, in his clinical writings (see, in particular, the preserved notes of the Rat Man case, 1909) he tended to invoke the concept only when there was a manifest allusion to himself or his family, and more rarely a reference to an obvious displacement figure. Such transference expressions were treated as isolated happenings within the patient and were seen as deriving from earlier genetic experiences; they were not considered to be embedded in the ongoing therapeutic interaction. These failings in listening and formulating led to conceptualizations that are unique to the communicative approach.

Findings and Hypotheses

It is possible here only to briefly summarize the most important contributions of the communicative approach to our understanding of resistances. Some of these postulates will be further clarified in the main body of this chapter. The following are most pertinent:

1. A distinction must be made between *gross behavioral resistances* and *communicative resistances*. Analysts (e.g., Glover 1958, Greenson 1967, Stone 1973, Blum 1981) have for some time recognized the existence of silent (i.e., unrecognized or subtly expressed) resistances, though they have had difficulty in formulating their nature and basis. The communicative approach reveals that there are actually two levels of resistance: one grossly behavioral, and the other defined in terms of the patient's communicative propensities. This insight helps to clarify the nature of previously unrecognized resistances and the techniques required for their resolution.

Gross behavioral resistances allude to patients' obstacles to the course of therapy, such as silences, absences, and lateness. By and large, the psychoanalytic literature on this subject has been restricted to this level of resistance.

Communicative resistances refer to the extent to which a patient provides a meaningful communicative network, with material that lends itself to interpretation or constructive management of the ground rules or framework of treatment. The communicative approach has shown that the patient is reacting unconsciously to the implications of the therapist's interventions. When there is a disturbance in the bipersonal field — and even after a validated intervention — the patient is motivated to work over the interactional issues between himself and the therapist. A meaningful communicative network therefore contains first, a clear representation or allusion to the adaptive context of the therapist's intervention, which is serving as the key stimulus for the patient's symptomatic fluctuations and unconscious (encoded or derivative) communications; and second, meaningful derivative material constituted first and foremost by valid unconscious perceptions of the implications of the therapist's interventions, meanings that are selectively represented through encoded or displaced images and narratives with the unconscious guidance of the patient's own madness. In addition to these valid encoded perceptions, the patient will also communicate meaningful responses to these perceptions — mainly efforts to cure or assist the errant therapist. A low level of communicative resistances is signaled by a well-represented adaptive context and rich derivative material; conversely, a poorly represented adaptive context and/or a relative absence of encoded perceptions indicate the presence of major communicative resistances.

2. The most important resistances in the course of psychotherapy and psychoanalysis are termed *relationship resistances*, and these in turn may be primarily transference- or nontransference-based. All resistances are to some extent *interactional resistances* in that they obtain inputs from both the patient and the therapist. Even though the obstacle to treatment is located for the moment in the patient, the *sources* of the difficulty tend to stem from both participants.

In general, transference resistances occur only when the therapist has secured the ideal ground rules of treatment and has adopted a basically interpretive approach. These conditions create an unconsciously perceived and dangerous claustrum for the patient with the mobilization of major death anxieties. Relatively distorted perceptions of the therapist are based mainly on the patient's own pathological unconscious fantasies and memories. These in turn lead to defensive operations designed to protect the patient from the fantasied dangers (along with their valid core), and to the development of both gross behavioral and communicative resistances.

Nontransference-based resistances arise in the presence of technical errors from the therapist in terms of both deviations from the ideal framework of treatment and departures from the use of sound interpretations. The dangerous qualities of these efforts may lead to gross behavior resistances and to communicative resistances as well—the latter in the form of essentially nonderivative (flat and empty) material. Quite often, the patient becomes resistant unconsciously in order to protect the therapist from encoded perceptions that would be disturbing for him to realize, for instance avoiding material that the therapist has unconsciously indicated to the patient he wishes to be set aside.

3. The distinction between resistances and defenses has been clarified. The communicative approach has demonstrated that intrapsychic and interpersonal defenses are always operating within the patient, while resistances are sporadic and intermittent. Thus, even in the presence of an ideal communicative network that is relatively resistant free, the patient is still making use of defenses through which he or she encodes and disguises the derivative level of expression. The familiar proposition that resistances are simply manifestations of the patient's defenses in the interaction with the therapist is therefore oversimplified and inadequate.

4. Among the many sources of resistance, it has been found that both patients and therapists are fearful of instinctual drive material, ground rule issues, and allusions to madness. Interactional resistances located in the patient often stem from defenses against the inevitable psychotic core in both patient and therapist. Resistances are also often an aspect of an effort to establish a pathological mode of relatedness with the therapist (Langs 1980, 1981, 1982).

RESISTANCES AND THE PSYCHOTHERAPEUTIC SITUATION

In all, the communicative approach has greatly widened our understanding of the concept of resistance. In order to further extend these insights, resistances will now be considered in terms of the seven dimensions of the therapeutic interaction, a process which I described in a recent work (Langs 1982). They are: (1) the state of the ground rules and frame of treatment; (2) the mode of relatedness between patient and therapist; (3) the mode of cure; (4) the mode of communication and other communicative issues; (5) the prevailing dynamics and genetics, including the person to whom these dynamics and genetics most cogently apply, therapist or patient (that is, whether they involve valid unconscious perceptions of the therapist or distorted unconscious fantasies and memories); (6) the area of self and identity (the realm of narcissism); and (7) sanity and madness.

State of the Ground Rules and Frame

The relationship between the ground rules and boundaries of therapy and the resistances of the patient is complex and extremely critical. The therapist's management of the framework of treatment is the single most important variable of the treatment experience and a major determinant of all other factors in therapy (Langs 1979, 1982). This particular aspect of the therapist's functioning is the means by which the core mode of relatedness is established, the holding and containing qualities of the relationship conveyed, and the conditions created for both trust and open communication—or mistrust and disturbances in expression.

In regard to resistances in the patient (and counterresistances in the therapist), it has been discovered that the vast majority of gross behavioral resistances are expressed through efforts to have the therapist modify the ideal therapeutic frame through behaviors that unilaterally modify the basic conditions of the treatment relationship, such as the set fee, time and length of sessions, and frequency of hours; the fundamental rule of free association; the therapist's neutrality, relative anonymity, and evenly hovering attention; the therapist's use of the couch, or more rarely, the face-to-face position; and the presence of total confidentiality and privacy.

For example, a patient may request a change in an hour or may simply miss a session. All such efforts to modify the therapeutic frame constitute gross behavioral resistances and disturb the pursuits of insight therapy. By and large, such deviations provide the patient with symptom alleviation through *framework deviation cures*, a form of uninsightful symptom relief that is, in part, a resistance against an understanding of the underlying truths of the patient's neurosis. With the

exception of acting out which takes place outside of the session, virtually all gross behavioral resistances involve some modification in the
ideal therapeutic frame.

A second proposition states that breaks in the frame by the therapist will tend to lead to gross behavioral and communicative resistances within the patient, and is a common cause of such phenomena.
In principle, when such deviations are carried out, the patient will respond with meaningful material that finds its most—often, *only*—
cogent implications in terms of the implications of the therapist's
alteration in the ground rules. It therefore follows that the patient's behaviors and associations must be conceptualized as Type Two derivative expressions in light of the particular deviant intervention context
at hand, and that all other issues are secondary. Thus, a deviation of
this kind will create communicative resistances regarding all issues except the break in the frame itself. Interpretive work, through which the
therapist explains the unconscious basis of these gross behavioral and
communicative resistances, must be organized around the counter-
resistance-based frame break by the therapist, lest the patient be encouraged to avoid this area and adopt an additional level of communicative and behavioral defensiveness and resistance.

Frame breaks by the therapist are a form of counterresistance, replete with specific unconscious meanings and functions defined by the
nature of the particular deviation. As such, they encourage resistances
in patients, including frame breaks of their own and acting out. They
are a major source of interactional resistances and should be considered when obstacles to therapy are identified within a particular patient. They are an important basis of nontransference resistances
stemming from valid unconscious perceptions of the therapist. Technically, they require *rectification* (a fresh securing of the frame to the
greatest extent feasible) as well as *interpretation*. In recognizing unconscious sources of patient-resistances in therapists, it follows that an important aspect of resolving such resistances entails the cessation of the
therapist's active, however unconscious, contribution.

Recent studies have indicated that a major reason gross behavioral
and communicative resistances arise in some patients is because of
their response to the ideal or secure frame which they unconsciously
request from the therapist. While patients will consistently validate the
secure-frame treatment paradigm on the derivative level, this particular form of positive holding and containment, though it establishes a

sense of basic trust in the patient, is also a cause of considerable anxiety. Central to these anxieties is the unconscious experience by the patient of a restrictive claustrum which mobilizes his death anxieties and basic vulnerabilities. On an unconscious level, patients experience threats of annihilation, blatant seduction and violence, and outbursts of madness under secure-frame conditions. Deprived of the therapist's countertransferences and madness, they fear the experience of their own subjective disturbance in a manner that would be psychically disintegrating. As a result, major resistances arise which must be interpreted in terms of the secure-frame interventions of the therapist.

Mode of Relatedness

The communicative approach has defined five modes of relatedness in psychotherapy (Langs 1982). These are:

The healthy symbiosis. For the therapist, this mode of relatedness entails securing the frame and maintaining an interpretive approach; for the patient, accepting the conditions of treatment including the ground rules and communicating meaningfully when necessary.

In principle, it is the healthy symbiosis that minimizes the counterresistances of the therapist and promotes the expression of transference-based resistances in the patient. By precluding pathological forms of merger and other types of pathological satisfactions, this mode of relatedness provides an optimal opportunity for understanding, interpretation, and insight. In the context of this type of relatedness, a patient will become resistant from time to time, but these resistances tend to be illuminated by his or her derivative communications and to therefore be resolvable and interpretable. Thus, the healthy mode of symbiosis implies a relative absence of counterresistances in the therapist and interpretable resistances in the patient. Further, this mode of relatedness tends to minimize the expressions of gross behavioral resistances in patients, though they may appear because of anxieties regarding the secure frame (based mainly on transference fantasies regarding phobic anxieties and fears of entrapment, and paranoid-like fantasies and expressions). This is therefore the realm of true transference resistances which lend themselves to interpretive intervention.

A pathological symbiosis. This mode of relatedness is constituted when a therapist modifies the ideal framework and/or adopts a noninterpretive approach. In this way, the therapist offers the patient unconscious but *real* forms of pathological merger, inappropriate narcissistic reinforcement, and the satisfaction of pathological instinctual drive and defensive and superego needs and expressions. The pathological mode of relatedness itself becomes a curative vehicle, and the quest for insight is set to the side.

In general, a patient will adopt but one mode of adaptation in dealing with a neurosis. As a rule, he will opt for the immediate satisfactions inherent in pathological modes of relatedness rather than experience the inevitable separation anxieties involved in a healthy symbiosis and the consequent and fearful expressions of his own psychotic core. Often, some form of therapeutic misalliance (Langs 1975) develops on this basis, and unconsciously shared resistances—both gross behavioral and communicative—are quite common. The central meaning of the patient's material is available only in light of these deviant intervention contexts as they illuminate the resistances created in the patient.

Many patients seek out a pathological mode of symbiosis with their therapist, hoping to alleviate their emotional pain through the pathological satisfactions obtained in this manner. When these wishes are thwarted, the patient will often respond meaningfully to the sound interventions involved. In addition, however, based on transference fantasies and wishes, the therapist's sound interventions may evoke resistance responses. These too prove interpretable as long as the therapist does not participate in the pathological symbiotic mode of relatedness. The effort by the patient to adopt this mode of relatedness is in itself an important form of resistance. Technically, the therapist, at the behest of the patient's own derivative communications, should not participate in this development, and should respond interpretively instead. Should the therapist fail to do so, the pathological mode of relatedness becomes the patient's source of relief and insight is set to the side.

Healthy autism. This mode of relatedness involves a relationship in which the therapist is silent (appropriately) because the patient's material does not call for an intervention. This is a period of holding, permitting the patient to "lie fallow," and to engage in self-interpretations. For the patient, healthy autism implies the absence of a meaningful communicative network at a time when there is no significant adaptive context for him or her to work over. Thus, the healthy autistic relationship is one of holding and being held in the therapeutic sense; it involves a lack of meaning in the absence of a need for its delineation. Thus, there is noncommunication though an absence of significant pathological resistances.

Healthy autism calls for a full evaluation of the communicative network in light of prevailing adaptive contexts. It is important to determine the relative absence of maladaptive resistances when the derivative complex is fragmented or relatively meaningless since no interpretation is called for under these conditions. It is here that the existence of strong defenses does not imply resistance or psychopathology, but instead signifies a period of nonmeaning and solidification.

Pathological autism. For the therapist, this mode of relatedness is reflected mainly in a failure to intervene when the material from the patient not only permits but is strongly indicative of the necessity for a framework management or interpretive response. It is also reflected in all erroneous interpretations since these derive mainly from the therapist's—rather than the patient's—needs. For the patient, this mode of relatedness exists in the presence of an activated adaptive context that calls for communicative responses, to which he nonetheless reacts without generating a meaningful communicative network. Thus, there is a failure to either directly, or with thin disguise, represent the adaptive context, and/or a fragmentation or flattening of the derivative complex.

Elsewhere (Langs 1978, 1982), this particular mode of communication has been termed the Type C mode to signify the destruction of meaning. The key factor is the destruction of the meaning link—the critical relationship link between patient and therapist (see Bion 1962; the other two links are love and hate). Thus, pathological autism implies powerful communicative resistances which may or may not be accompanied by gross behavioral resistances as well. Pathological autism in the therapist often leads to various types of resistances in patients, and especially to forms of acting out.

Parasitism. This is a mode of relatedness in which either participant to treatment exploits or attempts to harm the other. For the therapist, this involves self-serving deviations and interventions which tend to prompt gross behavioral resistances in patients. These are accompanied by either an increase or decrease in communicative resistances, depending on whether the patient wishes to work over the therapist's countertransferences meaningfully or to simply withdraw behind a defensive shield.

Patients who enter psychotherapy with intentions to parasitize their therapists usually do so by engaging him in a variety of inappropriate alterations in the basic ground rules of treatment. These efforts are *per se* a form of gross behavioral resistance. In addition, such patients may enter treatment with little true wish for understanding and may desire instead to exploit or misuse the therapist in a variety of ways. These ways include the development of pathological-relationship and instinctual-drive satisfactions, as well as the misuse of the therapist in the sense that the patient dumps into him (projectively identifies) his or her own pathology; much of this is a means of justifying the patient's own neurosis. All such efforts involve gross behavioral resistances, and they may become accompanied by either communicative resistances or by meaningful and interpretable (and rectifiable) material.

The combination of a parasitic mode of relatedness and a high level of communicative resistances is characteristic of patients who enter treatment in order to projectively identify into the therapist a variety of pathological contents and functions and to otherwise abuse the therapist and exploit the treatment situation. These patients are often agitated, rather paranoid, and quite demanding of pathological satisfactions. In the absence of meaningful material, their intention to mainly do harm to the therapist is in full evidence. As a rule, the therapist has no choice but to silently contain these pathological assaults until some glimmer of a meaningful communicative complex emerges. Therapists are often hard pressed to work with these patients and are sorely tempted to respond with countertransference-based interventions that reflect powerful counterresistances of their own.

On the whole, the establishment of a pathological mode of relatedness is a form of resistance that tends to preclude the pursuit of meaning and insight as it pertains to the unconscious basis of the patient's neurosis. The relationship satisfactions, which include pathological forms of merger, narcissistic reinforcements, instinctual drive satisfactions, superego gratifications, corruption of the superego and ego ideals, and the use of pathological defenses, tend to become the means of adaptation for the patient—and sometimes for the therapist as well.

Thus, there is an antagonism between pathological modes of relatedness and the pursuit of insight. In terms of resistance, pathological modes of relatedness are forms of gross behavioral resistance which are often accompanied by strong communicative resistances. At times, there will nonetheless appear meaningful expressions which virtually without exception find organization in terms of the therapist's errant interventions and deviations as they contribute to the prevailing pathological relationship itself.

Analyzable resistances require a healthy symbiosis, and, similarly, it is only when the therapist offers the patient this mode of relatedness that he or she is not on some unconscious level supporting the resistance tendencies of the patient. It is therefore critical to recognize that obstacles to therapy may be founded upon, and reinforced by, a pathological mode of relatedness which would render the resistances unanalyzable and unmodifiable until the pathological characteristics of the relationship itself have been modified. Here too, the principle of rectifying actual contributions by the therapist to the patient's resistances before or while interpreting their meanings comes into play. In addition, a patient's resistances when mainly intrapsychically and transference-based must be interpreted in light of both pathological relationship satisfactions and fantasy-memory meanings for insightful resolution to take place. The interplay between resistances and mode of relatedness is an important subject in need of further investigation.

Mode of Cure

There is a continuum regarding mode of cure which has true insight at one end and a combination of action-discharge, evacuation, and pathological forms of merger at the other. Genuine insight is defined in terms of Type Two derivative validation and requires interpretations that involve activated adaptive contexts and the patient's derivative responses as they illuminate therapeutic contexts—immediate expressions of his or her neurosis. The action-discharge mode of cure is uninsightful and involves the search for immediate relief through pathological defenses and forms of pathological satisfaction and superego sanction.

In general, the therapist's use of the action-discharge mode of cure tends to promote comparable pursuits within the patient, and therefore leads to an increase in both gross behavioral and communicative resistances. Nonetheless, from time to time the patient will attempt to meaningfully work over the adaptive contexts or interventions that reflect the therapist's tendencies in this direction. Should the therapist properly understand this material, he is in a position both to interpret its implications and to rectify these tendencies. Failure to do so creates a therapeutic relationship and setting in which uninsightful cure, such as that gained through a framework deviation or errant comment, is characteristic.

For the patient, gross behavioral resistances virtually always involve some means of action-discharge in the immediate moment. Nonetheless, an insightful understanding of these resistances in light of an adaptive context and a responsive derivative complex can render such behaviors an important source of insight for the patient. Failure to offer such interventions unconsciously promotes the patient's use of pathological modes of relief.

As for communicative resistances, their analysis may promote insight if there is an eventual shift to meaningful expression. On the other hand, long-standing communicative resistances tend to be utilized in support of action-discharge modes of cure and under such conditions they prove difficult to resolve. Here, the therapist is well-advised to seek out his own possible contributions to this form of resistance, and to rectify and interpret this aspect of the situation as the material from the patient permits. In the absence of a significant contribution from the therapist to this type of resistance, patient holding and containing is the only available intervention and should be applied. Communicative investigations have shown clearly that patients fluctuate spontaneously in their use of gross behavioral and communicative resistances, tending from time to time to show fewer of these tendencies in a quest for meaning and insight. The therapist can rely on these natural vicissitudes, shifts from relative defensiveness to relative nondefensiveness, as long as there is no unconscious input on his part that supports the patient's resistances.

Mode of Communication

Gross behavioral resistances may or may not be accompanied by a meaningful communicative network. If they are, the resistances prove analyzable and interpretable, and therefore contribute to insightful cure. In the latter case, the resistance may be used for uninsightful projective identification or for nonderivative defensiveness, creating temporary unmodifiable obstacles to insightful cure. Here too, the therapist must rely on his capabilities for holding and containing and on the patient's own need to eventually alter this level of resistance and defensiveness.

By definition, the existence of strong communicative resistances precludes intervention—interpretive or framework management. As noted, the basic technical approach to such resistances is one of silence and holding, during which the patient hopefully will rectify his own contributions to the defensiveness at hand. On occasion, a patient will represent a communicative resistance and so modify the obstacles involved, thereby providing a fragment of a meaningful derivative network—a briefly represented adaptive context and a small measure of derivative expression. At such interludes, the unconscious meanings and sources of the communicative resistances can be interpreted to the patient. Such an effort virtually always leads to an insightful alteration.

Dynamics and Genetics

Virtually any conflict, threatening (anxiety provoking) fantasy or memory, and disturbing conscious or unconscious perception, can be the source of the patient's resistances. Thus, virtually any psychosexual and aggressive, dynamic and genetic, constellation can be the underlying basis for a period of resistance.

As is well known, it is when these constellations are attached to the relationship with the therapist that resistances are at their greatest intensity. These obstacles may, as noted, involve either primarily transference constellations (under those conditions where the frame is secure and the therapist adopts an interpretive approach), or primarily nontransference constellations (under conditions of deviation and misintervention, and therefore in the face of expressed countertransferences). Thus, in tracing out the critical sources of resistance, the dynamics and genetics of both patient and therapist must be considered.

Because of the tendency of therapists to neglect this sphere, it is also important to note that instinctual drive expressions tend to evoke powerful resistances and counterresistances in patients and therapists alike. Every deviation enacted by a therapist creates an instinctualized image of himself because of the underlying pathological satisfactions involved. This level of perceptiveness tends to generate intense anxiety in the patient and to lead to considerable gross behavioral and communicative resistances. It is therefore critical to trace out the intrapsychic and interpersonal sources of all resistances, and to eventually identify their roots in instinctual drive-based conflicts, fantasies, memories, and perceptions.

Self and Identity

Since the publication of *Psychotherapy: A Basic Text* (Langs 1982), it has proven possible to add the dimension of narcissism, self, and identity to what was formally a five-part informational and observational schema, resulting in the seven-part schema presented in this paper. In this sphere, the therapist listens to images related to identity, sense of self (cohesive as compared to fragmented), themes of idealization and acceptance or confirmation, issues of ambition and aspiration, allusions to talents and skills, refrences to the affect of shame, control issues and tension states, and themes of exhibitionism-voyeurism and sado-masochism. This rather complex category touches upon the development of an individual's sense of identity and self, and issues that pertain to narcissistic satisfactions and pathology.

In general, disturbances in the self-identity sphere are interactional products with inputs from both patient and therapist even though the experience is that of the patient. Clinically, it has been shown that ongoing narcissistic difficulties appear in patients when the therapist deviates from the ideal frame or engages in errors of technique. Thus, the therapist's empathic sense, so important to listening in this sphere, must be attuned not only to the patient's conscious and direct communications, but also to his unconscious implications. Similarly, it is important to recognize sources of narcissistic disturbance that exist not only within the patient himself, but also through introjective identification with the therapist.

As for the connection to resistances, unconscious perceptions of narcissistic disturbances within the therapist will often lead to narcissistic disequilibrium in the patient and will be accompanied by gross behavioral and communicative resistances. Also of importance is the finding that manifest idealizations of the therapist are often a form of defensiveness and resistance in that they cover over, and defend against, underlying persecutory perceptions of, and fantasies about, the therapist. On still another level, both failures in empathy in response to the patient's unconscious expressions, and deliberate surface mirroring and other forms of narcissistic gratification of the patient, reflect counterresistances in the therapist; they will tend to evoke a mixture of resistance and communicative expression within the patient in response to these pathological intervention contexts. In all, a common source of resistance in the patient and disturbance in the therapeutic process derives from the therapist's own narcissistic (self-object or pathological symbiotic) misuse of the patient to satisfy his or her own pathological needs at the expense of the therapeutic needs of the patient. The interaction between disorders of identity and self and resistances is another area in need of further study.

Resistances and Sanity and Madness

The most recent dimension of the therapeutic interaction identified through communicative studies alludes to sanity and madness. The vicissitudes of this aspect of the treatment experience are such that, within certain limits, the intensification of mad expressions in the therapist tends to lead to the diminution of mad expressions in the patient. The presence of sanity in the therapist – conveyed through validated interpretations and frame-securing interventions – creates anxiety in the patient who is thereby deprived of the therapist's madness and must place his own madness to the forefront of the bipersonal field and therapeutic interaction. Such a prospect is extremely disturbing to the patient, and prompts many gross behavioral and communicative resistances. On the other hand, in the presence of a deviant and mad therapist, the patient's own subjective madness recedes to the background. Under these latter conditions, the patient will unconsciously work over the meanings of the therapist's madness, doing so in highly selective fashion in terms of his own – the patient's – madness. Still, it is a very different therapeutic experience to be working over unconsciously the madness of the therapist as a primary issue in the treatment field, as compared to working over the patient's own madness.

In the presence of therapist-madness – reflected in erroneous (nonvalidated) verbal-affective interventions (i.e., any intervention other than an adaptive context interpretation), and in framework deviations – patients at first feel a measure of relief, for the reasons just described. However, the errant therapist is also unconsciously perceived as dangerous in a number of ways: as unreliable, as incapable of maintaining proper interpersonal boundaries, as inviting pathological modes of relatedness, and as seeking out action-discharge modes of cure. As a result, the patient will often mobilize both communicative and gross behavioral resistances because he fears being harmed by the errant therapist. From time to time, however, the patient will communicate meaningful material in response to these adaptive contexts, thereby revealing the threatening encoded unconscious perceptions of the therapist that he is experiencing. Sound interpretations—and frame rectifications—are vital at such moments.

RESISTANCES AND DEFENSES

It has previously been shown that there are distinctions between resistances and intrapsychic and interpersonal defenses. Thus, the patient may show little in the way of gross behavioral and communicative resistances, while still maintaining relatively healthy (or pathological) levels of defense. These defenses are reflected in the encoding process through which the patient expresses himself through meaningful derivatives.

It is well known that the analysis of resistances is an important vehicle of insightful cure. This takes place on two levels: first, in terms of the insights and positive introjects accrued through this analysis; and second, through the revelation, usually in derivative fashion, of the constellation that underlies the resistance itself. It is here that the principle of the analysis of resistance before content applies.

Recent communicative studies have clearly established a hierarchy of intrapsychic and interpersonal motives for resistance. These investigations have supplemented the usual conception of intrapsychic sources of resistance with a full understanding of object-relational motivational systems. These efforts have been founded on fresh investigations of the use of defenses by patients and therapists alike.

It has been found, for instance, that human beings tend to be innately defensive and powerfully motivated to utilize defenses for both intrapsychic and interpersonal causes. These observations suggest that defensive needs have a primary autonomy and driving force of their own, though hypothetically they may well draw some of this power from underlying instinctual drive expressions. Nonetheless, it seems appropriate to indicate that in a metaphorical sense we have powerful and basic, almost instinctive, tendencies toward defensiveness and self-protection. This formulation brings us back to Freud's (1905) first instinct theory, in which he distinguished the ego instincts from the sexual instincts. The ego instincts were seen as self-preserving and therefore as defensive and fundamental.

Clinical observation indicates that all patients (and therapists) have powerful defensive needs which are expressed automatically in the face of anxiety and danger. At times, these defensive structures, which may be derivative or nonderivative (based on the use of repression or on denial and lie-barrier systems), often take precedence over the gratification of instinctual drive needs. In regard to resistances, these findings and formulations suggest that the development of obstacles to treatment is an automatic response in patients, that it is both self-protective and self-preserving, and that it is strongly motivated by both intrapsychic and interpersonal needs. This line of thought lends further support to the importance of the analysis of resistances as a means of dealing with a fundamental human tendency in and of itself.

Resistances and Technique

To summarize the technical implications of the communicative approach to resistances, we may identify the distinctive techniques to be used in the presence of gross behavioral and communicative resistances. In the case of gross behavioral resistances, it is important that the therapist *rectify* any error or gross alteration of the frame which is contributing to the patient's resistances. In addition, gross behavioral resistances are critical indicators and expressions of the patient's neurosis. As such, they also call for interpretation in terms of activated intervention contexts and the available derivative complex—with a primary emphasis on unconscious perceptions of the therapist in light of his interventions, and the patient's subsequent fantasies and other reactions. As a rule, gross behavioral resistances lend themselves to this type of interpretation; the main exception occurs when a patient is endeavoring to develop a pathological mode of relatedness and cure with his or her therapist, with a strong emphasis on framework deviation relief and action-discharge.

With communicative resistances, the therapist by definition has no recourse but to remain silent and to hold the patient, while quietly rectifying any contribution that he or she has made to the patient's state of resistance. Then, as the patient modifies his own level of communicative defensiveness, the communicative resistance itself can be interpreted in light of activated intervention contexts and the available derivative complex.

Clinical Example

The communicative viewpoints offers a rather systematic approach to the identification of both gross behavioral and communicative resistances, and the investigation of their *sources*. The first step—that of recognizing the existence of resistances—is founded on the listening-formulating-intervening process or schema (Langs 1982). As noted, this entails an evaluation of the patient's material for the presence of patient indicators (including gross behavioral resistances), represented adaptive contexts, and the existence of a meaningful and coalescible derivative complex. Since gross behavioral resistances are manifest phenomena, they are usually identified quite directly. The evaluation of communicative resistances is based on the extent to which the patient's material fulfills the necessary recipe for intervening—that is, provides significant patient indicators, well-represented activated intervention contexts, and a meaningful and coalescible derivative complex. Failures in any of these spheres imply the existence of communicative resistances.

When gross behavioral or communicative resistances are identified, the key clinical question is: *What are their sources?* The answer can be provided systematically by an investigation of the seven-part informational schema that has been discussed in this paper. The sources of resistances lie in seven spheres: the state of the ground rules and frame, the mode of relatedness, the mode of cure, the mode of communication, the dynamics and genetics and the person to whom those dynamics belong and apply, the area of self and identity, and the sanity and madness of the patient and therapist. Throughout the present discussion, the manner in which pathological expressions in one or more of these spheres can become the sources of resistances in the patient have been identified. Sound functioning in these spheres may at times lead to transference-based resistances as well.

To confine ourselves to one brief illustration, we will consider Miss

A., who was in therapy with Dr. B. She was being seen once weekly in face-to-face psychotherapy. The patient had been referred to the present therapist by another therapist who had provided some form of psychotherapy and who had eventually shifted to a social relationship with the patient that included sexual intercourse.

The present therapist had set an initial fee of fifty dollars, but the patient soon introduced an insurance policy that would pay for half the fee. When the material from the patient indicated on a derivative level that the therapist's completion of this insurance form (which he carried out the first two months of treatment) was highly destructive to the therapeutic process, the therapist had intervened by pointing out the derivatives that revealed these detrimental effects. He then proposed (however, without derivatives from the patient) that she no longer utilize the insurance policy to cover any part of her psychotherapy. While the patient agreed that the insurance was infantilizing and was making her suspicious and fearful of communicating to the therapist, she stated that she could not afford the therapist's fee. The therapist then immediately proposed a reduction to a thirty-dollar fee which he felt the patient could handle on her own. While the patient objected to this fee as well, she agreed to continue treatment on that basis.

In the hour prior to the one that will be abstracted, the patient spoke about not using her insurance, and then of a new job that offered her fresh opportunities. The therapist suggested that the elimination of the insurance had offered her a fresh chance at therapy. The patient responded that she supposed so and that the insurance was no longer a problem—that she had taken care of that at the office. After a period of silence, the patient then ruminated about her new job in a rather empty fashion. The therapist then asked the patient if she could change the day of her hour from Thursday to Friday in order to accommodate certain revisions he had to make in his schedule about four weeks hence. The patient said this would be no problem, and then fell silent until the end of the session.

The patient had entered therapy because of brief episodes of hysterical blindness, strabismus, and other somatic difficulties. She began the following hour of therapy by stating that her eyes were getting worse and that she was really unable to see clearly. She then fell silent for a long period of time. She went on to say that the therapist did not seem to understand. After another long silence, she said that it made her angry to see that way. After still further silence, the therapist pointed out to Miss A. that she had stated that her eyes were getting worse, that he didn't understand her, and that seeing things this way made her angry.

After a brief silence, the patient said that she had indeed said just that. All she wants to do is to be able to see like a normal person. Is that too much to ask? After a long silence, she said that she didn't want to have to go to the eye doctor and visit all sorts of other doctors and specialists. She had been in treatment for four months and was still unable to make a decision as to how to handle her eye problem, which is why she came to her sessions in the first place. After another period of silence, as the hour drew to an end, the therapist said that the patient seemed to be talking about people who were supposed to be helpful but were not helpful at all. He suggested that this was contributing to the patient's silence since it appeared to be her view of him. They should explore this problem further in the next hour.

To apply the listening-intervening schema to this material, the main *patient indicator* in this hour is the gross behavioral resistance of the patient's long silences (a break in the frame—nonconformity to the fundamental rule of free association). There is a background context in the possibility that the patient was in some way submitting insurance forms herself. There is also the fact that her eye symptoms are continuing, and her discontent with treatment—the latter also has a sense of gross behavioral resistance. There is, as well, a hint that the patient may be thinking of quitting therapy—another possible resistance and break in the frame. In all, then, there is a significant level of patient disturbance, much of it in the form of gross behavioral resistances, that require interpretation (if possible) in light of activated intervention contexts and the patient's derivative material.

As for the main *adaptation-evoking contexts*, there is the therapist's intervention in the previous hour which did not obtain validation, as well as his request that the patient change the day of the sessions. An important background adaptive context is the therapist's reduction of the fee and elimination of the insurance form. As can be readily seen, none of these adaptive contexts are represented manifestly or in thinly disguised derivative form. There is thus a high level of communicative resistance in regard to representations (portrayals) of intervention contexts.

As for the *derivative complex*, it too is quite thin and reveals a high level of communicative resistance. The patient's comment that her eyes are getting worse and that she is seeing more poorly may well be an unconscious perception of the therapist's blindness and technical errors—his unconfirmed intervention and his own request that the frame be modified. The comment that the therapist does not seem to understand the patient is direct and manifest, and her sense of anger appears to be a direct response to the difficulties perceived in the therapist. All of this material, which emerged before the therapist's intervention, is rather straightforward and flat, with a minimum degree of derivative implication.

The material that follows the therapist's intervention may, on a derivative level, reflect the patient's wish for a more normal and adequate therapist, though it appears to contain little else in the way of derivative meaning. We may therefore conclude that the therapist's intervention did not at all modify the patient's communicative or gross behavioral resistances, and that his comment did not obtain any form of Type Two derivative, encoded and indirect, psychoanalytic validation. The material throughout the hour remains flat and empty in terms of its function as carrier of derivative meaning. In all, then, there is a high level of communicative resistance in respect to both the representations of the adaptive context and the patient's derivative responses—perceptions and reactive fantasies.

We may conclude, overall, that this is a session with a high level of both gross behavioral and communicative resistances. What, then, are the sources of these obstacles to therapy? To answer, we will apply the seven-part observational schema to this treatment situation and relationship in an effort to identify the most significant factors.

First, in regard to the state of the frame, the therapist has modified the ground rules of therapy in several ways: first, and particularly, by unilaterally suggesting that the insurance be eliminated; second, by reducing the patient's fee; and third, by asking her to change the day of her hour. The first modification is manipulative, while the second is highly seductive and self-sacrificing; the third is distinctly exploitative (parasitic) in that it serves only the therapist's needs. The patient herself may have further modified the framework of this therapy by secretly submitting insurance forms to collect part of her fee.

In all, then, there are several major breaks in the ground rules of this therapy. We may propose that these deviations on the part of the therapist (and patient) have created a sense of threat and uncertainty; the patient is protecting herself from the implications of these frame breaks by invoking resistances that will help her to distance herself from the therapist and to maintain a relationship relatively devoid of meaning. Further, the therapist's alterations in the frame become a model for the patient, leading her—based on an introject of the therapist and on her own propensities—to modify the framework of the treatment herself through her silences.

Next, in terms of mode of relatedness, the therapist has offered this patient a mixture of pathological symbiosis and parasiticism. The patient herself may also be expressing pathologically symbiotic and parasitic needs of her own because of the possibility that she has secretly contacted the insurance company. There is a further parasitic quality to this hour, since the patient appears to be making it very difficult for the therapist to respond interpretively to her material—this in face of her complaints that she is getting nowhere. Finally, the patient's feeling that she is not understood suggests an autistic mode of relatedness in that the critical relationship link between patient and therapist is certainly that of the meaning-link (Bion 1962).

In all, the therapist appears to be contributing to both levels of resistance via his offer of pathological symbiotic satisfactions, and his efforts to parasitize the patient. The patient protects herself against the therapist, and attempts to establish a pathological mode of relatedness similar to the one he has generated.

As for mode of cure, the therapist's deviations speak for action-discharge and merger; they detract from the quest for understanding and insight. Similarly, the patient's use of silence and the general absence of meaning in her material suggest that she too hopes for cure in this fashion. This type of cure always involves both gross behavioral and communicative resistances, as evidenced here.

As for mode of communication, the patient is clearly destroying meaning and is therefore by definition utilizing the Type C mode (Langs 1978). There is some quality of the B-C communicative means of expression (pathological dumping, without cognitive meaning). However, the therapist, through his deviations and previous erroneous intervention, is also making use of the B-C communicative mode; his deviations constitute disturbing pathological projective identifications into the patient as well as defensive barriers to insightful therapeutic work. All deviations by therapists involve the B-C communicative mode to some extent, and they therefore promote the use of gross behavioral and, especially, communicative resistances in patients; the resistances, in turn, are designed to maintain the relative absence of meaningful expression in the therapeutic interaction.

The dynamics and genetics reflected in this material are quite thin. There are no genetic allusions, but there are expressions of bodily concern, bodily damage, hostility, and obsessive uncertainty. The most evident quality is that of aggression. For the moment, erotic aspects are deeply repressed and split off or denied.

Functionally, these qualities appear to apply most meaningfully to the therapist for the moment, for it was he who expressed his hostility in the request to change the day of the hour. Whatever aggression lies within the patient, this level of perceptiveness must be taken into account before turning to the patient's own needs and conflicts. In addition, the underlying erotic and aggressive dynamics contribute to the patient's resistances, which serve in part as defensive barriers against submission to the therapist's aggression and to his seductive deviation.

In the main session excerpted here, there is evidence of concerns of self and identity in the patient's comments regarding the deterioration of her eyes. Her feeling that the therapist did not seem to understand her could imply some measure of empathic failure, while the patient's response to the therapist's intervention—that she wants to see like a normal person—could constitute a wish to achieve a stable sense of identity.

These indications of pathology in the area of narcissism and self seem to derive mainly from the therapist's exploitative deviations, through which he inappropriately used the patient as a self-object or in pathological symbiotic ways. A therapist's technical errors are unconsciously perceived by the patient as reflecting a disturbance in sense of self—as nonconfirmation of her personal self and narcissistic needs—and as conveying the therapist's own fragmentation of identity and loss of control. Erroneous interventions therefore reflect disturbances in narcissism and self in the therapist which are consistently introjected by the patient and alluded to through her own self-allusions. These perceived disturbances in the therapist contribute to the patient's gross behavioral resistances.

In regard to sanity and madness, once again the clinical data is thin. When a therapist engages a patient in sexual intercourse, as had the patient's previous therapist, we are probably dealing with a major form of therapist madness and a form of patient madness as well. In general, physical contact of this kind is an extreme form of therapist madness that is likely to produce temporary or even lasting madness in a patient.

With respect to the present treatment situation, securing the ground rules of treatment and eliminating the insurance tends to reflect the sanity of both patient and therapist. However, the therapist's decisions to decrease the fee, and to change the day of the patient's hour, tend unconsciously to be viewed as expressions of therapist madness and countertransference. Derivatively, this may be one factor in the patient's allusion to her eyes getting worse, and the image seems especially pertinent to her wish that she could see like a normal person. It is in this latter allusion that the patient most clearly indicates her unconscious wish that the therapist would behave in a sane fashion rather than madly. In all, it seems likely that the patient is responding to expressions of therapist madness with a form of madness herself— her use of silence, which runs counter to the fundamental rule of free association. By and large, gross behavioral resistances are indeed reflections of patient madness, though their interactional sources in interventions from the therapist must be identified and eventually interpreted.

Finally, it is well to note that in general a patient has far less opportunity and need to behave in a mad fashion during the actual therapeutic session than does the therapist. It is usually relatively easy for a patient to follow the ground rules of treatment and to thereby behave in a sane fashion. On the other hand, the therapist is required to maintain the framework of treatment, and to establish a claustrum which is unconsciously perceived as dangerous by both participants to treatment. Furthermore, he has a responsibility to put together a sound interpretation, a cognitive act that mobilizes many issues related to madness and one that is easily carried out incorrectly—that is, in mad fashion. For these reasons, it is often the therapist's madness that is the prime mover for gross behavioral and communicative resistances rather than the madness of the patient.

Based on this analysis, we can propose that the therapist's deviations, especially the reduced fee and the request to change the patient's hour, have created the atmosphere for the intensification of Miss A.'s resistances. In response, the patient engages in her own framework deviation, efforts at cure through action-discharge, a continuation of a pathological mode of relatedness, and the use of a defensive and dumping manner of communication. There are also defenses directed against the expression of underlying erotic and aggressive dynamics and genetics, and a sense of narcissistic despair. In the area of sanity and madness, the patient expresses the wish for rectification of the situation and a shift toward normality.

The patient's resistances can be traced mainly to the therapist's deviations and their ramifications. In essence, they are interactional resistances with a significant input from the therapist. The patient herself seems prone to the use of resistances of this kind, in that she could, if she so chose, work over by means of derivatives the therapist's deviations, guiding him toward rectification and interpretation. Instead, she tends—because of her own pathological needs—to join the therapist in the pathological mode of cure and relatedness that he offers her, and in the state of relative noncommunication. It is here, in the face of countertransference-based inputs from the therapist, that the patient *responds selectively* in keeping with her own needs.

Thus, while these are primarily nontransference-based resistances with highly significant vectors derived from the therapist's efforts, the patient's contribution can be identified through her own mode of defense and defensiveness. In this way, even under conditions of nontransference-based resistances, aspects of the patient's own propensities can be identified, interpreted, and modified. Nonetheless, it is well to recognize that the first responsibility of a therapist under conditions of this kind is to rectify his or her contributions to the patient's resistances as a foundation for interpretive work. Whatever other failings in the therapist's efforts reported above, the absence of such rectification proved critical in the continuation of the patient's defensiveness.

FINAL COMMENTS

This paper has focused on the contributions of the communicative approach to the investigation of the nature, function, and sources of resistances. Prior analytic investigations have focused almost entirely on gross behavioral resistances, and have used the patient's manifest material as the basis for formulations related to these obstacles to treatment. In contrast, the communicative approach distinguishes between gross behavioral and communicative resistances, and accounts for their manifestations in terms of the patient's encoded or derivative expressions. Further, it has shown an intimate relationship between resistance phenomena and seven critical areas of experiencing, observing, and formulating: the state of the ground rules and frame, the mode of relatedness, the mode of cure, the mode of communication, the prevailing dynamics and genetics, including the person to whom they are primarily applicable, the area of self and identity, and sanity and madness. It is hoped that the adaptational-interactional approach to resistances will deepen and enrich our understanding of this critical phenomenon and lead to a far more sensitive technical approach to resistance problems.

REFERENCES

Bion, W. (1962). Learning from experience. In W. Bion, *Seven Servants*. New York: Jason Aronson, 1977.

Blum, H. (1981). Some current and recurrent problems of psychoanalytic technique. *Journal of the American Psychoanalytic Association* 29: 47–68.

Freud, S. (1900). The interpretation of dreams. *Standard Edition* 4/5: 1–627.

———— (1905). Three essays on the theory of sexuality. *Standard Edition* 7: 125–243.

———— (1908). Hysterical phantasies and their relation to bisexuality. *Standard Edition* 9: 155–166.

———— (1909). Notes upon a case of obsessional neurosis. *Standard Edition* 10: 153–320.

———— (1912). The dynamics of transference. *Standard Edition* 12: 97–108.

———— (1914). Remembering, repeating, and working-through (further recommendations on the technique of psycho-analysis II). *Standard Edition* 12: 145–156.

Glover, E. (1955). *The Technique of Psycho-Analysis*. New York: International Universities Press.

Greenson, R. (1967). *The Technique and Practice of Psychoanalysis*. Vol. 1. New York: International Universities Press.

Langs, R. (1975). Therapeutic misalliances. *International Journal of Psychoanalytic Psychotherapy* 4: 77–105.

———— (1978). *The Listening Process*. New York: Jason Aronson.

———— (1979). *The Therapeutic Environment*. New York: Jason Aronson.

———— (1980). Some interactional and communicative aspects of resistance. *Contemporary Psychoanalysis* 16: 16–52.

_____ (1981). *Resistances and Interventions: The Nature of Therapeutic Work.* New York: Jason Aronson.

_____ (1982). *Psychotherapy: A Basic Text.* New York: Jason Aronson.

Stone, L. (1973). On resistance to the psychoanalytic process: some thoughts on its nature and motivations. In *Psychoanalysis and Contemporary Science,* Vol. 2, ed. B. R. Rubinstein, pp. 42–73. New York: Macmillan.

CHAPTER 8

Resistance: A Misnomer for Shame and Guilt

Helen Block Lewis

This chapter takes the position that the psychoanalytic concept of resistance ought to be abandoned because its use is harmful to the therapeutic enterprise. Like all the other theoretical concepts in Freud's metapsychology, the concept of resistance is embedded in his individualistic view of human nature. In contrast to voluminous work on transference, resistance has been relatively neglected in psychoanalytic literature. I think this neglect reflects the profession's tacit agreement that the concept of resistance is not useful because it often excuses and obscures therapeutic difficulties. Transference and countertransference, although equally a part of Freud's metapsychology, manifestly refer to a social transaction. Resistance, in contrast, focuses on the person's unbalanced internal economics, which resist the forces of health. Resistance is thus even more deeply embedded in Freud's metapsychological instinct theory than transference and countertransference, and therefore readily lends itself to the notion that intractable psychiatric problems are reflections of the intractable power of Thanatos. This chapter provides the reasons why I think the concept of resistance takes us into a theoretical and a therapeutic dead end.

SOME HISTORICAL CONSIDERATIONS

Looking at the historical background helps to explain why Freud's metapsychology evolved as it did. Freud's fundamental clinical discovery was that psychiatric symptoms somehow develop out of forbidden sexual longings. What at first caught Freud's attention was an exploration of the sexual instinct. For nearly twenty years after his great discovery about forbidden sexual longings, Freud was content to label the forbidding agency simply "disgust, shame and morality" (e.g., 1905, p. 176). It was not until *Totem and Taboo* (1913) that Freud undertook an inquiry—rather belatedly, as he himself acknowledged—into the origin and nature of guilt. By that time, Freud was already deeply committed to his individualistic concept of human nature in which primary narcissism is a fundamental premise.

At the time Freud made his fundamental discoveries not only about psychiatric symptoms but also about dreams and about sexual development, there was no better materialist-theoretical framework available to him than the Darwinian concept of individual instincts geared to species survival as the driving force in human adaptation to life. Human sexuality was therefore embedded by Freud in a Darwinian framework. Since anthropology was only nascent as a science, the universality of human culture and its primacy in human development was not clearly understood. It was not known, for example, that all human cultures, even the most "primitive," are systems of moral law, however variable the content of these laws (Edel and Edel 1968). Since Freud's time, anthropologists have found it useful to postulate that human culture is our species' unique evolutionary adaptation to life (e.g., La Barre 1954). More recently, sociobiologists (e.g., Barash 1977) have likewise suggested that "culture is a major biological adaptation of Homo sapiens" (p. 319).[1] In this framework, human sexuality is

---

[1]It is instructive to observe in passing some of the political implications of a Darwinist position about human culture. Anchoring culture in biology can readily become social Darwinism; that is, a doctrine that rationalizes the inequities, oppression, warfare that characterize many cultures, including our own. But human culture is Janus-faced: it *sometimes* comprises institutionalized oppression, warfare, and the subjection of women, but it *always* involves the institutionalized nurturance out of which morality arises. Anchoring morality in biology calls attention to the profoundly social nature of our species, as well as to the destructive capacities that are unleashed when social bonds are threatened. Calling attention to the biology of nurturance can thus be a tool for the critique of particular cultures' institutionalized oppression and war.

embedded in human culture. This is a concept toward which Freud was reaching in *Totem and Taboo* when he saw humanity's morality as an advance over Darwin's primal horde. But Freud's theorizing postulated the origin of guilt in a way that virtually ignored the role of mothers' nurturance in the process of forming guilt. This is only one illustration of the difficulties in starting with the premise that human nature is individualistic rather than social by biological origin.

At the time Freud made his clinical discoveries, little or nothing was known about infants or about mother–infant interaction. Studies by the Harlows and by Spitz, Bowlby, and Mahler were undertaken in response to Freud's inspired observation that "what we call affection will unfailingly show its effects one day on the genitals as well" (1905, p. 233). We now know also that infants are much more competent and organized creatures than Freud had any way of knowing. James's (1890) big, buzzing, blooming confusion as a description of infancy is simply not correct, but it was the prevailing notion in Freud's time and it is clearly the model of the id. Studies now show that infants 36 hours old are capable of imitating expressions of primary emotions (Field, Woodson, Greenberg, and Cohen 1982).

Studies of the mother–infant interaction strongly support the concept of the social nature of human nature. Bowlby (1969), whose work grew out of the questions Freud asked, postulates a biologically-given system of attachment that parallels the affectional system that the Harlows demonstrated for primates. Studies of the mother–infant interaction suggest that a "secure self" develops out of what Ainsworth and Wittig (1969) call "mutual delight" in each other's company. Current theorizing suggests, moreover, that the problem of human development is not, as Freud put it, how infant polymorphous perverse creatures (governed by the id) become social creatures, but how narcissists develop out of originally sociable human beings (Hogan 1975). Hoffman (1981), for example, suggests that altruism is an intrinsic part of human nature, and is mediated by empathy, a universal human response.

The issue of the nature of human nature has been central in the writings of the psychoanalytic revisionists, beginning with Adler and including Horney, W. Reich, Fromm, and Sullivan, all of whom criticized Freud for his individualistic theory. None of these critics, however, explicitly formulated the theory that human nature was social by reason of its cultural nature. A theory of psychiatric symptoms based on the cultural nature of human nature sees symptoms as the means by which people try to remain acculturated in the face of threats to their basic affectional ties. This theoretical framework rests on Freud's *description* of "primary process" transformations of emotional conflict into symptoms, but it abandons his theoretical account of "primary process" and his theory of "primary narcissism." The framework includes Freud's descriptive accounts, in which unresolved shame and guilt are always the immediate precursors of symptom formation. It places these two affective-cognitive states as givens of human cultural nature, by means of which we all maintain our affectional ties. "Resistance" to therapeutic intervention is, like the symptom itself, an expression of shame and guilt. Resistance is a social transaction, even though it may sometimes have the apparent strength of a physical force. Furthermore, resistance, although it often appears to be irrational, always represents (like the symptom it maintains) some emotional truth about threatened affectional ties as these are represented by the patient– therapist relationship.

FREUD'S INADEQUATE THEORY OF EMOTIONS

Freud's clinical descriptions of his patients' emotional conflicts focused on shame and guilt as the forces inhibiting sexual longing. But in dealing with guilt as a psychological phenomenon he was invading the domain of religion. Indeed, he was secularizing guilt. In 1923, for example, he published the case of Christoph Haizmann, a 17th-century painter, about whom the church fathers had preserved an autobiographical account of his possession by the Devil and his miraculous cure by the intervention of the Virgin Mary. Freud's purpose in publishing his interpretation of the case (which bears many resemblances to the Faust story), was to show how psychoanalytic concepts could supplant Church doctrine. In such an atmosphere, relying on the scientifically acceptable concept of instincts rooted in evolutionary biology was more comfortable than relying directly on emotional conflict as a theoretical base.

There is a long intellectual history behind this discomfort. Murphy (1978), in a historical review of depression, tells us of a defense offered by a 16th-century physician, Johannes Weyer; accused witches, he said, were suffering from an exaggerated conscience, and so not responsible. Weyer had to withdraw the defense on pain of excommunication. Characterizing guilt as a mental illness, rather than as a result of actually trafficking with the Devil, was a dangerous crack in Church control.

Thus, although Freud (1913) vividly described the conflict between (the son's) affection and hatred as the source of guilt, his reliance on the science of evolutionary biology precluded his acceptance of emotions as "realities," and as an adequate base on which to build theory. In his materialist view, the emotions were somehow insufficiently anchored in reality to be credited with their own powers. Freud thus refused to accept the primal deed as an allegory that reflected universal human emotions. Even though he later (1930) retracted his insistence on the reality of the primal deed, he accompanied his retraction by suggesting that guilt was a conflict between two instincts, Eros and Death – and once again entangled emotional conflict in a theoretical obscurity.

Freud used Darwin's concept of the emotions as legacies of our ancestors' adaptive responses as a scientific framework for his theories on the emotions. Darwin (1872) proposed three principles of adaptation to account for emotional expressions: some were originally "serviceable," became habitual and persisted in the animals' repertory; other emotional expressions were understandable as attempts to control these useless habits; still others were direct products of the action of the nervous system. Intrinsic in at least the first two of these principles of adaptation is the idea that emotions are inevitable but useless remnants of our primitive heritage, requiring control by higher order rational processes. Research since Freud's time has suggested that emotions are not only disruptive, but that some play an important part in organizing, motivating, and sustaining behavior (Leeper 1948, Schachtel 1959, Tomkins 1962, 1963, Izard 1971, 1977).

We now know also that both "positive" and "negative" emotions, such as happiness, surprise, sadness, disgust, anger, and fear are similarly apprehended (from facial expressions) by people in different cultures (Izard 1971), including nonliterate, isolated cultures (Ekman, Friesen, and Ellsworth 1972). While the precise role of the face in emotions is still a lively research topic, there seems to be general agreement that beginning with the social smile of the three-month-old infant, the face is a primary communicator of emotions. The smile is thus both an instigator and resultant of fundamental social interactions.

Several consequences follow from Freud's Darwinian theory of emotions. While affects are primary motivators, the affects on which the model focuses are the "negative" affects—those that are disorganizing to the smooth functioning of the individual's behavior. From this emphasis one can easily slip, as Freud did, into the hypothesis that *all* affects are inherently disorganizing or "primitive," and that the task of the developing human being is to change affects into "cognitive signals."

Another chain of theorizing is set in motion by a model which starts from the disorganizing negative affects. Because the threatened aggressions in the model imply real dangers, the cognitions that accompany the negative affects are understood as valid representations of real world events, including those arising within the organism, as, for instance, hunger. But if the cognitive representations are valid and, by implication, the negative affects appropriate, how do these veridical cognitions and appropriate affects arise out of disorganization? A tortuous question thus arises—one that also plagued Freud (1926). What is the primary force in the development of valid cognition? Negative affect?

To answer this question, two theoretical models developed within the Freudian movement. In both theoretical models, Freud's own (1900, 1926) and the similar model expounded by Anna Freud (1946), all cognitions originate in the negative affect associated with physical danger. By implication, the positive emotions are unknowable.

It was to correct the concept that all cognitions are born out of negative affect that Hartmann (1951) offered a second model which included a concept of the "conflict-free" ego-sphere. In a compromise position, Hartmann offered the thesis that some veridical cognitions arise in direct adaptive response to what Hartmann specified as the "average expectable environment." Had Hartmann's formulation explicitly specified an average expectable *benign social* environment, Freud's major thesis that all cognitions derive from affects might have been maintained. As it was formulated, however, Hartmann's correction continued to assume the individualistic nature of the organism, and a dichotomy between affect and cognition. It assumed also that affect influences cognition only if it is "negative" and by implication equates affect with "disturbances" of cognition.

Hartmann's correction also left intact that aspect of Freud's theoretical view of the relation between affect and cognition in which the former is specified as primitive and the latter as an advanced form of human behavior. Rapaport's (1968) effort to systematize psychoanalytic theory by distinguishing between a special clinical theory and a general theory of human behavior rested on this emphasis in Hartmann. In fact, Rapaport, following Hartmann, equated primary-process and secondary-process models of functioning with primitive and more advanced thinking, respectively. Yet when Freud was describing clinical phenomena, whether it was symptom, dream content, everyday mistakes, or jokes, it is clear that primary-process transformations are not primitive but often very sophisticated ways in which thought symbolizes feeling and vice versa.

It is instructive to speculate (with hindsight) on how Freudian theory might be formulated had the adaptive exigencies of the nurturant mother and her infant been the guiding principle of evolution. Smooth emotional bonding would then become the primary motivation of behavior. Positive and negative affects would be equally geared to affectional maintenance. Cognition would not be opposed to affect, but assumed to work coherently with it in order to maintain bonding. This coherence of cognition and affect is what Freud actually assumed in his clinical descriptions of emotional states but ignored theoretically.

An important consequence of viewing human nature as fundamentally social is that the emotions, which bind and separate people, become primary motivational forces in human behavior. This is a modern-day view of emotions which was not available to Freud. It is a view espoused only by some investigators, notably Tomkins (1962, 1963) and Izard (1971, 1972, 1977) and is still controversial. It was the view that was implicit in Freud's descriptions of the formation of symptoms, but not in his theoretical account of those events. We can now see more clearly than he could that the emotions, which originate in the social matrix, always comprise both an individual arousal and a communicative function. It is their communicative aspect that makes emotions very complex cognitive operations which offer feedback and control of affective states. As in the case of the self, which always involves experiences of significant others even at its most narcissistic, so emotional states always involve implied communication to others even when individual arousal is at its height.

Freud's clinical description of the resistance always directly involved shame and guilt as its source. But in the absence of an adequate theory of these primary moral attachment emotions, the tenacity of peoples' attachment emotions could not be postulated as the foundation of resistance. The rationale of resistance was thus obscured.

CLINICAL ILLUSTRATIONS

Let us turn now to some illustrations of the way in which the concept of resistance has obscured the operation of shame and guilt in the therapeutic situation. A first example comes from Freud's (1909) case of the Rat-Man, in which the resistance was successfully overcome and the obsessional symptoms yielded after only nine months of treatment. Freud gives a vivid clinical description of the agonies Paul experienced as he first tried to tell Freud about his obsessive thoughts that rats would bore their way into the anuses of both his fiancée and his (long-dead) father.

> Here the patient broke off, got up from the sofa, and begged me to spare him the recital of the details. I assured him that I myself had no taste whatever for cruelty and certainly no desire to torment him, but that naturally I could not grant him something that was beyond my power. He might just as well have asked me to give him the moon. The overcoming of resistances was a law of the treatment, and on no consideration could it be dispensed with. . . . I went on to say that I would do all I could, nevertheless, to guess the full meaning of any hints he gave me. Was he perhaps thinking of impalement? — "No, not that . . . the criminal was tied up. . . . " He expressed himself so indistinctly that I could not immediately guess in what position . . . — "The criminal was tied up . . . a pot was turned upside down on his buttocks. . . . some rats were put into it . . . and they . . ." — he had got up again and was showing every sign of horror and resistance. . . . "bored their way in . . . " into his anus, I helped him out.

Although it is clear that Paul was experiencing the agonies of shame, and that Freud was empathically aware of the state he was witnessing, nowhere does Freud explicitly label Paul's state as shame.

He does call the state he is witnessing "horror and resistance." Let us examine the consequences of focusing on the affective state of "horror" rather than on the technical metapsychological concept of resistance. We may speculate that it was out of empathy and sympathy with the "horror" of Paul's situation that Freud volunteered to "help him out" by guessing as many of the abominable details as he could. Freud's response reflected his intuitive knowledge that Paul would experience Freud's accurate guesses about the content of sadistic fantasies as evidence that such thoughts could be generated by Freud as well as by Paul. From this demonstration of shared guilt comes the relief of personal shame, which is what Freud meant by doing all he could to help Paul out. Present-day analytic technique vetoes such direct, generous attempts as Freud was making to help overcome the patient's shame. But the therapist's stance in the face of a patient's shame is a question of therapeutic technique that requires a focus on the nature and function of the shame state. Indeed, it is possible that Freud's spontaneous helping response, with its implied emotional closeness of therapist and patient, was more helpful to Paul than present-day classical analytic theory would allow.

It is perhaps in transference behavior that we get the clearest picture both of the extent of the shame with which he had to cope and of the complexity of the psychical operations connected with shame. Freud describes the "deep depression" (p. 281) which the patient suffered when he was obliged to tell Freud "frightful" thoughts about Freud. The theme of almost all of the fantasies which the patient found so acutely shameful to tell was that of Freud's humiliation. For example, one fantasy was that Freud's daughter was practicing fellatio. Another was of Freud being ordered by the patient to bring his daughter into the room so that he could "lick the Miessnick" (the ugly one). Still another was of the humiliation Freud's mother would feel at witnessing the hanging of her son as a criminal. The patient had a dream in which he was marrying Freud's daughter for her money, not for her beautiful eyes. Still another fantasy was of copulating with Freud's daughter by means of a stool from her anus.

> His demeanor as he repeated these insults to me was that of a man in despair. "How can a gentleman like you, sir," he used to ask, "let yourself be abused in this way by a low, good-for-nothing fellow like me? You ought to turn me out, that's all I deserve." When he talked like this, he

would get up from the sofa and roam about the room—a habit which he explained at first as being due to delicacy of feeling; he could not bring himself, he said, to utter such horrible things while he was lying there so comfortably. But soon he himself found a more cogent explanation, namely, that he was avoiding my proximity for fear of my giving him a beating. If he stayed on the sofa, he behaved like someone in desperate terror trying to save himself from castigations of terrific violence; he would bury his head in his hands, cover his face, jump up suddenly and rush away, his features distorted with pain, and so on. He recalled that his father had a passionate temper and sometimes in his violence had not known when to stop (p. 209).

Let us examine in some detail why Paul should be in such a state of acute despair as he tells of his insulting thoughts about Freud. The "delicacy of feeling" that Paul first reports involves the discrepancy between Paul's being so comfortable on the couch (while he is humiliating Freud) and Freud's (presumed) discomfort on being humiliated. In Paul's ethical system, repaying acceptance and kindness by insults is unfair and thus brings Paul into an immediate state of guilt. The acute shame, however, which has accompanied Paul's recital of his obsessive thoughts to Freud requires retaliatory fantasies in order, as folk wisdom puts it, to "get even." Being even with the other, however guilt-evoking, is a more comfortable state than being humiliated by the other. On the one hand, the idea that Freud suffers humiliation brings with it some relief; on the other hand, it brings guilt and fear of retaliation. No wonder the patient is in despair. It is, of course, the acceptance of unavoidable pleasure in the humiliating "other's" humiliation that patients find so hard to manage because it evokes such guilt.[2] The fear of retaliation (guilt), which both Freud and Paul knew would *not* happen, made Paul seem much more irrational than he actually was in his despair, a despair which reflected his insoluble dilemma between states of shame and guilt. Analyzing both the cognitive messages in shame and guilt, as well as the effort at maintaining affectional ties, thus clarifies the emotional rationale of the patient's "resistance," instead of regarding it only as part of his or her pathology.

Freud very clearly conveys the complexity of Paul's state when he

---

[2]The reader will observe that this is a reformulation of humiliation in its affective-cognitive terms rather than as a representation of the partial instinct sadism. See Lewis (1981) for a fuller treatment of this issue.

describes the "strange, composite expression on [Paul's] face [as he was telling about the rat punishment]. I could only interpret it as one of *horror at pleasure of his own of which he was unaware.*" (Italics are Freud's.) We can now understand the unavoidable pleasure in the humiliating "other's" humiliation as part of a complex set of attachment emotions. When Paul emphasized his guilt, that is, his fear of retaliation from Freud, he was taking a position that was less damaging to Freud's feelings than to his own. The transference connections to fear of his father's beatings emphasize Paul's helplessness rather than Freud's.

Another example of shame and guilt masquerading as "resistance" comes from Freud's account of the fourth and fifth hours of Paul's treatment, the two hours immediately following Paul's agonizingly shameful recital of his rat fantasies. In this example, we see the development of Paul's doubt about the correctness of Freud's theory, and the sequence from this doubt into a dread thought that Paul himself is very crazy. Paul had begun the hour immediately following his disclosures by telling Freud that he had been pursued by relentless self-reproaches for being absent at the moment of his father's death. "The only thing that had kept him going at that time had been the consolation given him by his friend who had always brushed aside his self-reproaches as idle on the ground that they were grossly exaggerated." Hearing this, Freud says, "I took the opportunity of giving him a first glance at the underlying principles of psychotherapy" (p. 175). Freud contrasted the attitude of the analyst with that of the lay person, who says that affect is exaggerated, therefore the inference that the patient is a criminal is false. The analyst knows better than this: "The affect is justified. The sense of guilt is not open to further criticism. But it belongs to some other content" (by which Freud means some childhood act). Freud concluded by admitting that this way of looking at the matter gave rise to some hard problems, "for how could he admit that his self-reproach of being a criminal toward his father was justified when he must know that as matter of fact he had never committed any crime against him?" (p. 175).

In the next (fifth) hour the patient "ventured to bring forward a few doubts" about Freud's theories. Specifically, the patient wondered why "knowing that self-reproach was justified could have a therapeutic effect" (p. 176). If the sense of guilt is not open to further criticism, how can Freud's method work any better than a friend's consolations? But if

Freud is right, then the patient must be suffering from a *"disintegration of personality"* (italics are Freud's), and it is doubtful he can be helped. The session ended by Freud's reminding him that his "youth was very much in his favor, as well as the intactness of his personality. In this connection I said a word or two upon the good opinion I formed of him and this gave him visible pleasure" (p. 178).

Let us trace the sequence that leads from the patient's acute shame into a doubt about the correctness of Freud's ideas, and thence into a frightening thought that he, the patient, is crazy (which evokes a reassurance from Freud but leaves the patient's shame unanalyzed). Let us suppose that the patient was attempting to convey, in the session following his most shameful fantasies, the "consolation" that is implied in a friend's sensible reassurance that such self-reproaches are exaggerated. It is not that the patient does not himself know that his self-reproaches are exaggerated. But his knowledge is inadequate to counter the force of his obsessive thought about being a criminal, just as it was inadequate to prevent his acute shame at his humiliating fantasies. Let us suppose further, that the patient was miffed by Freud's explicit derogation of the therapeutic effect of the consoling friend's ideas. In structure, the affect toward Freud is the same as that toward his friend: a kind, sensible listener says that Paul's self-reproaches are exaggerated, as Freud himself appeared to convey in his accepting attitude toward Paul's fantasies. But now Freud is saying that Paul's guilt was justified, although admitting that this view gave rise to some "hard problems" logically. In the patient's logical difficulties about therapy for a sense of guilt not open to further criticism, we may discern not only the patient's excellent mind, which seized upon a real theoretical difficulty, but the subtle working of his sense of shame at being helped by Freud. This feeling drives him to wish for Freud to be in theoretical difficulties. Having stated a doubt of Freud's powers, however, the patient quickly shifts the burden of difficulty back upon himself with the idea of having a disintegration of personality, thus evoking reassurance from Freud. We know, from Freud's daily account of the case, that whenever Freud praised him, he (Paul) was pleased, but also had the thought "I shit on it" (p. 315). We may suppose that in this instance, as well, Paul retaliated against condescending reassurance. The sequence from unanalyzed shame into the recollection of exaggerated guilt was not analyzed by Freud. Freud, instead, appeared to be saying that Paul's guilt was justified. This was succeeded by Paul's doubt about

Freud's therapy and was immediately followed by Paul's dread that he was even crazier than he appeared, thus returning to the position of the shameful patient. As I have shown elsewhere in the transcripts of psychotherapy sessions, this current of unanalyzed shame which the patient experiences vis-à-vis the therapist, is likely to be transmitted into derogatory thoughts about therapy, and thence back into the formation of new shameful images of the self as a patient (Lewis 1971).

We come next to an example of resistance in the form of chronic doubt, behind which it is possible to discern the effects of bypassed shame, apparently inaccessible to both parties in the therapeutic interaction. Freud tells us that the Wolf-Man (1918) was "unassailably entrenched behind an attitude of obliging apathy. His unimpeachable intelligence was cut off from the instinctual forces which governed his behavior" (p. 11). Specifically, what evoked Freud's impatience with the Wolf-Man's behavior as a patient was his attitude of doubt.

> We know how important doubt is to the physician who is analysing an obsessional neurosis. It is the patient's strongest weapon, the favorite expedient of his resistance. The same doubt allowed our patient to lie entrenched behind a respectful indifference and allow the efforts of the treatment to slip past him for years together. Nothing changed, and there was no way of convincing him (1918, p. 75).

It was under the press of this exasperation that Freud set a termination date for the analysis, without first obtaining the patient's consent.

> Under the inexorable pressure of this fixed time limit his resistance and his fixation to the illness gave way, and now in a disproportionately short time the analysis produced all the material which made it possible to clear up his inhibitions and remove his symptoms. All the information, too, which enabled me to understand his infantile neurosis is derived from this last period of the work, during which resistance temporarily disappeared and the patient gave an impression of lucidity which is usually obtainable only under hypnosis (1918, p. 11).

Many years later, Freud (1937) pronounced his insistence on termination to have been a technical mistake which contributed to the Wolf-Man's several relapses as well as paranoid symptoms. Freud's explanation of these relapses was that some aspects of the transference had not been resolved. As I have shown (Lewis 1971), one unresolved

aspect of the transference is bypassed shame; this can easily be overlooked, especially if it becomes absorbed in analytic zeal to reconstruct
the past. The Wolf-Man's "lucidity" under the press of bypassed shame
may have been such an instance.

The patient's attitude of obliging apathy or doubt is also easily understood as an (unconscious) retaliatory posture of hostility toward the
therapist's ideas. The "indifference" which Freud confronted is inherently insulting without being anything more overt than an emotionally neutral attitude. It is, however, inevitably humiliating to the
therapist's investment in his own wisdom. Freud was so irritated by it
that when he encountered it again in his brief analysis of a young homosexual woman (Freud 1920) that he called it "Russian tactics."
"Once, when I expounded to her a specially important part of the [psy-
choanalytic] theory, one touching her nearly, she replied in an inimitable tone, 'How very interesting', as though she were a *grande dame*
being taken over a museum and glancing through her lorgnon at objects to which she was completely indifferent" (1920, p. 163).

The affect of indifference is, on the face of it, a contradiction in
terms. In this respect it is on a par with "unconscious ideas" in the logical puzzle it appears to represent. Freud struggled patiently to clear up
the contradiction between an idea and unconsciousness of it. The affect of indifference was never subjected to a similar analysis. As we
think about it, it forces us to realize that an emotion can be conceptualized in at least two categories: the category of individual arousal, and
the category of communication to others. An emotion can be conceptualized as occurring simultaneously in what Hartvig Dahl (1979)
would call the Me category (arousal), and what he would call the It category (communication to others). In a failure to be impressed by the
other's wisdom, we do not necessarily feel overtly scornful or hostile
but simply not aroused. In that state (zero affect in the Me category),
we are simultaneously communicating a bundle of hostile and derogatory affects (high value in the It category)—depending, of course, on
the emotional state of the recipient. My understanding of the affect of
indifference is that it bypasses shame. It succeeds in warding off feelings
of humiliation in the self and it can succeed in evoking them in the
other.

I come finally to the way in which the concept of resistance has
made it easier to conceptualize a group of difficult patients as borderline or narcissistic personalities, a diagnosis that reflects a relatively se-

vere degree of pathology. In this formulation, the patients' narcissism is seen as the core of resistance to forming a stable transference, thus impeding a successful analysis. It is in this respect that these patients are thought to be different from the "classic" patients observed by Freud, and they are therefore said to need new parameters of treatment. As will be apparent, Kohut's (1971) Mr. A was very reminiscent of the Wolf-Man in his overtly indifferent attitude.

It is clear that Kohut's formulation of the narcissistic personality is based on an individualistic concept of human nature. In this respect, Kohut follows Freud. Kohut puts it this way: "I am inclined to believe that imputing to the very small child the capacity for even rudimentary forms of object-love (not to be confused, of course, with object-relations) rests on retrospective falsifications and adultomorphic errors of empathy" (p. 220). As Kohut conceptualizes it, "the equilibrium of primary narcissism is disturbed by unavoidable shortcomings of maternal care" and the child then replaces previous perfection by grandiose, exhibitionistic tendencies. Two separate developmental lines are postulated: one which leads from autoeroticism via narcissism to higher forms and the other to pathological transformations of narcissism. In both developmental lines, the assumption is of the primary narcissism of human nature.

From Kohut's case account we learn that Mr. A had a tendency to feel vaguely depressed, lacking in zest and energy, and this mood was triggered by the vulnerability of his self-esteem, that is, by his sensitivity to criticism, to lack of interest shown him, or to the absence of praise from the people he experienced as his elders or superiors. Thus, although he was a man of considerable intelligence who performed his tasks with skill and creative ability (let me here interject that obviously Mr. A's ego was not defective), he was forever in search of guidance and approval. At slight signs of disapproval, however, or of loss of interest in him, he would feel drained and depressed, would tend to become enraged and then cold, haughty, and isolated, and his creativity and work capacity deteriorated. Kohut tells us, further, that Mr. A was ashamed of his father's failures, that is, of his father's inability to withstand the impact of defeat. Kohut describes the patient as also being unable to enjoy his own powers.

As we read Kohut's account of Mr. A, it seems that the patient was far from being narcissistic in the conventional sense of the term. Narcissists, in the common meaning of the term, are people who are so overtly conceited, arrogant, and thick-skinned that it is virtually impossible to insult them; they are usually impervious to anything so mild as disapproval. If anything, Mr. A fits the description of a "moral masochist," with the masochist's familiar readiness to experience himself as inferior and to suffer dreadfully under the resulting humiliation. For example, the fact that Mr. A was ashamed of his father presumably also involved feelings of superiority vis-à-vis his father. It is a good guess that he was unable to enjoy his own powers, that is, unable to feel gratification in his own superior achievements, because this would mean having bested his father. His mechanism for warding off shame in the patient–therapist relationship where he confronted a "superior" therapist was to appear to be without transference feelings, that is, indifferent to the analyst. The mechanism he used would most closely fit the mechanism I have described as bypassing shame.

Narcissism is clearly a very slippery term. Most observant people are aware that narcissists are actually vulnerable to humiliation or shame, and that they are warding it off with their airs or their detachment. What psychoanalysts since Freud have known is that being in a chronic state of guilt (or shame) is a defense against forbidden pleasure in others' humiliation (sadism); that some patients unconsciously cultivate a sense of their own worthlessness because they cannot bear their own triumph over the significant others in their lives. Reik's (1941) description of the forbidden narcissism in masochism remains a classic.

In summary, converting "resistance" back into the affective cognitive states of shame and guilt has a number of advantages for therapeutic technique. The first of these is a less pejorative atmosphere for the analysis of states of pride, triumphant pleasure, and shame. Adopting the viewpoint that shame is a normal state which accompanies the breaking of affectional bonds allows shame to take its place along with guilt as a universal, normal human state of being. Analyzing shame reactions in an atmosphere in which their natural function is taken for granted makes analytic work considerably easier. Pride and shame are, of course, states in which one is aware of an incongruity between the self's subjective reaction and objective circumstances. Explain either to yourself or to someone else just what your *ego-ideals* are, and, unless you are a hopeless prig, you will see how quickly you become ashamed of your ego-ideals, that is, your "grandiosity." Because shame and pride involve strong affect, it can seem for the moment as if the ego was defective. Thus, Kohut (1971), in a footnote (p. 181), rather cavalierly dismissed the well-documented idea that shame results from a failure to meet ego-ideals. He regards shame as a result of the flooding of the ego with "unneutralized exhibitionism." But what is flooded in shame is *not* the ego, but the self. If the ego were not simultaneously registering an awareness of an incongruity there would be no shame. In recent years, I have been much impressed by the rational components in shame reactions which tell one that shame is *only* about the self, therefore about objectively "trivial" events. Most important of all, however, reconverting resistance into shame and guilt focuses on the affectional ties, for the sake of which our patients have so often formed their symptoms.

REFERENCES

Ainsworth, M., and Wittig, M. (1969). Attachment and exploratory behavior of one-year-olds in a strange situation. In *Determinants of Infant Behaviour IV*, ed. B. F. Foss. London: Methuen.

Barash, D. (1977). *Sociobiology and Behavior*. New York: Elsevier.

Bowlby, J. (1969). *Attachment and Loss*. Vol. I. New York: Basic Books.

Dahl, H. (1979). The appetite hypothesis of emotions: A new psychoanalytic model of motivation. In *Emotions in Personality and Psychopathology*, ed. C. Izard. New York: Plenum.

Darwin, C. (1872). *The Expression of Emotions in Man and Animals*. London: John Murray.

Edel, M., and Edel, A. (1968). *Anthropology and Ethics*. Rev. ed. Cleveland: Western Reserve University Press.

Ekman, P., Friesen, W., and Ellsworth, P. (1972). *Emotions in the Human Face: Guidelines for Research and Interpretation of Findings*. New York: Pergamon.

Field, T., Woodson, R., Greenberg, R., and Cohen, D. (1982). Discrimination and imitation of facial expression by neonates. *Science* 218: 179–181.

Freud, A. (1946). *The Ego and the Mechanisms of Defense*. New York: International Universities Press.

Freud, S. (1900). The interpretation of dreams. *Standard Edition* 5.

———— (1905). Three essays on the theory of sexuality. *Standard Edition* 7: 123–243.

———— (1909). Notes upon a case of obsessional neurosis. *Standard Edition* 10.

———— (1913). Totem and taboo. *Standard Edition* 13.

———— (1918). From the history of an infantile neurosis. *Standard Edition* 17.

———— (1920). The psychogenesis of a case of homosexuality in a woman. *Standard Edition* 18.

_____ (1923). A seventeenth century demonological neurosis. *Standard Edition* 19.

_____ (1926). Inhibitions, symptoms and anxiety. *Standard Edition* 20.

_____ (1930). Civilization and its discontents. *Standard Edition* 21.

_____ (1937). Analysis terminable and interminable. *Standard Edition* 23.

Hartmann, H. (1951). Ego psychology and the problem of adaptation. In *Organization and pathology of thought*, ed. D. Rapaport. New York: Columbia University Press.

Hoffman, M. (1981). Is altruism a part of human nature? *Journal of Personality and Social Psychology* 40: 121–137.

Hogan, R. (1975). Theoretical egocentrism and the problem of compliance. *American Psychologist* 27: 533–540.

Izard, C. (1971). *The Face of Emotion*. New York: Appleton, Century, Croft.

_____ (1972). *Patterns of Emotion: A New Analysis of Anxiety and Depression*. New York: Academic Press.

_____ (1977). *Human Emotion*. New York: Plenum.

James, W. (1890). *Principles of Psychology*. Vol. 1. New York: Holt.

Kohut, H. (1971). *The Analysis of the Self*. New York: International Universities Press.

La Barre, W. (1954). *The Human Animal*. Chicago: University of Chicago Press.

Leeper, R. (1968 [1948]). A motivational theory of emotions to replace 'emotion as disorganized response'. In *The Nature of Emotion*, ed. M. Arnold. Middlesex, England: Penguin Books.

Lewis, H. (1971). *Shame and Guilt in Neurosis*. New York: International Universities Press.

_____ (1981). *Freud and Modern Psychology*. Vol. 1. New York: Plenum.

Murphy, H. (1978). The advent of guilt feelings as a common depressive symptom: a historical comparison of two continents. *Psychiatry* 44, 229–242.

Rapaport, D. (1968). The psychoanalytic theory of emotions. In *The Nature of Emotion*, ed. M. Arnold. London: Penguin Books.

Reik, T. (1941). *Masochism in Modern Man*. New York: Grove Press.

Schachtel, E. (1959). *Metamorphosis*. New York: Basic Books.

Tompkins, S. (1962, 1963). *Affect, Imagery and Consciousness*. Vols. 1 and 2. New York: Springer.

CHAPTER 9

Object Relations and Transference Resistance

Althea J. Horner

The term *object relations* refers to the nature of self- and object-representations, and to the dynamic interplay between them. These mental *structures* become manifest in interpersonal relationships, particularly in the transference. The more central object-relational issues (i.e., pathology of the character structure) are to the patient's problems, the more they will be expressed transferentially and the more they will stand as a source of significant resistance.

The concept of acting out in the transference, rather than remembering, is especially relevant to the treatment of the patient where the early object-relations situation is still dominant in the inner representational world, and is played out with the therapist. The psychic dangers and the infantile wishes associated with this representational world will be experienced in treatment and will either be played out or defended against in the transference. To the extent that this acting out is not analyzed, it will constitute a major resistance to change. The timing of such interpretation, however, is critical in the face of significant structural psychopathology.

Freud (1914) reminds us that we must treat illness, "not as an event of the past, but as a present-day force" (p. 151). This is especially relevant to the treatment of the patient with structural pathology. It is the here and now of the treatment relationship and what it tells us of the patient's here and now character structure, of his still active early representational world, that is a major force in treatment. Interpretations that have a genetic focus are likely to bring an intellectual defense into action, or lead to a disillusioned, "So what?" What is being experienced now in the transference is experienced as real. The capacity to maintain the observing ego and the working alliance in the face of the activation of this prototypical interpersonal situation is not to be counted on with such patients, especially in the earlier stages of treatment. Only while working in the here and now, on the structural as well as on dynamic issues which are manifest in the transference, can we expect that some connection with the past will probably take place. However, even here, the route to the past will have to be through the present, through the analysis of the individual's here and now way of relating with significant others as well as with the therapist. He must come to understand both the structural and dynamic importance of rigidly maintaining these patterns of interaction.

Freud (1912) tells us that in analysis there is a tendency toward the activation of unconscious fantasy and that this process is a regressive one and revives the subject's infantile imagos (p. 102). It is this regression and this reactivation that will at times confuse us with respect to the character diagnosis. Are these the emergent repressed imagos of a well-differentiated individual; or are they the imagos, the self- and object-representations, that are still central to the character organization and pathology of object relations which constitute, not memory, but experienced reality?

Freud (1912) notes that when a person's need for love is not entirely satisfied by reality, he tends to approach every new person he meets with anticipatory ideas, and that these are directed toward the analyst. He comments that "this cathexis will have recourse to prototypes, will attach itself to one of the stereotype plates which are present in the subject . . . " (p. 100).

The analogy of stereotype plates lends itself well to the concept of self- and object-representations as structure, and the manner in which these representations are played out in the treatment situation. To the extent that the patient must cling to this stereotypical manner of relating for one reason or another, the transference will be a powerful source of resistance.

OBJECT RELATIONS AND PSYCHIC STRUCTURE: THEORETICAL CONSIDERATIONS

What do we mean by psychic structure? What evidence do we have for the validity of the concept? We all have direct evidence of a structured self inasmuch as we know who we are every morning when we wake up. The sense of self-sameness over time, from day to day and from year to year, tells us that there is an aspect of the mind that we call self which is enduring. Fairbairn (1931) referred to an "arrangement of mental phenomena into functioning structure groups . . . " (p. 218). A mental structure is an enduring organization of psychological elements which function as a unit, *enduring organization* being the key phrase. Although we do not know what the actual brain correlates of mental structures are, we have to assume that they are there. These are Freud's "stereotype plates." It is useful to think of these structures in terms of Piaget's (1936) schema. The schemas we refer to as the self- and object-representations have not only cognitive elements, but incorporate affect, impulse, and perception as well.

And what is the relationship between this self-structure and the ego? According to Beres (1956) the functions of the ego are (1) relation to reality; (2) regulation and control of instinctual drives; (3) object relations; (4) thought processes; (5) defense functions; (6) autonomous functions; and (7) the synthetic function. A shift from the ego psychology of Hartmann (1964) and others to an object-relations theory comes with the emphasis on the central role of object relations development in the overall structuring of the ego.

Of these functions, the synthetic function is the link between the biological organism and the psychological person, and it is manifest in the innate tendency and capability of the organism (of the infant) to assimilate, organize, and integrate its experiences from the very beginning. Although this tendency is innate, even in an organically competent infant these capabilities can be overwhelmed by excessively chaotic or disruptive environmental conditions.

So far as the remaining functions are concerned, the emerging organization and patterning of the self- and object-representations provide the matrix within which they unfold; that is, all aspects of ego functioning become organized *within* the self-representation in healthy development and cannot be separate from it. They are all experienced and understood as aspects of an integrated self. The failure of such organization is viewed as a manifestation of pathology of the self. Object-relations theory is a particular approach to understanding the organization of the ego.

Jacobson (1964) defines the self as the whole undifferentiated psychophysiological self—essentially the organism, both mental and physical. Hartmann defines the self-representation as the unconscious, preconscious, and conscious endopsychic representations of the bodily and mental self in the system ego. Jacobson further notes that the establishment of the system ego occurs with the discovery of the object world and the growing distinction between it and one's own physical and mental self.

In effect, the ego as structure is the *composite* of enduring mental structures, including the self- and object-representations. Pathology of ego structure implies a deficit in the organization, differentiation, and integration of various islands of self- and object-representations. When we speak of ego strength, we refer first to the degree to which all aspects of the psychophysiological self are assimilated into and organized within the self-representation; then, the degree to which the self is fully differentiated from the object; then, the degree to which various early self-representations have become integrated with one another (and the same for the various object-representations); and, finally, the degree to which identifications with the object are firmly secured within the self-representation and are experienced as part of the self rather than as an introject which is neither part of the self nor outside it.

IDENTIFICATIONS AND IDENTITY

We need to clarify the term identification and to distinguish the primary identifications of early object-relations development from later identifications. Identification as a process leading to a change in the structure of the self-representation must be distinguished from the kind of gross identification that serves as an ego defense against object loss or other dangers to the ego. The internalizations that allow one to *give up* the object—as with the completion of the separation-individuation process (Mahler, Pine, and Bergman 1975), and with the resolution of the Oedipus complex (Freud 1924)—are not the same as the identifications that *defend against* the anxiety and depression of loss.

One woman, whose mother died when she was a young adolescent, essentially *became* her mother—a defense that propelled her into an incestuous relationship with her father. Defensive identification does not lead to a structural change in the self-representation. Developmental identifications do.

Primary identifications are those that are the outcome of the separation-individuation process, at the end of which identifications with the primary attachment object lead to the intrapsychic autonomy of a fully differentiated self. Through this process of internalization, aspects of the early undifferentiated object-representation become part of the self-representation, even as the self is being differentiated from the object.

Beyond separation and individuation, with the achievement of identity and object constancy, later identifications *continue* to modify the self-representation throughout life. Identifications with the later mother of reality and with the father, or with other important models, contribute to continued change. Identification is an important aspect of analytic treatment, insofar as functions and attitudes of the analyst are taken into the self, and eventually enable the individual to become his or her own therapist.

As this differentiated and psychically autonomous self-representation continues to be modified throughout life, it is the basis for our identity as both a changing yet enduring self. The term identity relates to the conscious aspect of the self-representation. Jacobson speaks of that awareness of the self as a differentiated but organized entity which is separate from one's environment. This conscious awareness finds emotional expression in the experience of personal identity. A split in the self-representation will, in consciousness, be experienced as a split in identity.

STRUCTURE AND TRANSFERENCE RESISTANCE

What are the organizational desiderata of a mature self-representation? In my view they are cohesion, reality-relatedness, and object-relatedness.

The cohesive self is characterized by an adequate integration of affect, impulse, perception, and cognition; it is not subject to fragmentation or disorganization. Deficits of cohesion, in my view, characterize the borderline personality. In a more evolved character structure, under the impact of intrapsychic conflict, integrated feelings, wishes, or thoughts may become subject to repression. However, their reemergence into consciousness will result in guilt or anxiety and not in disorganization. The borderline's deficits in cohesion are the basis for the excessive dependency upon the object. The sense of connection with the object has an integrating effect; that is, the object serves as an intrapsychic prosthesis for a structurally vulnerable self. It is because of this excessive dependency that differentiation and object loss are traumatizing for the borderline patient; that is, they result in the dissolution of the self.

Because of severe separation anxiety and the potential panic that goes with loss, the borderline patient will have to protect his connection with the analyst. This situation can lead to a pervasive transference resistance that has, as its motive, the sense that survival depends upon maintaining the optimal status quo. Obviously managing, handling, and interpreting this resistance will take tact, skill, patience, and much preparatory work.

A reality-related self not only has adequate reality testing; but also a firm sense of a real self in contact with the external world, and particularly with the interpersonal environment. In the false-self organization described by Winnicott (1965) there is a deficit in the reality-relatedness of the true self. The false-self identity is consolidated around the child's *reactions to* the other who may be either abandoning or impinging. The false self may also be consolidated around parental projections. The true self identity is consolidated around that which originates from within and to which the object responds empathically. Thus, the responding other is a bridge between the inner world of experience and the outer world of reality. A self-representation that is cut off from reality-relatedness and is in autistic isolation is potentially a delusional self.

When the false self is brought into the therapeutic alliance, what appears to be a therapeutic process is, in fact, an acting out. To the extent that the therapist participates in the alliance with the false self, he is either consciously or unconsciously in collusion with the resistance. The positive transference may be at one and the same time both an aspect of the alliance and a manifestation of transference resistance. When the therapist is seduced into playing out the role of helper, rescuer, or encourager, for instance, he is probably participating in the acting out.

The false self, in such instances, may be that which has been consolidated around the maternal projection of her inadequate self, allowing the mother to realize her idealized, perfect, mother-self in her interaction with her child. Later, as a patient, this child brings the inadequate self into the treatment relationship and often quite subtly manipulates the therapist into playing out the corresponding superadequate object role.

The object-related self is characterized by internalizations and identifications that, in optimum development, lead to libidinal object constancy; to a well-secured identity with the capacity to regulate one's narcissistic equilibrium from resources within the self; to the capacity for signal anxiety (Horner 1980); and, finally, to the structuring of the superego.

Failure of object-relatedness characterizes autism in the extreme, as well as schizoid detachment in which a pathological self and its corresponding pathological object are split off and repressed early in development. With pathological detachment there can be no achievement of object constancy and its desired correlates. Since the individual who uses these character defenses is thrown back into a state of excessive emotional reliance upon an essentially impoverished self, the pathological grandiose self takes on important defensive and compensatory functions.

Detachment and denial of the significance of the therapist as a person also constitute a transference resistance. When what is being defended against is the severe object-relational pathology, the loss of a separate self, and the dangers of overwhelming negative affect, the management of the resistance is quite critical. I have written (1984) of resistance as an ally in the service of structuralization. Working directly on structural issues hopefully brings about a greater degree of ego strength, which then makes it possible to move toward the dangers which have been defended against with the detachment in the therapy relationship.

What happens to the early object representations? To the extent that they are essentially a composite constructed by the very young child out of preverbal experience and with immature cognitive abilities, they may bear only a slight resemblance to reality. We have to keep this in mind and not assume we are being presented with a true picture of the real mothering person: it is the mother as perceived and personified by the very young child. In healthy development, the early, primitive object-representations become subject to repression, but may be manifest later in dreams, fantasy, and in regression with developmental or situational stress or in the analytic situation. They will be replaced in consciousness by the specific images of the specific mother and father, and by more closely reality-dominated perceptions and memories of others.

With the more evolved character, interpersonal issues and transference issues will spring largely from relationships with the real mother (the mother of reality), with a father who is clearly differentiated from mother, and with siblings who are differentiated from others, and so on.

When the object-representation has not been fully differentiated from the self-representation, it remains as part of the ego—as an unassimilated introject (Giovacchini 1979). It will later be projected in the interpersonal situation with a considerable distortion of reality. This, of course, will become evident in the transference. To the extent that self and other come together from the start of life in characteristic kinds of interaction, the early representations are derived from these interactions and bear the imprint of their characteristic quality. Later on, we find that a particular self-representation tends to be associated with a particular object-representation along with characteristic affect, impulse, and later ideational elaboration. To the extent that the patient has an emotional investment in a particular experience of self, he will need the other—the therapist—to be the embodiment of the corresponding object so as to enable that self to be realized. This situation will be one which stands as a formidable resistance. Interpretation made precipitously will be experienced as a danger to the loved self.

These transference reactions emerge rapidly at the start of treatment when there is significant pathology of object relations. With a more mature character structure, although the early situation is still present in the unconscious and manifest in dreams and fantasies, it is not likely to emerge in the transference until later in treatment (with the regression inherent in the analytic process), if at all.

In general, object-relational issues—remembering that object relations refers to the structures we call the self- and object-representations—will be evident with patients, and manifest in the transference with individuals who have failed to negotiate the early attachment process and the subsequent separation and individuation processes satisfactorily. The inner representational world will still be characterized by failures to organize certain affects and impulses within the self, by a lack of full differentiation of self from object, and by the failure to integrate disparate self- and object-images. The immature representational world will be externalized in the transference and will generate certain resistances which can be characterized as transference resistance. There may be massive defenses against the dangers to the survival of the valued self, to the identity which is the conscious experience of a positive self-representation. The dangers are particularly those experienced in the affectively colored interpersonal situation. We must remember that resistances are defenses and not merely annoyances to be done away with. We need to ask ourselves what the dangers are in object-relational terms.

If the therapist makes a careful structural diagnosis and understands both the defensive and gratification functions of the transference resistance, he or she can make a measured decision with respect to their management, handling, and eventual interpretation.

THE THREAT TO THE SELF

The dangers facing the self in the interpersonal situation will be directly related to the specific nature of the developmental pathology. When affect or impulse have not been structured within the self-representation, their activation will pose the ever-present threat of disorganization. In a more evolved character, where ego and superego structuralization has taken place, the threat may be due to the sense of consonance and internal harmony of that structure—the structural and dynamic basis of neurotic conflict. Basch (1976) comments: "Emotions are subjectively experienced states and always related to a concept of self vis-à-vis some particular situation" (p. 768). When that situation is an interpersonal one, affect will be related to the self in interaction with the other.

We need to distinguish the traumatic state from signal anxiety. Krystal (1978) describes psychic trauma as the outcome of being confronted with overwhelming affect: that is, the ego is overwhelmed. With signal anxiety, adequate defenses can be mobilized and trauma prevented.

Khan (1963) attributes what he calls cumulative trauma to the failure of the mother to function adequately as a protective shield for the child. This may be due to lack of empathy, or it may be due to illness and pain in the child which she is powerless to alleviate. The child is then subjected to repeated traumatic states which interrupt and interfere with the budding organization of the ego and the synthesizing of a cohesive self-representation.

Krystal notes that in adult life the fear of affect may represent a dread of the return to the infantile type of trauma. There is not only a dread of the return to the traumatic state; there is an *expectation* that it will occur (p. 98). Winnicott (1974) views the fear of breakdown in a similar way. The fear of death may represent the fear of nonbeing which is experienced when this breakdown occurs.

How does this relate to transference and resistance? When fear and rage carry the threat to disorganize the self and lead to a state of psychic death, they will have to be warded off in the interpersonal situation, and particularly vis-à-vis the therapist. This may be carried out by an assiduous clinging to a positive attitude, along with detachment when that attitude cannot be maintained. As always, we must deal with the danger behind the defenses before the defenses can be relinquished. Inexperienced therapists will often push for the anger in a confrontational manner. The outcome too often is an overriding of the ego and an emergence of the traumatic state once again. The indiscriminate "going for affect" before the structural deficits are tended to is the basis for many unfavorable reactions to treatment.

When differentiation of self from object is not secure, the danger to the boundaries of the self will be experienced in the transference. Whatever the therapist says or does may have to be rejected to safeguard those boundaries.

CLINICAL EXAMPLES

A 28-year-old married professional woman, with predominant schizoid defenses and complaints of severe death anxiety, was experiencing disgust and revulsion associated with her sexual response to a seductive colleague. As her therapist attempted to explore further, she said she did not want to tell her thoughts. She was certain the therapist wanted her to think something in a particular way. "I don't want to say anything to make you think you're right." She accused the therapist of having some preconceived notion, and felt she had to carve room for herself either with silence and withholding, or by not letting herself have the feelings or thoughts she believed the therapist was demanding.

The revulsion was experienced not only in a sexual context, but in a cognitive one as well, and was a reaction to felt impingement and demand for sameness. There was generally a wish element in all these situations that the patient described, and they were experienced primarily with mother, father, brother, and her therapist, who was a woman. The wish for oneness, sexual or nonsexual, led to the same annihilation anxiety. Revulsion — a reaction formation — defended against the danger of sexual attraction and physical annihilation, while silence defended against the danger of cognitive annihilation. Referring to her "crush" on her colleague, she said, "When he reacts as though we think the same it drives me nuts!"

Although the interpersonal and intrapsychic dangers of the oedipal situation were clearly operative, the more fundamental danger to the boundaries of the tenuously differentiated self was the major determinant of her resistance in the transference. It was manifest in the transference, and in her need to maintain her sense of differentiation vis-à-vis the therapist through silence and withholding.

It is in this kind of clinical material that we can see so clearly how object-relational issues are central, and how sexual and aggressive impulses are experienced, expressed, or defended against in a manner that is determined by the structural, object-relational situation. In this instance, the patient's oedipal strivings threatened her psychic survival and this danger played a major role in her retreat from them. She could not understand her pull to her mother, but when we see the importance of the mother as the external and primary internal organizing object, this begins to make sense. With differentiation comes a further danger, that of the rapprochement crisis. At this point in development, at about eighteen months of age, the illusion of infantile omnipotence is lost and the self is experienced as weak, dependent and helpless, and generally devalued vis-à-vis the now idealized object. The shared omnipotence of the symbiotic period now clearly belongs to the other. With this awareness of psychic as well as physical separateness that is central to the rapprochement crisis comes the emotional dangers of anxiety and shame.

This patient continued to struggle with the conflict between her wishes for closeness and her drive towards individuation. The wish for closeness carried the danger of the annihilation of the separate self. The wish for individuation carried the danger of object loss. She continued to express her discomfort about discussing her feelings with her therapist. If Dr. M. did not mirror her—that is, if she defined herself as separate from the patient—the patient felt stupid and dismissed; that is, she once again felt the shame and anxiety of the rapprochement crisis with its painful confrontation of the realities of separateness. But, "it's no good if we *are* the same!" she emphasizes. Withholding and silence were her reactions to this danger. She said she no longer brought up her crushes, which were associated with the revulsion, because she felt her therapist was not interested in hearing about them. A denial of sameness—that is, that they are *both* interested—protects separateness and further embellishes the rationale for acting out the transference resistance by withholding.

At the same time, she noted the fear of nothingness, and the ever-present underlying panic continued to haunt her. Object loss carried the threat of the dissolution of the self, of a terrifying level of nonbeing. Structurally, the failure to develop a cohesive self-representation made her intrapsychically dependent upon the internalized object which was still part of the undifferentiated self. The internalized object served as a psychic prosthesis for the tenuously organized self. The crush, for her, was a manifestation of the sexualized wish for the idealized other. It was experienced in her oedipal strivings for her father, but the interpersonal dangers vis-à-vis an angry mother were there, made even more lethal because of the object-relational situation. The anxiety then led to further retreat and regression.

In her work with this woman, Dr. M. became caught up in the issues of power and control, a focus that did not go anywhere. In general, it is my view that the pathology of structure (the object-relational issues) has to be tended to before the dynamic interpretations can take hold. As long as there is a structural danger inherent in the therapy relationship, the interpretive work must be focused here.

Elsewhere (1984) I have reported on my work with another patient with similar object-relational pathology. Her detachment was understood and interpreted as a way to maintain her sense of separateness and to maintain her psychic survival. She spoke of her detachment in her relationship with her boyfriend as follows: "With Carl it's a wall that he would come up against and would have to acknowledge. It would force him to do something. It would make him aware of me."

The relevance of the wall to the transference came up when we talked about her need to screen out any reaction to me. I suggested, "Perhaps you want a wall for me to come up against." She replied, "I guess there's that and also the sense that having a more personal involvement would mean opening up and the more precious elements would run out. I'm not sure there would be anything left when I wanted to close." (Tears.)

Over time there was an ongoing focus on the structure of the self-representation — on issues of boundaries, integration of various aspects of herself, and on the defenses that protected her from the dangers to her psychic survival. During this time I accepted the defense as necessary, essentially, and at no time did I push for affect or for fantasies relating to me. I understood that such insistence would be experienced as a gross violation of her boundaries and would lead to overwhelming anxiety. During her 136th session — now experiencing the solidity of a more cohesive and integrated self — she commented: "What I don't understand is that you haven't existed very long, and all I've read about transference. Now it seems that it was very important that there was none — whether because I refused to allow it, or the essence of my problem precluded considering you as a person. I want an intellectual answer for that more than I need an answer emotionally." I explained that there had indeed been transference, at the start of our work, when she expressed the feeling that I had put up a certain picture just to draw a reaction from her, that she had experienced me as the intruding and impinging mother. I explained that the transference was manifest negatively, by its absence, by what its absence protected her from. With the structuralization that took place in this context, she was now able to let herself experience me as a person, and to deal with transference issues at this more evolved level.

Giovacchini (1972) reminds us that analysis of resistance is not the same as overcoming resistance (p. 291). The analysis of resistance must not become an exhortative struggle to make the patient give up something in the interest of analysis. This is especially so when the transference resistance lays bare the object-relations pathology. Under these conditions our interventions should be aimed *first* at correcting these deficits of psychic organization. Our interpretation of resistance should enhance structuralization: to say to the patient in effect, "I fully understand and appreciate the necessity of making me not be — that right now your sense of survival as a self is what is most important."

With this attitude on the part of the therapist, the basic trust that is built up will eventually enable the frightened patient to move closer to relationship issues.

THE FALSE SELF AND RESISTANCE

Thus far, I have described how problems of cohesion and of object-relatedness are manifest in the transference resistance. The third desideratum of the self-representation – reality-relatedness – becomes an issue when there is a false-self identity and false-self self-representation that is brought into the treatment relationship. Winnicott (1965), in his analysis of this kind of problem, became aware of a disturbance in identity that he referred to as the false self. With such patients, the working alliance may be with the false self and, as a result, the work of therapy is not experienced as real and cannot be integrated or sustained. The mobilization of the real self is crucial to the effectiveness of treatment.

Through her empathic responses to the child, the mother becomes a bridge to reality. She is the link between the child's inner world of experience and the outer world. When she fails in this capacity, and instead is experienced by the child as an impingement, the child's inner representational world, and thus his identity, becomes consolidated around *reactions to* the other. The real self remains cut off from external reality; and a split-off, emotionally isolated, sometimes autistic self may exist alongside the false self through which the individual relates to others. When the patient relates to the analyst through the false self, the transference resistance permeates all that goes on in the treatment situation.

A therapist in training was working with a 30-year-old woman who seriously abused drugs, often endangering her life. There were frequent hospitalizations. It was clear that she related to the therapist as "good patient" and that this identity constituted a major transference resistance. For her own reasons, the therapist was not able to follow through on her superviser's recommendation that the false self alliance should be a focus of work. Instead, she simply attempted to handle the resistance by reassuring the patient that she could say whatever was on her mind or in her feelings. This reassurance led the patient to feel that she was not being a good enough patient. In one session she had reported that she was unable to go to her daughter's father for money anymore because he had developed a sexual problem, and she could not be of any use to him anymore. The therapist was advised to explore the implications for treatment. Did she miss appointments when she thought she had failed to meet the therapist's needs, whatever she imagined them to be?

One day the patient reported the following dream.

> It was about my stepfather, mother, and sisters. I'm living with them. They want me to stay in. I went out against their wishes. My stepfather brought me home and beat me. My mother beat me. Everyone said how much she loved me and wanted to help me and I didn't respond. Then my mother said she would stop beating me and let me be, let me do what I wanted. But my stepfather said I can't because I blew his image of himself. I hurt his ego.

Then she commented that her stepfather never beat her. She was angry in the dream. She couldn't understand how they could say they loved her. Her sisters were angry at her for hurting her mother. She was angry at the mother for not meeting her needs and was punished because she did not meet her mother's needs.

In supervision there was a discussion of how the patient attempted to meet her therapist's narcissistic needs, how when she was a "bad patient" she blew the therapist's image of herself. At the same time, her own needs were suppressed, leading to frustration and anger. This activated the image of the bad-self representation which was tied to the image of the bad object. She defended against the bad-self image with projection, and then reported that she was afraid to go outside.

The following week the therapist was ill and canceled, and the patient called back saying she was suicidal and had gotten high on drugs. The therapist interpreted that she tried to cover up her negative feelings with pills or thoughts of suicide and that she needed to explore these feelings. The patient then said contritely, "I really try in therapy. I really do the best I can." She said she felt like a failure.

In treatment the patient played out the immature object-relational situation. She desperately clung, like an insecure rapprochement child who is afraid that if she does not meet the needs of the important other she will be abandoned. The way to maintain the attachment with the good object is to meet the narcissistic needs of the object. But then there is an annihilation of the real self. Furthermore, the sacrifice does not pay off and she is enraged. Then she feels that she is bad, and when this is projected she becomes fearful. There is a *wish* to have the total love and devotion of the important other. There is a *belief* that the way to get this is to meet the needs of the other. The *reality* is that no matter how hard she tries, the other is still separate and has a life apart from her. The *consequences* are that she is angry and bad and feels she has failed and that she is inadequate. The use of drugs is both a rebellion and, in a roundabout way, a self-affirming (albeit self-destructive) act. At the same time, the drugs wipe out the threatening rage. The problems that the therapist now has to manage in the treatment of the patient concern the aftermath of the failure of the fantasy, which she tries to play out in the treatment situation.

As long as the core transference and character resistance are not interpreted, everything the therapist says is taken in by the false good self, and is experienced as something else she has to try to do right if she is not to be abandoned.

THE NEED FOR PERFECTION

A positive transference is essential to the therapeutic alliance. However, this becomes a contaminated alliance when the positive transference is also a source of resistance. This will be the case when the fantasy of a special relationship with the therapist is maintained, often secretly. In the following clinical example, the transference resistance—the wish to be the "preferred child"—was latent through most of treatment, whereas the need to maintain the image of the perfect self was most conscious.

The patient was a 30-year-old professional woman whose presenting problem related to marital dissatisfaction, and who was clearly developing an acute anorexia nervosa at the time. She was troubled by a pervasive detachment and "deadness" that had also developed. She was concerned that all she really wanted to do was sit around and eat bonbons—what came to be understood as a metaphor for her passive dependent yearnings. She was the oldest of five children; her sister was born when she was 18 months old—the height of the rapprochement crisis. She recalled that as a small child she experienced severe anxiety relating to fantasies of anything or any person—be it a green pea or one of her dolls—being lost and alone.

Her major character defense rested on her identification with her idealized intellectual father, with a corresponding devaluation of her "bumbling" mother. The father was not only the object of oedipal strivings, but, more important, was the recipient of the displaced feelings and wishes for the pre-oedipal idealized omnipotent early object. A moral perfectionism, Calvinistic and stoic, was the fabric of this identification, and its heir was an idealized perfect self. This was not the ego ideal of a mature superego, but an ego *identity*, the self-representation of the prematurely individuated and intellectually precocious child as it came to be further elaborated in her identification with father.

A major resistance throughout treatment was the protection of this image of the self inasmuch as any deviation from it threatened the sense of self. At the height of the anorexia, the number of the scale which indicated her weight also became a statement of her identity in a sense.

Therapy focused primarily on the identity issue, although oedipal and sibling rivalry dynamics were also dealt with. The transference resistance (the need to have me see her as she wanted to see herself) came more into focus and discussion in the termination phase of treatment. Just prior to my summer vacation, and after a termination date four months hence had been set, she brought in a long and complex dream. One aspect related to the sibling rivalry issues vis-à-vis the therapist and her other patients. Another related to abandonment rage. A dream about an invisible thing that ate people and made pasta from their blood was readily understood as related to cannibalistic castration fantasies with respect to her envied baby brother, oral sex, and her loathing of anything "icky." Other imagery related to the female genitalia and fantasies of castration. What is notable is how this difficult, repressed material could emerge and be reported at the same time as the transference resistance was being dissolved after long and diligent interpretation.

After she reported the dream and her associations to it, I wondered about her competitiveness with my other patients. She thought she was competing for who could be the most interesting—not pathetic or needing help, but "struggling nobly and not whiny." Here we see the rejection of the passive-dependent yearnings and the idealized self-representation which was the product of the defensive, schizoid, grandiose self as elaborated by her identification with her father.

I inquired about the boarded-up school in her dream and its relation to my vacation. "This is like a school. You go to learn and to be judged on your performance. Then you graduate." She noted that in her dream, when she came back to the boarded-up school, she had to make it habitable. I commented on her fear that it wouldn't be the same and she acknowledged that now I wouldn't be worried about her because she would be a "short-termer."

> T: Now you'll be displaced by the other patients—by all the brothers and sisters.
> P: By *Donna*! (The next youngest sibling.)
> T: So now there's the danger of the horrible thing.
> P: Me in my coat (referring to the dream).
> T: An *aspect* of you.
> P: The angry dangerous one that would hurt my sister.

At this point the cannibalistic associations and fantasies, going back to witches in fairy tales, emerged, as well as their relation to sexual and eating inhibitions.

In this session she commented that she was, in fact, the only one in the competitive race, and that what was important was that she persevered and finished. Then she noted, "I'm not detached today and I can talk about this and not feel it's so farfetched. And I'm not bothered because I'm not so unusual and I'm not so terribly evil."

I noted that as she experienced therapy less as a competition for my love, she could bring out these things without fear that they might alienate me. She agreed that they could alienate but thought I was used to stuff like this. Then she dealt further with the persisting wish to be at least near the top of the list when it came to my feelings for my patients. It was especially important now that I knew all these secret and real things about her.

So as the defenses of perfection yielded to the therapeutic efforts, the underlying transference resistance emerged into consciousness in the form of a wish. As it was interpreted and was in the process of being dissolved, repressed unconscious material related to the symptomatology was able to come into consciousness and be reported.

The specific object-relational issue here was the defense against remembering and reexperiencing the rage and object loss that was evoked by the birth of the sister when the patient was 18 months old. The defensive character structure which came into play was that of the pathological grandiose self. The need for both physical and moral perfection were aspects of this defense. The perfect body that needed nothing from the outside—the wish and fantasy associated with the anorexia—was a further elaboration of this defense. The anorexia had abated by the time we moved into the termination phase of treatment. As we began to talk about ending, she reported buying two cookbooks. The compulsive purchase of cookbooks is part of the anorexia syndrome. The regressive and defensive nature of this behavior and its relevance to ending was interpreted and she was able to accept the interpretation.

TIMING OF INTERPRETATION OF RESISTANCE

It is my feeling that when the patient is unable to experience the transference without losing the observing ego or without destroying the therapeutic alliance, the defenses manifest in the transference resistance should be left alone until later on when working around these specific defenses has achieved adequate structuralization. A 35-year-old married woman with a young daughter described how she could not let herself be aware of anything about me. If I fell short of at least 97 percent perfection she would no longer be able to work with me. We worked for a long time on the transference reactions of daily life: on projection, boundary structuring, the defensive grandiosity, and on her struggle against her identification with the hated mother. The transference resistance was manifest in regular lateness. She had to come at *her* time and not mine, as a way to act out the definition of separateness. After long and hard work on these issues, and with structuralization increasingly apparent, she started to come on time.

> P: I had the vision of you not minding when I canceled, of your not feeling personally rebuffed. For the first time I recognized the degree to which this arrangement is mine officially. I habitually see that if I don't come to your party, you'll be upset. I fail in my obligation to you and I see you as *really* hurt. It's like, "Mommy, I don't want to play with you." It occurred to me here especially and in the world at large, that I operate as though there's a bunch of feelings at the end of the telephone. More often it's not so. Even if it were so it shouldn't determine what happens.

(Laughs.) I can't injure you by not coming. It is true? Have I gone too far? You won't be injured, hurt, crippled. You will survive and lead your full life. I'm laughing but almost crying (Cries.) The enormity of the idea! It's not that people don't have feelings, but they're not crippling. I have to turn the situation into one in which I and the other do not feel anything – neutered.

    T: Not dangerous.

    P: I know! I dove 100 feet and wonder if I really did it! It's the counterpoint of not being special. As I gradually learn I have no greater rights by virtue of being born a goddess princess, I also have no greater power to destroy.

As structure building proceeded, she could look at the frightening fantasies behind the transference resistance and subject them to reality testing.

In the face of object-relational pathology, the management, handling, and interpretation of the transference resistance will be the key to treatment. Its timing, tone, and precision are exquisitely important. With a basic understanding of and concern for the structural issues, one can make these clinical decisions in a more appropriate and correct manner, and therefore with a higher level of expected outcome.

REFERENCES

Basch, M. (1976). The concept of affect: a re-examination. *Journal of the American Psychoanalytic Association* 24: 759–778.

Beres, D. (1956). Ego deviation and the concept of schizophrenia. *Psychoanalytic Study of the Child* 11: 164–235.

Fairbairn, W.R.D. (1954). *An Object Relations Theory of the Personality.* New York: Basic Books.

Freud, S. (1912). The dynamics of transference. *Standard Edition* 12: 99–108.

———— (1914). Remembering, repeating and working-through (Further recommendations on the technique of psychoanalysis II). *Standard Edition* 12: 145–156.

———— (1924). The dissolution of the oedipus complex. *Standard Edition* 19: 72–79.

Giovacchini, P., ed. (1972). *Tactics and Techniques in Psychoanalytic Therapy.* New York: Jason Aronson.

———— (1979). *Treatment of Primitive Mental States.* New York: Jason Aronson.

Hartmann, H. (1964). *Essays on Ego Psychology*. New York: International Universities Press.

Horner, A. (1984). *Object Relations and the Developing Ego in Therapy.*2nd ed. New York: Jason Aronson.

———— (1980). The roots of anxiety, character structure, and psychoanalytic treatment. *Journal of the American Academy of Psychoanalysis* 8: 565–573.

Jacobson, E. (1964). *The Self and the Object World*. New York: International Universities Press.

Khan, M.M.R. (1963). The concept of cumulative trauma. *Psychoanalytic Study of the Child* 18: 286–306.

Krystal, H. (1978). Trauma and affect. *Psychoanalytic Study of the Child* 33: 81–116.

Mahler, M., Pine, F., and Bergman, A. (1975). *The Psychological Birth of the Human Infant*. New York: Basic Books.

Piaget, J. (1936). *The Origins of Intelligence in Children*. New York: International Universities Press, 1952.

Winnicott, D.W. (1965). *The Maturational Processes and the Facilitating Environment*. New York: International Universities Press.

———— (1974). Fear of breakdown. *International Review of Psycho-Analysis* 1: 103–107.

CHAPTER 10

Transference and Resistance as Psychic Experience

Benjamin Wolstein

> Any line of investigation, no matter what its direction, which recognizes these two facts (transference and resistance) and takes them as the starting point of its work may call itself psychoanalysis, though it arrives at results other than my own.
>
> *Sigmund Freud, 1914*

The study of resistance has not, until recently, fared at all well in psychoanalytic research and discussion. Along with some other equally difficult issues, it does not stand up to a careful exposition of its historical development as a major defining term of clinical psychoanalytic inquiry. As though to cover up some secret and unacceptable historical origins, up to now its examination has usually earned the dubious status of deferment to some indefinite date in the future. But now, perhaps because current psychoanalytic research is already moving beyond the adaptive and consensual point of view, and as new meta-

---

Extended discussions of some conceptual and clinical issues related to the theme of this chapter can be found in the following:

Wolstein, B. The psychic realism of psychoanalytic inquiry. I and II. *Contemporary Psychoanalysis* 17:399–412, 595–606.

Wolstein, B. The psychoanalytic theory of unconscious psychic experience. *Contemporary Psychoanalysis* 18:412–437.

psychology is also manifesting a far greater concern with the psychology of the self, that future may finally be here.

Compare, for example, the limited study of resistance with the many and extensive studies of transference carried out since the matured statement of the classical id model of psychoanalysis of 1915–1917. Or, as further example, compare it with the many and extensive studies of anxiety carried out since the full envisioning of the modern ego-interpersonal and object-relational models of the 1930s. For reasons that I shall outline in hypothetical form, resistance has to date escaped the empirical and systematic treatment that one might expect so basic a definition of clinical psychoanalytic inquiry deserves.

The notion of resistance is first defined in the classical id model as a function of the positive and the negative transference of the instinctual-libidinal derivatives under direct clinical observation. Later, in the modern id-ego model, it is further defined, for those in the biological wing, as a function of the anxiety accompanying, in their terminology, the defense mechanisms of the adaptive ego. For those in the sociological wing, resistance is similarly and also defined as a function of the anxiety accompanying—in their terminology—the security operations of the consensual self-system. However, even though the study of resistance is, from the very beginnings of psychoanalysis, a major theme of the actual clinical inquiry, the history and development of that study have yet to be examined with focal energy. That, in itself, is a matter of considerable interpretive interest.

Only in the late 1920s, with the rise of character analysis, did resistance become a serious topic of direct clinical psychoanalytic inquiry. That new development is clearly anticipated by Rank and Ferenczi's innovative but long-neglected collaborative monograph, *The Development of Psychoanalysis* (1922). Later in the 1920s, in the groundbreaking Reich seminar at the Vienna Psychoanalytic Institute, the institute's members began to discern ways to carry out the clinical psychoanalytic study of resistance in depth for the first time. Using the terminology of character analysis, Reich published his and the institute's findings under the title *Character Analysis* in 1933. But throughout the radical and changing decade of the 1930s (not only for the individual in psychoanalysis but for society at large), the clinical study of resistance matured into a genuinely new approach to psychoanalytic procedure, reconstructive and without precedent. Witness, as already noted, the new psychoanalytic therapy of the id-ego's defense mechanisms, represented by such as A. Freud, Hartmann, Kris, and Loewenstein in the biological wing of ego-interpersonal psychoanalysis; or, in its sociological wing, the new intensive psychotherapy of the interpersonal security operations, represented by such as Fromm-Reichmann, Horney, Sullivan, and Thompson.[1]

Even so, prior to those new id-ego and interpersonal developments in both interpretive metapsychology and in direct clinical procedure, the manifestations of resistance were not simply ignored. But while they were duly observed, they were not deemed worthy of psychoanalytic inquiry in depth, nor worth the care and detail given to psychoanalysis of the manifestations of transference.

In other words, resistance was to be "overcome" and "conquered" instead. In Freud's id model, the therapeutic aim was different: to make the interpretation of transference straightaway, especially of its oedipal manifestations. (Which, in fact, reflects the unilateral decisions of the classical psychoanalyst who encounters resistance in the application of his interpretive work.) Freud still had not, in 1915–1917, sighted a structural view of the id-ego and its defense mechanisms, nor had he yet considered the id-ego and its defense mechanisms part of the actual field of inquiry with the patient. The procedures of the first model of therapy were already completed in the 1915–1917 *Introductory Lectures*, especially in the 27th and the 28th; so the first model remained, as clinical inquiry, strictly a therapy of the id.

During that early period, however, the id-ego and its defense mechanisms are not yet sighted and formulated within the domain of interpretive metapsychology; consequently, as perspective, not yet capable of guiding and governing the conduct of direct clinical inquiry into that sector of personality. But since the 1930s ego-interpersonal (or biosocial) models of psychoanalytic inquiry, that early practice to "overcome" and "conquer" resistance (originally the standard procedure of the id, or biological, model), sharpen the issue I am raising to open this discussion. Namely, that the historical and clinical study of the psychoanalysis of resistance has for so long remained hidden and

---

[1]These brief historical comments are being sketched here as background for discussing the relation of both transference and resistance to the psychoanalytic theory of unconscious psychic experience. Readers interested in a somewhat more detailed historical commentary on the work of Freud, Reich, A. Freud, and others in the biological wing of ego-interpersonal therapy are referred to the introduction of this book.

even lost. The reason for this is not hard to see. Among the salient themes pursued to clarify the terms and sustain the conditions of psychoanalytic inquiry, the patient's resistance obviously stood in the way of the classical psychoanalyst's efforts at interpretation; and so, until the 1930s, the obvious thing to do about resistance was to get it out of the way. But is it also reasonable, then, to infer that Freud's metaphors of interpretation manifested his own unnoticed and undefined counterresistance? Either way the answer was not critical at that time, for resistance was not yet a matter of direct psychological inquiry in its own right.

SOME COMMENTS ON TERMINOLOGY

This paper clears the ground for a working definition of resistance in its own right, against the background of its relation to that of transference, and shows how both may be stated in terms of the theory of unconscious and preconscious psychic experience. I comment first on the use of established terminology in psychoanalytic inquiry; go on to suggest a basis for the psychic realism of transference and resistance; then discuss the creative approaches made to the study of resistance during the 1930s in such diverse, yet compatible, perspectives as character analysis, ego psychology, interpersonal relations, and object relations, with a special commentary on object-relations theory; and conclude with a delineation of transference from resistance on the basis of the threefold psychoanalytic theory of conscious, preconscious, and unconscious psychic experience.

Considering the terminology needed for the discussion of this topic, I am singularly aware of the awkwardness with which it envelops my theme. However, I fully accept it along with its limitations and strengths. Even to those who well know its history, from the late 19th century hypnocathartic and autohypnotic therapies to the present, it is somewhat cumbersome and needs *very* careful articulation. Nonetheless, I do not expect to carry the argument in favor of this terminology to the uninitiated, but shall, instead, suggest why I still value its communicational power.

The use of psychoanalytic terminology here serves a number of purposes. First, it marks out a line of continuity in both the historical and the systematic development of psychoanalytic theory and practice.

Also, the continuity points to how our predecessors once could – as we now can, and our successors still may – rework that terminology in line with the ongoing changes in psychoanalytic inquiry. Moreover, that terminology records both similarities and differences between the clinical procedures in use when a psychoanalytic term is first introduced, and the clinical procedures it is modified to represent in later usage.

Finally, because of a continuity in terminology, similarities and differences in clinical procedure do not simply become the artifacts of language and metaphor; nor do they simply reflect the private and arbitrary belief systems of their originators. Rather, they depict real features of the evolution of psychoanalytic inquiry: that is to say, the historical development of clinical psychoanalytic inquiry comprising matters both of empirical observation and definition, and of systematic transformation and explanation.

Over the long run, terminology has proved capable of guiding the discussion of the developing similarities and differences in clinical procedure. Most important of all, it has proved itself capable of articulating how, for example, the major models of therapy evolve from one another:

(1) from the pre-classical hypnotic therapies, the biological model of transference and resistance;

(2) from the classical id therapies, the sociological model of transference, resistance, and anxiety;

(3) from the modern ego-interpersonal or object-relational therapies, and psychological model of transference and resistance, anxiety and self; and

(4) from the post-modern experiential therapies.

In the various stages of this evolution, from the pre-classical to the classical, to the modern, to the post-modern, our terminology has so far been both firm and flexible. It has been firm enough to represent the basic terms and conditions that endure, yet flexible enough to support the later enlargements and modifications that were unanticipated and unprecedented.

One last point about the terminology of transference and resistance. From a strict psychological point of view, there is no difference in definition between transference and countertransference, between resistance and counterresistance, or between transference-resistance and countertransference-counterresistance. Empirically, they refer to the same sorts of process and pattern; and systematically as well they are subject to the same sorts of transformation and explanation. Consider, therefore, that the point of "counter" in countertransference and counterresistance is only to name the particular coparticipant in the inquiry, the one who possesses the particular process and pattern being observed and defined. So it is by common agreement that we say the psychoanalyst countertransfers and counterresists, and the patient transfers and resists.

From a strictly psychoanalytic point of view, the working relationship of psychoanalyst and patient, however, is not social but psychic, not hierarchical but symmetrical, not manipulative but exploratory. Now, if we take seriously as an irreducible dimension of their relationship that the psychoanalyst and the patient both possess such processes and patterns of human psyche quite naturally and ineluctably, we may also seriously propose that the two are capable of full engagement with one another to the extent of their endowed capacities. They are both, without external reservation, equally capable of transferring and resisting, becoming anxious, and having and expressing a center of self, and so on through the overall structure of psychoanalytic inquiry. It is, then, in the interest of our own terminological clarity that we use the prefix "counter" to set off statements about the psychoanalyst from those about the patient.

But this usage is, finally, arbitrary and conventional. One can easily imagine a psychoanalytic frame of reference in which the reverse were true: the psychoanalyst's participation being described as transference, resistance, and so on, and the patient's described as countertransference, counterresistance, and so on. Because our usage has by now become a well-established convention of the psychoanalytic community, arbitrary though its acceptance of this convention may—in psychic fact—be, there is, in my opinion, no plausible reason to abandon it. Far from being arbitrary or conventional, the empirical and clinical reference of this terminology is in fact objective and substantive. It is, therefore, evidence for psychic realism. So while it continues to serve us well, with the field and focus of psychoanalytic inquiry changing, its specific terms of reference may be reconstructed and redefined.

DISTINCTION BETWEEN PSYCHOLOGY AND METAPSYCHOLOGY

In a most general philosophic metapsychology, the notions of transference and resistance (including countertransference and counterresistance) may be viewed as universal traits of the human psyche. From the standpoint of psychoanalytic inquiry, they may also be viewed as generic, pervasive, and ultimately irreducible in all fields of therapeutic experience, individual and shared. Here I focus on aspects of transference that relate it to resistance, and on aspects of both transference and resistance that relate them to unconscious and preconscious psychic experience.

In addition, I view these notions of transference and resistance in terms larger than is usual in psychoanalytic metapsychologies, and then, in psychoanalytic psychology, in terms narrower than usual. Metapsychology fundamentally differs from psychology along the ineradicable line drawn, as in all structures of science, between the interpretive and speculative on one side, and the empirical and systematic on the other. That is how it is in psychoanalysis, too. The metapsychology and the psychology of transference and resistance do not, however, mark out two separate and disparate fields of inquiry, nor do they demand two radically incompatible kinds of theory. Rather, I prefer to treat them in their quite distinct ways as the coordinated orders of a single structure of psychoanalytic inquiry. They are copresent; for in experienced fact, at some indefinite points of the organized inquiry, the two tend to coalesce and become integrated in the psychic uniqueness of the individual coparticipant, psychoanalyst and/or patient. For those doing the psychological inquiry, psychoanalysis has room for a pluralism of beliefs, values, and ideals.

There is, it should be noted, a two-theory view developed by Rapaport (1960), G. Klein (1969), and others (Gill and Holzman, 1976). They propose to split the structure of psychoanalysis into two virtually distinct disciplines: first, a clinical psychoanalytic theory of therapy and, second, a general psychoanalytic theory for psychology in general. They are, in addition, explicitly committed to one particular perspective on metapsychology – that of the instincts or drives, or the libido – without, however, opening their structure to the interpretive and speculative strivings of the other perspectives in use at present.

But that, in my view, is not the major difficulty with their proposed construction. The two-theory approach stems from a fundamental fact—that all psychoanalytic inquiry takes place on a variety of levels, or in a sequence of orders, so that it coordinates its unitary orders of empirical and systematic psychology on the one hand, with its pluralistic order of interpretive and speculative metapsychologies on the other. The two-theory approach to this fundamental fact may be somewhat misleading. For it proposes to develop an empirical and systematic clinical psychology side by side with a single-factor, interpretive, and speculative metapsychology without a structural or experiential linkage between the two. Yet neither logically nor empirically need a clinical psychoanalytic theory be constructed so far apart from a general theory: unitary psychology and pluralistic metapsychology belong together, coexisting and cooperating in one and the same body of knowledge.

I stress the importance of this distinction between psychology and metapsychology here for two further reasons. First, the interpretive and speculative metapsychology of transference and resistance, once freed from any exclusive tie to the libido metaphor, opens up far more varied metaphors of beliefs, values, and ideals. Second, the psychology of transference narrows down to far more sharply defined processes and patterns in which clinical psychoanalytic inquiry is governed by the theory of unconscious psychic experience distinct from the psychology of resistance whose clinical psychoanalytic inquiry is governed by the preconscious dimension of that theory. Let us consider these two points in greater detail.

The first and more open interpretation of transference occurs at the order of psychoanalytic metapsychology. Generally transference is a direct emergence of the human psyche that moves forward the psychic endowment of unconscious, uniquely individual experience into conscious, social, and ego-interpersonal behavior. For a perspective of pluralism of metapsychology, it follows that any such emergence of uniqueness is, in strictly psychological terms, nothing more nor less than the inbuilt striving to make the unconscious conscious, to make the irrational rational, to make the dissociated associated. But most important, however else one may describe it, implicitly it is the inbuilt striving of the human psyche to individuate its uniqueness in social and ego-interpersonal relations. For that after all is what the unconscious becoming conscious really means—in effect, making the individual social. There is, of course, much more to say about the psychoanalytic view of the socialization of the individual, especially as to whether the process of making the unconscious conscious "shrinks" or "expands" the stream of consciousness, or does both; but that theme extends beyond the scope of this paper.

When put in the context of the striving for individuation, transference, arising from within the individual's unconscious psychic experience, seeks the external and social conditions for that individual's unique and creative resources, which, because they are "uncon-scious" in a most literal sense, were never before known to their possessor, nor to any social and ego-interpersonal other. The psychic experience of making them "con-scious" is, again in a most literal sense, making them known to both self and other together. Transference, therefore, represents the striving to become known – and public – to both self and other through the unconditioned "sponses" expressing original, and private, psychic experiences, as distinct from adapting to the derivative "responses" of social and ego-interpersonal conditioning.

It is worth noting that the distinction of *sponse* from *response* further refines the terminology of psychoanalytic thought. We may use it to call the original and unconditioned process "sponsive," as distinct from calling the adaptive and consensual pattern "responsive." It also prepares the ground for differentiating transference from resistance more sharply. And, in addition, it runs parallel with a number of other important distinctions: active process and reactive pattern; generative sources and distributive context; inner experience and outer behavior; (self)-individuation and (other)-relatedness; and, of course, the deep unconscious from the surface preconscious aspects of psychic experience.

As to the second, and narrower definition at the order of psychoanalytic psychology, transference – in the actual workings of psychoanalytic inquiry – defines at the very least some sort of activity in relatedness and communication toward the emergence of love and attachment at the growing edge of psychic experience. To speak of transference-love is therefore a tautology, for transference in the present view is, strictly speaking, nothing else but the dynamic of love in its most general sense of human psyche opening out into the world. It is the unconditioned, self-generated, and self-moving desire of psychic origin to know the world (potentially always from the innermost depths of human psychic being) through active curiosity about the self and other, about the natural and nonhuman, about the superhuman and transcendent, or about practically anything at all, in wonder or openness, with a capacity to find, coordinate, and make intelligible, so as to have the experience both for its own sake and for transmitting it from one field to another.

As distinct from resistance, then, transference always arises in the psychic experience of curiosity. Seeking the novel, and bearing the precarious, it therefore "sponds" during psychoanalytic inquiry in search for self-knowledge by psychological means. Resistance, on the other hand, arises in such "responsive" patterns as the armoring of character, the mechanism of defense, the operation for interpersonal security, the internalized object relation in defense. The line of distinction between transference and resistance reflects the critical difference in psychic experience between, so to speak, moving outward from within and moving inward from without.

The transference of resistance is, from this point of view, the dynamic of transference turning back on itself. A clinical development of unexpected complexity, it places transference at the service of resistance, and resistance at the service of transference, and that is why it is most difficult to psychoanalyze. Transference-resistance, moving in a circle, brings the therapeutic inquiry to a standstill: when transference looks forward, resistance moves backward; and when resistance looks backward, transference moves forward. It indicates a conflict between seeing the other through self (which manifests transference), as against seeing the self through other (which manifests resistance), or between the anxiety of self-individuation as against the anxiety of other-relatedness. Unlike the triggering of transference by a significant psychic event from within, resistance is triggered by a significant ego-interpersonal event from without.

TRANSFERENCE RESISTANCE AND COUNTERTRANSFERENCE

The distinction between the dynamic of transference and the transference of resistance is obviously not without precedent in psychoanalytic thought. But it has not been spelled out adequately in accordance with the psychology of the self now emerging, as distinct from either the biology of instinctual-libidinal drives, or from the sociology of ego-interpersonal or object relations. For, without a psychology of the self, the vital dialectic of transference and resistance breaks down; from this breakdown, I suggest, arises the widespread occurrence of schizoid, borderline, and characterological disorders, and, particularly, the present-day ubiquity of pathological narcissism. Clearly transference and resistance need one another—to sustain the one's substantive dynamic in vital dialectic with the other's operational mechanism. Yet the two also need a center of psychic self to guide them through unfolding, conflicting, and coalescing. Otherwise, without the first-personal experience of their dialectic, the mechanism has no dynamic from within to move it, and resistance cut loose from transference tends to persist on its own through the patterning of character armor, ego defense, or interpersonal security, and becomes increasingly sucked into the vacuum of its psychic vacancy and boredom, resourceless greed and envy, inner deadness, and so on.

Unlike the ego-psychological structuralists and the interpersonal relationists (who both, in their special ways, sidestep the problems and the possibilities of the immediate experience of self and individuality), we are attempting to work with this dialectic of experience, and to draw into our programmatic picture of consciousness the important line between the deeply personal unconscious and the surface ego-interpersonal preconscious in psychic experience. It then becomes possible to view transference itself as manifesting the unconscious become conscious, and resistance as manifesting the preconscious become conscious.

Freud very early observed that transference itself is capable of becoming resistance. But from our current vantage point, I think it reasonable to observe that the transference he saw turning into resistance was a response to his own psychoanalytic procedure of mirroring interpretation. In fact, the transference-resistance that he described may even be considered now as a conditional response under the specific conditions of his psychoanalytic approach; that is to say, a patient's response to the classical psychoanalyst's private wish (from behind the mirror) to receive the patient's dynamics of transference, without, however, permitting either coparticipant the open acknowledgment of any evidence for the dynamics of his countertransference. He does this in accordance with the id model—in point of historical fact during the decade before ego psychology. At that time Freud did not allow any study of countertransference to take place within the field of psychoanalytic inquiry in which the countertransference first occurred. The reason? Exclusively committed to the id (without ego) model as he then was, Freud would have had to consider manifesting libidinal instincts directly with a patient; proper Victorian doctor and dedicated psychoanalyst that he was, he would not indulge in an acting out of his sexual impulses.

Even so, any such interlocking of openly expressed transference and covertly withheld countertransference marks the point in classical psychoanalytic inquiry at which transference-resistance arises. For it is at that point that the patient, blocked in fear and frustration, brings the working therapeutic relationship to a standstill. In that interlocking of transference and countertransference, the dynamic of transference turns away from its generative sources and backs into the mechanism of resistance instead. And that, in clinical fact, hits the classical psychoanalyst where he is the most vulnerable—both in theory and in practice. Namely, in the failure (because of his metapsychological limitations at this point) to study the counterresistance to exploring countertransference directly with the patient; not to mention, in this complex of countertransference-counterresistance, the counter-anxiety about exploring it as well; nor the first-personal point of origin from which to make this sort of decision during the actual psychoanalytic inquiry.

In this connection, note the recent work by Chertok and de Saussure, *The Therapeutic Revolution* (1979). In contrast to the above view, the authors seek to root this aspect of Freud's clinical procedure in the idiosyncracies of his personal psychology; they even consider the use of the notion of transference itself as his intellectualized defense against a particular female patient's direct sexual moves toward him. They do not see it as a limitation of his id metapsychology, but rather place it in a larger historical perspective of psychotherapy that runs from Mesmer through Bernheim and Charcot to Freud. In other words, from animal magnetism through hypnosis to psychoanalysis to ego psychology. That history, they suggest, may be interpreted by "the 'prophylactic lineage' which has hitherto haunted the unconscious of every practitioner" (Chertok and de Saussure 1979, p. 128), including Freud. Psychotherapists from Mesmer onward, say the authors, had to defend themselves against manifesting any direct sexual response to the patient's positive transference (typically a woman's), never a man's, nor, of course, to a child's of either sex.

This is a very interesting historical/biographical interpretation, and it reopens what has until now been a closed—and, in the primary sources of sanctioned biography, even a foreclosed—chapter in the early development of Freud's contribution. For that alone, of course, we are indebted to these authors.

But, at the same time, theirs is a questionable piece of psychogenetic analysis, reducing as it does the empirical psychoanalytic definition of transference to the defensive pressures of Freud's personal psychology. It should suffice to note that in the id (without ego) model through Freud's 1915–1917 *Introductory Lectures*, there is still lacking a structural view of the ego coherent and coordinated with both the id on one side and with the superego on the other. So why go along with Chertok and de Saussure's views that the genesis of the notion of transference came from Freud's own personal defensive system when, with at least equal historical probity, it is possible to consider it as a genuinely innovative effort of creative magnitude? Then, too, it is possible to trace back to a general limitation of the 1915–1917 perspective Freud's insistence on keeping any evidence for countertransference out of the actual psychoanalytic inquiry. He, of course, took care of his limitation in perspective during the 1920s with the new tripartite metapsychology of id, ego, and superego, as did so many others in their respective variations in perspective and terminology during the 1930s, such as Rank, Ferenczi, and Reich; A. Freud, M. Klein, and Horney; Hartmann, Sullivan, and Thompson. New clinical procedures to encompass the study of countertransference in the actual field of its occurrence, however, were not attempted until the 1950s.

THE 1930S MOVEMENT OF PSYCHOANALYTIC THOUGHT

In the 1930s psychoanalysis evolved into character analysis, ego psychology, interpersonal relations, object relations, and so on. But they were more or less all different names for the same development of perspective. Historically, psychoanalytic metapsychology did not, of course, suddenly erupt into its 1930s study of the patient's social, cultural, and ego-interpersonal environment. We may sketch out that line of development as follows: From around 1900 until the early 1920s, the classical model of id therapy emphasized the genetic study of the depth dynamics of transference, and treated resistance as a negative obstructing factor merely to be overcome (the psychoanalyst's participation was depicted as being that of a mirror). Through the 1930s to the late 1940s, the modern model of ego-interpersonal or object-relational therapy emphasized the functional study of the operating mechanisms of resistance and anxiety that appear in transference, with the psychoanalyst's contribution being depicted as being that of a participant observer and/or interpreter. I discuss some aspects of object relations theory later, to illustrate both the strengths and the limitations of this environmental chapter in the history of psychoanalytic metapsychology.

The early 1950s to the present marks the post-modern period of individual and shared experience. In various perspectives and procedures, this model emphasizes both the genetic and functional study of transference and resistance, anxiety and self, and the psychoanalyst's contribution is now one of direct involvement in a coparticipant inquiry. For the first time, during this inquiry there arises the empirical and systematic study of countertransference, counterresistance, and counteranxiety from the new standpoint of the uniquely individual self—both the psychoanalyst's and the patient's, howsoever they meet in the therapeutic experience with one another. In this last model, the principle of pluralism in perspectives on metapsychology becomes a necessary commitment. Since the interpretation of countertransference and counterresistance, and so on, is a matter of deeply ingrained individual differences in beliefs, values, and ideals, I do not expect that all psychoanalysts can now, or in the foreseeable future, reach full agreement on precisely how the study of the subject be carried out in any particular case.

Let us now consider some strengths and limitations of the theory of object relations. It became part of the larger movement of psychoanalytic thought during the 1930s which assumed the social, cultural, and ego-interpersonal environment of the human psyche as a major therapeutic concern, and marked a radical and innovative departure from the dominant concern with biology until the early 1920s. The 1930s movement of psychoanalytic thought is made up of many diverse perspectives and terminologies, and at the time, of course, held out great future promise. Clinical psychoanalytic inquiry, for the first time, directly connected with the beliefs, values, and ideals of the environment. As new therapeutic emphasis, it became other-related to outside conditioning.

Even so, looking at the theory of object relations from the clarity of our current vantage point, we see something that is not strictly speaking a theory but a perspective, an approach, or framework of psychoanalytic metapsychology. We see an "object" that is not capable of actively objecting. We see "relations" that are not capable of spontaneously relating. Here the relations to the object are not active, direct, and externalizing, but passive, controlled, and internalized; not enlivened by the uniquely individual self but instead enacted from the standpoint of the object-relational other. In sum, "I" do not define myself at all; my object relations define "me" instead.

Within the perspective of object relations, it is, nevertheless, hard to see how the object can possibly relate in fact. Consider the object relation: somehow already in existence, it may, in some way, become internalized. Yet a subjective dimension by which to actively internalize the object is missing from the scope of its working perspective. The object on its own is somehow unaccountably capable of making the relation, and does so without evidence of a subject relating, or even capable of appearing, in a perspective of the object solus. By so constricting the scope of its defined field of inquiry, the theory of object relations effectively cuts itself off from the missing subject relations. The object of object-relations theory, then, resembles the objective of continental existentialism—an existence in search of its essence; or, in deontologized terms, an ego-interpersonal relation (the object) in search of its self (the subject).

No less than ego psychology or interpersonal relations, therefore, does object relations lack the genuine dynamics of psychic uniqueness, as an active, spontaneous, self-generating experience of psychic origin that moves itself outward from within. There is, however, one unexpected result of the convergence of these perspectives on the social, cultural, and ego-interpersonal environment of the human psyche. They tend, clinically, to block out the unconscious psychic reality of the dynamics of transference, and overemphasize instead the preconscious ego-interpersonal reality of the mechanisms of defense, or the operations for security.

Those 1930s perspectives are, of course, all deeply affected by the great economic depression of the period. When psychoanalysis began to reject, modify, or simply drop the biology of instinctual determinism in favor of the conditioning sociology of beliefs, values, and ideals, the classical analysis of transference was no longer enough. Analysts had to look elsewhere for the major therapeutic tool with which to go beyond it. Each focused, in his or her own way, on the distribution of the ego's mechanisms of defense, or the interpersona's operations for security, or the object internalized from relations with others. In that way, they also focused the attention of their clinical psychoanalytic inquiry onto the environment of resistance, and, by that token, onto the preconscious—as distinct from the unconscious—sector of psychic experience.

In so doing, however, they also blocked out the origin in immediate experience of first-personal psychic processes generated at first hand, in the singular and active. The human psyche generates inbuilt processes that are capable of moving spontaneously on their own, from one field to another, from one context to another, from one situation to another, from one relation to another. Such first-personal processes are, I am suggesting, essential features of the unconscious psychic reality of transference. The human psyche, by dint of its own self-supporting resources, by means of its own self-defining dialectic, runs its course between its bipolar limits: externalizing the dynamics of "sponse" from within, internalizing the mechanisms (or operations) of "response" from without.

CONSCIOUS, PRECONSCIOUS AND UNCONSCIOUS PSYCHIC EXPERIENCE

Recall, once again, Freud's early distinction between the dynamics of transference and the mechanism of resistance in the perspective of id metapsychology. Terminology aside, the empirical basis of that distinction still holds, I believe, though we may now prefer to place its interpretation in some larger, even completely different, perspective. While transference and resistance may both become conscious, they each, in their own distinct ways, arise from different qualitative sectors of psychic origin and function beyond awareness. They compare as follows: transference of unconscious psychic experience, resistance of preconscious psychic experience; transference of unconscious processes of individual psychic origin, resistance of preconscious patterning of social, cultural, and ego-interpersonal or object-relational functions; the one, potentially, innermost private experience, the other, outermost public behavior; anxiety of self-individuation in one, of other-relatedness in the other.

But we are dealing with far more than a topological view of consciousness. In the comparison between transference and resistance, we learn something important about their respective origins and functions. While both are, by defined observation, found to persist outside the conscious field of awareness, the preconscious functions of resistance, once having become conscious, are capable of becoming conscious again, but the unconscious origins of transference were never conscious. In "A Note on the Unconscious in Psychoanalysis," Freud wrote:

> We are accustomed to think that every latent idea was so weak and that it grew conscious as soon as it became strong. We have now gained the conviction that there are some latent ideas which do not penetrate into consciousness, however strong they may have become. Therefore, we may call the latent ideas of the first type *preconscious*, while we reserve the term *unconscious* (proper) for the latter type which we came to study in the neuroses. The term *unconscious* . . . designates not only latent ideas in general, but especially ideas with a certain dynamic character, ideas keeping apart from consciousness in spite of their intensity and activity (Freud, 1912, p. 25).

Put in other terms, the difference between the two may be used to point up the basis of two principles of unconscious psychic experience. On the one hand, transference, arising from the innermost reaches of unconscious psychic experience, emerges into awareness by transcending the previous limits of conscious experience; this we may call, first, becoming transconscious. On the other hand, resistance is directly related to the previous conditions of conscious experience, and it instead reemerges into awareness by derepressing those previous conditions; and this we call, second, becoming reconscious. Hence, the transconscious and the reconscious—the two sides of psychic experience beyond awareness. Making the transconscious conscious is truly a creation of something new; making the reconscious conscious is always a discovery of something already in existence.

Given these two principles of unconscious psychic experience, the difference between transference and resistance is the difference between a creation and a discovery. The one gives the internal process of the subject and generates the self from its unconscious point of origin, the other gives the external pattern of the object and distributes the ego-interpersona or object relation along the preconscious lines of its function. The one originates the psychic process moving outwardly and integratively, and directly receives everything; the other derives the ego-interpersonal or object-relational pattern moving inwardly and defensively, and directly accepts nothing. We say one is separateness; the other, relatedness.

In closing this discussion of transference and resistance, I propose the following definition of transference in its most general empirical sense: it is the movement of unconscious psychic origin from one situation to another. It is, always, an instance of psychic movement that is self-generated—or, as a neologism, automotivated—process in the first person, singular and active. What it carries, however—and that may be anything from the gracious dynamic of love to the defensive mechanism of fear—depends on what the analysis of the particular transference shows it to be carrying. So it is that a genuine experience of transference expresses a petition, a literal seeking, a process initiating its own function, a self in search of the other—therefore, the immediate experience of first-personal self-knowledge, with the makings of psychic individuality. The genuine experience of resistance is, rather, a repetition, a literal reseeking, a pattern researching its own functions, an other in search of the self—therefore, a reflective experience of characterological, egoic, interpersonal, object-relational defense and security, with the makings of ego-interpersonal sociality. The former moves forward in openness, arising from the psychic dynamics of love; the latter moves away in defense, arising from the ego-interprsonal mechanisms of fear.

In that famous seventh chapter of *The Interpretation of Dreams*, Freud (1900) emphasizes that "the unconscious is the true psychical reality" (p. 613). No matter whether we accept his instinctual-libidinal metaphor as the foundation of a universal metapsychology with which to interpret this "true psychical reality," the enduring truth of his emphasis still stands. For the foreseeable future, moreover, this view promises to remain, namely, that the origin of transference itself, whether it carries love, resistance, anxiety, or anything else, takes hold in that unconscious reality of psychic experience. The psychic realism of unconscious experience remains to this day the central organizing concern of all psychoanalytic inquiry—Freudian, post-Freudian, post-

post Freudian—and the effort to make it conscious still best characterizes the special exploratory and scientific focus governing the structure
of that inquiry.

So that is what psychoanalysis does best—study both unconscious
and preconscious psychic experience in relation to conscious psychic
experience. It wholeheartedly accepts the psychic realism of unconscious experience, from which deeply private and unalienable sources
originate transference and countertransference, both of which may, in
turn, carry resistance and counterresistance, both of which may, in
turn, carry anxiety and counteranxiety, and so on. It works its creative
therapeutic magic by twilight, seeking a center point of psychic origin
at which both transference and resistance may come together, inter-
fuse, conflict, and, of course, integrate. It runs its clinical course
through inner space and time, extending the light of awareness among
the shadows cast by the originals of current subject (or first-personal)
relations in transference, and by the facsimiles of past ego-interpersonal or object relations in resistance, and, of course, countertransference and counterresistance as well.

REFERENCES

Chertok, L., and de Saussure, R. (1979). *The Therapeutic Revolution.* New
York: Brunner/Mazel.

Freud, S. (1900). *The Interpretation of Dreams.* New York: Basic Books, 1956.

———— (1912). A note on the unconscious in psychoanalysis. *Collected Papers.*
Vol. 4. London: Hogarth Press, 1950.

———— (1914). On the history of the psychoanalytic movement. *Collected Papers.* Vol. 1. London: Hogarth Press, 1950.

———— (1915–1917). *A General Introduction to Psychoanalysis.* Garden City:
Doubleday, 1943.

Gill, M., and Holzman, P. (Eds.). (1976). *Psychology versus Metapsychology.*
New York: International Universities Press.

Klein, G. (1969). Freud's two theories of sexuality. In *Psychology versus Metapsychology,* eds. M. Gill and P. Holzman. New York: International Universities Press, 1976.

Rank, O., and Ferenczi, S. (1922). *The Development of Psychoanalysis.* New
York: Nervous & Mental Disease Monographs, 1925.

Rapaport, D. (1960). *The Structure of Psychoanalytic Theory.* New York: International Universities Press.

Reich, W. (1933). *Character Analysis.* New York: Orgone, 1945.

CHAPTER 11

Resistance to Countertransference

Robert Mendelsohn

This paper examines the concept of resistance to countertransference, and explores their mutual interaction in the psychoanalytic setting. As Goldman and Milman, the editors of this volume, suggest, resistance seems to have been a long neglected concept in psychoanalysis. Since mid-century, however, there has been an increasing interest in countertransference (Goldman and Milman this volume, Epstein and Feiner 1979, Kernberg 1976, Langs 1976, 1979, Searles 1979a, b, Spotnitz, 1969, 1979).

COUNTERTRANSFERENCE AND RESISTANCE AS SYNONYMOUS

Historically, only brief mention has been made of countertransference resistance (Fleiss 1953, Greenson 1967, Racker 1968). In fact, this may be because many analysts view the two as synonymous; that is, they view countertransference as an inherent resistance to the experiencing of the patient's clinical material, and believe that the analyst's resistance must usually have its source in his or her countertransference.

Menninger (1958) seems to hold to these views. He cites some of the common ways in which countertransference appears, that is, "*becomes an interference,*" [italics mine] such as an inability to understand certain of the patient's material "*which touch on the analyst's own problems*" [italics mine]: for instance, carelessness regarding arrangements for the pa-

tient's appointments, persistent drowsiness, increase of interest or decrease of interest in a certain case, arguing with the patient, and so on.
Menninger discusses these and other countertransferences, which he
believes by definition are impediments (resistances) to the treatment.
He also touches on the belief that countertransference and resistance
are synonymous when he suggests that countertransference by definition is unconscious, but that it "is dangerous only when it is forgotten
about" (1958, p. 90). Menninger suggests a training analysis,
and continual self-scrutiny, as answers to the "problem" of countertransference resistance. Thus, Menninger sees countertransference as
primarily negative, as an impediment to psychoanalytic treatment. As
Goldman and Milman (this volume) suggest, resistance is also usually
seen as inherently negative, as an impediment. From the classical point
of view then, it appears that analysts often find themselves in a "Catch
22" kind of situation. That is, an analyst should never be resistant to
his countertransference, but his countertransference is something
which he shouldn't have in the first place! Eissler (1953), who seems to
typify this view, suggests that psychoanalysis is analogous to many
other scientific-medical procedures. Eissler uses the example of the
medical technique of surgery when he suggests that analysts ought to
operate under 'antiseptic' conditions. The analyst should not "infect"
his patient with the analyst's own unconscious conflicts. Thus, from
this point of view, all clinical material should come from the patient,
and the focus should remain exclusively on diagnosing and treating
the patient's "disease" (see Mendelsohn 1982, for a further elaboration
of this issue).

One manifestation of the patient's disease is his transferences; another is his resistances. The analyst must "cure" himself of his own
countertransferences and resistances. Further, the analyst must never
be resistant to the awareness of how he may be "infecting" his patient.
Yet, for an analyst to be aware of his "infecting," he must also be willing
and able to tolerate a self-image which goes counter to his ego-ideal, an
ego-ideal of a good and helpful person. This ego-ideal, a product of every analyst's own childhood, is later reinforced during the analyst's
training, and during his training analysis, particularly if his transferences to his own "perfect parent" analyst have not been completely resolved. Margaret Little (1951) suggests that there are two childhood
motives for becoming an analyst: curiosity and reparation. It would
appear from the above, that an analyst must be continuously curious

regarding his "badness," (that is, his countertransferences and resistances) and his attempts at reparation for his "badness," so that he may continue to "forgive" himself for these countertransferences and resistances. In any case, the result here is that many analysts see countertransference and resistance as both negative and synonymous.

Issacharoff (1979) clearly sees countertransference and resistance as the same. He suggests that the analyst's countertransference is one of his "barriers to knowing": "Like the patient, with his basic and profound resistance to becoming an observer of his own transference distortions, we analysts require a constant reawakening of interest in and observing our own countertransference and in studying its implications . . . " (Epstein and Feiner 1979, p. 30). Greenson (1967), Fine (1971), and Racker (1968), like Menninger (previously cited), suggest that the analyst's countertransference may often be inferred by his resistance to the uncovering of certain of the patient's material.

Only Spotnitz (1969, 1979) specifically isolates and discusses, albeit briefly, the concept of "countertransference resistance." Spotnitz (1979) suggests that the terms "countertransference" and "countertransference resistance" can be considered reciprocals of the terms "transference" and "transference resistance." Spotnitz differentiates between what he calls a subjective countertransference and objective countertransference. Subjective countertransference is defined by Spotnitz (1979, p. 331) as those responses "attributable to insufficiently analyzed adjustment patterns in the therapist," while objective countertransference is defined as "those responses that are realistically induced by the patient's transference feelings and attitudes."

Spotnitz encourages the "analyzing out" of subjective countertransference, and agrees that subjective countertransference can itself lead to resistance (called, perhaps, subjective countertransference resistances). However, Spotnitz (1979, p. 332) suggests that objective countertransference should be fully experienced by the analyst in order to help "maximize the empathic understanding of his patient." While Spotnitz's classification of objective and subjective countertransference seems on the surface to be a clear-cut one, such distinctions are probably considerably cloudier. Thus, while many "normal" analysts, of a particular personality type and temperament, might react to a patient's personality characteristics similarly, not all "normal" analysts would. What type of analyst, with what type of countertransference reactions, would be having an objective countertransference in this instance? And, further, "objective countertransference" might consist at times of the therapist's feelings toward the patient's realistic reactions to the therapist's actual characteristics. Thus, it would appear that an alternative to Spotnitz's objective-subjective countertransference dichotomy, would be to view all countertransference reactions as having both objective and subjective aspects, and to suggest that it is the interaction of both the analyst's and the patient's objective and subjective transferences which fuel the therapy's wellspring of creativity. In any event, Spotnitz is the one analyst, up to the present, who has attempted to clearly and directly define countertransference resistance.

A CHANGING VIEW OF COUNTERTRANSFERENCE AND HOW IT RELATES TO COUNTERTRANSFERENCE RESISTANCE

Epstein and Feiner (1979) suggest that historically there have been two theoretical strands with regard to the psychoanalytic concept of countertransference; countertransference as a hindrance, and the analyst's use of his own unconscious transference derivatives to understand the patient. Further, Epstein and Feiner feel that these two strands have intertwined "like a double helix throughout the historical development of psychoanalytic conceptions of countertransference" (1979, p. 1). Milman and Goldman (this volume) suggest that countertransference is no longer a neglected nor denigrated concept in psychoanalytic treatment. In fact, as I have said previously, since the 1950s there has been increasing interest in countertransference, and attempts have been made to integrate this "two-strand conceptualization." Thus, as Epstein and Feiner suggest, many analysts now respect the antitherapeutic aspects of countertransference while they also believe that by studying it we may gain a deeper understanding of the therapeutic process. Further, increasing study of countertransference has expanded our understanding of transference as well. These conceptions have been applied not only to psychoanalysis, but to analytic work with particular clinical populations (schizophrenic and borderline patients, see Searles 1979a, 1979b, Spotnitz 1969, and Mendelsohn 1981); to other kinds of analytically oriented therapy, such as short-term therapy (Mendelsohn 1978) and group therapy

(Mendelsohn 1981); and even to the use of countertransference data in the initial interview (MacKinnon and Michels 1971; Billow and Mendelsohn 1982). However, with increasing interest in countertransference, there appears to be a need to more fully examine the concept of countertransference resistance. Further, if countertransference is no longer to be considered inherently negative, then perhaps countertransference resistance can now be considered as a major source of valuable clinical data. Such data's value may lie in its leading one to his countertransferences, and thus to a deeper understanding of his patient. Thus, countertransference resistance is the analyst's resistance toward material which stimulates countertransference reactions: that is, countertransference resistance is the analyst's resistance to the experiencing of his own transference.

From the classical point of view, Menninger (1958, p. 81) defines transference as "the unrealistic roles or identities unconsciously ascribed to a therapist by a patient in the regression of the psychoanalytic treatment, and the patient's reactions to this representation derived from earlier experience." For Menninger, transference resistance is the resistance that the patient has to the experiencing of transference; the resistance to his own ascribing of unrealistic roles or identities, and the resistance to his own reactions to these representations. But the analyst's reactions are more than that. It is perhaps clearer that the analyst is subject to a more complete reaction to the patient, which contains both subjective and objective aspects. This more complete reaction is the analyst's countertransference, and his resistance to experiencing the totality of the patient, including the totality of the interaction between himself and the patient, can now be defined. This resistance is the countertransference resistance. In order to help make this definition clearer, let us look at a clinical example.

CASE EXAMPLE

Mr. D, a 30-year-old white single male, entered psychoanalytic therapy with a competent, experienced, 45-year-old male analyst. Mr. D's presenting problems were feelings of inadequacy, and a fear of intimacy, particularly with women. After the initial several months of therapy (at three sessions per week), during which time the patient had been prompt, Mr. D began coming late for his hours. While this lateness was never more than three or four minutes, it was consistent. The analyst's questioning of the patient's feelings and fantasies regarding this lateness seemed to lead nowhere. After a time the analyst stopped questioning the lateness and "accepted" it as this patient's "characterological resistance to intimacy." The analyst's reasoning here was that this chronic lateness was probably related to the patient's testing out of authority, and perhaps of autonomy, and that any further questioning might promote the establishment of a sadomasochistic relationship. In such a relationship, the analyst believed, the patient would sadistically withhold "time" by being late. The therapist would then "sadistically" question and probe the patient. Thus, each member of the dyad would be attacked, each would then masochistically submit, and each would then attack again. While the therapist's explanations seemed reasonable enough, after a few more weeks he brought this case to supervision, as it began to be clear to him that the case was not going well. The patient had now "lost interest" in the therapy, and was questioning whether or not to continue with it.

In the supervisory sessions, examination of the patient's resistances soon led to an exploration of the therapist's resistance to the uncovering and understanding of this patient's slight yet chronic lateness. Further, the therapist's own associations led him to memories of his own childhood, and of his "dawdling" in the morning while his mother was attempting to rush him off to school so that she could be on time for her own employment. Further associations led the analyst to old angers at his mother, "she would never let me stay home unless I was *really* sick. I couldn't be late, ever, so I guess that I'd go slow." As the therapist continued to associate, he realized that he himself had been experiencing a repetition of an earlier personal childhood experience in his patient's chronic lateness. The patient was unconsciously acting out his own, as well as the analyst's, "dawdling child" transference, while the analyst was able to act out the role of an "accepting mother," who would tolerate (secretly accept and collude with) this patient's "dawdling defiance." Thus, the analyst was engaged in a repetition compulsion of his own past which led him into a concomitant identification (Racker 1968) with the patient. Now it was the patient who could be "too sick" (too resistant) to "grow up" and face his responsibilities, while the analyst could live vicariously through this conflict.

It is important to emphasize, at this point, that I am not suggesting that this analyst was dysfunctional. In fact, he was a creative and highly capable individual. Moreover, it seems evident that most analysts would have some sort of reaction to a patient's chronic lateness. In such a situation, for example, an analyst's countertransference reactions might range across the psychosexual stages; from feeling abandoned and then reunited (oral level) to feeling competitive and assertive (phallic level). Or, an analyst might react to this patient's chronic lateness with characteristic defenses (resistances) to the patient's acting out resistance. Thus, an analyst might be overly accepting, supportive, and mothering (denying his own orality and oral rage). Or the analyst might be overly polite (in reaction-formation against anal-sadistic impulses toward the patient). Or an analyst might be overly passive (turning his own phallic-aggression into its opposite). The point to be made here is that this patient's acting out resistance (which was the result of his transferences) led his analyst to certain countertransference reactions. Further, the analyst then resisted his own countertransference reactions *in his own characteristic ways.* Thus, it was the interaction of the patient's transferences and resistances with the analyst's transferences and resistances, which led to the current therapeutic impasse.

Following the supervisory work, the analyst reported changes in himself, changes in the patient, and changes in the therapy. No longer resistant to the exploration of his patient's lateness (a covert, subtle resistance), the analyst was now able to work with his patient's total range of feelings. Thus the analyst began to work more effectively with the patient. The patient's presenting conflicts had centered on his fear of intimacy. In fact, the patient saw all intimate relations as smothering, destructive, life-taking experiences, where he would be used and exploited, as he had felt himself to have been used and exploited by a clingingly depressed mother. Therefore, this patient's lateness had been an expression of hopelessness about his inability to give up an exploitative, "fused-mother" transference. But it had also been a desperate attempt by the patient to help his analyst cure him, by "curing" his analyst. Searles (1979a, p. 382) suggests that each patient has an inherent need to "cure" his analyst. Further, he suggests that stalemates in treatment always result from the analyst's having received a kind of therapeutic support from the patient to maintain the status quo, while successful change always seems to involve some unconscious "curing" of the analyst by the patient:

Thus ironically, and in the instance when this status quo does not become resolved, one can say indeed tragically, in those very instances wherein the analyst is endeavoring most anguishedly and unsuccessfully to help the patient to resolve the tenacious symptom, or the tenaciously neurotic or psychotic modus vivendi, at an unconscious level the analyst is most tenaciously clinging to this very mode of relatedness as being one in which he, the analyst, is receiving therapy from the patient, without conscious knowledge of either of them.

The patient in the case history discussed was trying to provoke his analyst into activity, and out of what the patient perceived to be his analyst's passive depression. The analyst, however, had perceived his patient's "defiance" through the eyes of the analyst's own character, that is, his own resistances and his own transferences. When the patient's acting-out resistance became a treatment-destructive resistance, the analyst was able to overcome his "barriers to knowing" (Issacharoff 1979) and to therefore uncover the transferences that these barriers concealed.

THE ANALYST'S INTERNAL WORK SPACE AS A PROTECTION AGAINST TREATMENT-DESTRUCTIVE COUNTERTRANSFERENCE RESISTANCE

As has been suggested, analysts are often placed in a no-win "Catch-22" situation: they feel that they should never be resistant to countertransference, but they also feel that countertransference is something which they should not have too much of (any of) in the first place. And to have either too much countertransference or too much resistance would seem to go against an analyst's idealized self-image, an image of himself as a sane, good, and helpful person.

In several other contexts, I have suggested (Mendelsohn 1982, Billow and Mendelsohn 1982) that an analyst needs to create an "internal work space." In this internal work space, the analyst takes the patient in and works on him "like a sculptor works on marble, creating new structures from the surface. The analyst then projects his creations back into the patient" (1982, p. 48). This work space provides the analyst with an opportunity to "work on" the patient internally, and to "create" a good-mother, benevolent, patient-therapist interaction. This process, I believe, creates what Searles (1979a, p. 174) has called a "therapeutic symbiosis," where the patient can be loved and accepted by his analyst, even while the patient is hateful and resistant to the therapy, ". . . before significant increments of hate have come to intrude into this oneness and transform the emotional matrix of it into one of pervasive ambivalence." And even while the analyst is also hateful and resistant as well. As Epstein and Feiner (1979), Searles (1979a, b), Winnicott (1958), and others (previously listed), have suggested, an analyst must be aware of and be able to work with his total range of reactions to his patient—both his positive reactions and his negative reactions. By creating an internal work space where the analyst can work with his patient, the analyst will, hopefully, protect himself and his patient from treatment-destructive resistances. Such new and broader conceptualizations of the analyst's work should most certainly lead us to a greater ability to understand and effectively treat our patients.

SUMMARY

An attempt has been made to examine the concept of countertransference resistance. This concept has not been widely examined, perhaps because of the inherently negative conceptualizations of both countertransference and resistance. Also, many authors seem to hold to the view that countertransference and resistance are synonomous. Thus, many analysts view countertransference as always being a resistance. Using the new and broader conceptualizations of countertransference which have been recently introduced, I have defined countertransference resistance as the analyst's resistance to experiencing the totality of the therapeutic interaction, including his resistance to the experiencing of his own, and the patient's, transferences. I have also suggested that the analyst must create for himself an "internal work space." In this work space, both the analyst and his patient can be protected from the hateful and resistant parts of each member of the therapeutic dyad.

REFERENCES

Billow, R.M., and Mendelsohn, R. (1982). Intimacy in the initial interview. In *Intimacy*, ed. M. Fisher and G. Stricker. New York: Plenum.
Eissler, K.R. (1953). The effect of the structure of the ego on psychoanalytic technique. *Journal of the American Psychoanalytic Association* 1:104–143.

Epstein, L., and Feiner, A.H. (eds.) (1979). *Countertransference*. New York: Jason Aronson.

Fine, R. (1971). *The Healing of the Mind*. New York: McKay.

Fleiss, R. (1953). Countertransference and counteridentification. *Journal of the American Psychoanalytic Association* 1:268–284.

Greenson, R.R. (1967). *The Technique and Practice of Psychoanalysis*. New York: International Universities Press.

Issacharoff, A. (1979). Barriers to knowing. In *Countertransference*, ed. L. Epstein and A.H. Feiner. New York: Jason Aronson.

Kernberg, O.F. (1975). *Borderline Conditions and Pathological Narcissism*. New York: Jason Aronson.

Langs, R. (1976). *The Bipersonal Field*. New York: Jason Aronson.

———— (1979). The interactional dimension. In *Countertransference*, ed. L. Epstein and A.H. Feiner. New York: Jason Aronson.

Little, M. (1951). Countertransference and the patient's response to it. *International Journal of Psycho-Analysis* 32:32–40.

MacKinnon, R.A., and Michaels, R. (1971). *The Psychiatric Interveiw in Clinical Practice*. Philadelphia: Saunders.

Mendelsohn, R. (1978). Critical factors in short-term psychotherapy: a summary. *Bulletin of the Menninger Clinic*. 42:133–149.

———— (1981a). Active attention and focusing on the transference/countertransference in the psychotherapy of the borderline patient. *Psychotherapy, Theory, Research and Practice* 18(3):386–393.

———— (1981b). When groups merge: transference and countertransference issues. *International Journal of Group Psychotherapy* 31:139–15.

———— (1982). Intimacy in psychoanalysis. In *Intimacy*, ed. M. Fisher and G. Stricker. New York: Plenum.

Menninger, K. (1958). *Theory of Psychoanalytic Technique*. New York: Basic Books.

Racker, H. (1968). *Transference and Countertransference*. New York: International Universities Press.

Searles, H.F. (1979a). *Countertransference and Related Subjects*. New York: International Universities Press.

———— (1979b). The analyst's experience with jealousy. In *Countertransference*, ed. L. Epstein and A.H. Feiner. New York: Jason Aronson.

Spotnitz, H. (1969). *Modern Psychoanalysis of the Schizophrenic Patient*. New York: Grune and Stratton.

———— (1979). Narcissistic countertransference. In *Countertransference*, ed. L. Epstein and A.H. Feiner. New York: Jason Aronson.

Winnicott, D.W. (1958). Hate in the countertransference. In *Through Paediatrics to Psycho-Analysis*, ed. D. W. Winnicott. New York: Basic Books.

CHAPTER 12

Resistance to Dream Analysis

Donald Meltzer

The shift in the view of the transference, which Klein's conception of the "concreteness of psychic reality" introduced into psychoanalytical thought, raised the analysis of dreams to a new level of meaningfulness. Not only were dreams to be viewed, after Freud, as the high road to the unconscious, but actually as a visual record of the transactions of narcissism and object relations in the depths of the mind. The transference in this sense, as an externalization of the immediacy of these events in the depths of the mind, imposed a new task on the analyst, beyond that of searching for transference phenomena functioning as resistance to analytical exploration. It made possible a view of the analytical method as a living process in addition to its established role as a vehicle of scientific inquiry into unconscious events.

This new dimension, the geographical aspect of metapsychology (Meltzer 1978) that so enthralled Klein's followers, has been put into a clearer perspective vis-à-vis the totality of mental functioning by the work of Wilfred Bion. He sees the level at which the Kleinian formulations operate as basic, at the level of dream and myth, Row C in his "grid" (Bion 1965), but only as the starting point for processes of rational thought. Nonetheless, it is seen as the level at which the emotional experiences are given a symbolic form so that the processes of thought may operate. If this initial step (which he calls alpha-function) fails (Bion 1963), the fragments of the emotional experience cannot be used for thought or memory, but can only be evacuated as meaningless fragments of behavior to "unburden the psyche of accretions of stimuli," as Freud would say.

In this framework of thought the concept of resistance – namely, the evasion of mental pain – becomes observable as an economic factor in the patient's relation to pain, and loses its meaning as resistance to insight, which, in turn, becomes transformed into the concept of "denial of psychic reality." It is this aspect of the transformed general concept of resistance, whose original weakness in operation lay in the facility with which responsibility could be shifted from analyst to patient, that the reference to dream analysis finds its most incisive place in our technical armory. In this area it is very clear that the patient's responsibility for reporting dreams finds its counterpart in the analyst's responsibility to make use of them. As Bion puts it, many patients find it much simpler to mobilize the analyst's resistance to understanding the transference, rather than to offer direct resistance to the process of investigation themselves.

I therefore divide my inquiry into this area into its two appropriate compartments: the patient's resistance to remembering and reporting his dreams, and the analyst's resistance to making use of them in the analytical work. I hope to describe the analytical situation vividly so that I need not employ particular clinical examples.

THE PATIENT'S RESISTANCE TO REMEMBERING AND REPORTING DREAMS

A theoretical discussion of dream life is necessary in order to introduce a systematic discussion of this problem area. Following Klein's and Bion's formulations about mental functioning, we are inclined to see the dream process as a continuous transaction in the "space" of psychic reality, probably interrupted only during non-REM periods of sleep which may interrupt dreams temporally but do not disrupt their continuity. The Kleinian "unconscious phantasy" and the Bionic "Row C" of dream and myth may be taken as substantially equivalent. The "emotional experiences" that the waking and sleeping individual is having (we must not exclude "sleeping experiences" any more than prenatal ones as a possibility, although we have difficulty in documenting such a supposition) must be transformed through the mysterious processes of symbol formation in order that they may be represented in psychic reality as what I have called "the internal theater where meaning is generated" (Meltzer, in press). If this is not accomplished, the experience remains at the level of disturbing stimulation, devoid of meaning, and must be discharged either in behavior or in somatic innervations (this bears on Bion's concept of the "proto-mental apparatus" and its relation to "Basic Assumption Groups," and constitutes his theory of the interrelation of primitive group mentality and psychosomatic disorder [Bion 1962, 1968]).

Once the experience has been thus transformed, further transformations are required in order that the meaning generated may be scrutinized and elaborated to abstract levels for integration with other experiences, for generalization, and for the purpose of growth in the self and in the view-of-the-world. For these purposes, verbal transformation, while not absolutely essential, is certainly potentially the most precise and memorable method. This view has a certain overlap with Freud's ideas about the relative position of word- and thing-representations in the system's conscious and unconscious (Freud 1900). A certain amount of transformation into language certainly can occur in the dream process itself, a fact that Freud was quite unwilling to recognize. Experienced patients even reach a stage in their relation to their dream-life in which the observation and interpretation of the dream process is indeed part of the sleeping experience of dreaming. This fact can only be understood if the rigid differentiation of conscious and unconscious (in the descriptive sense) is relinquished in favor of viewing consciousness as what Freud called "an organ for the perception of psychic qualities" and therefore equivalent to "attention."

This takes us back to the Kleinian concept of transference as a ubiquitous tendency to deny psychic reality, and externalize internal processes as relationships and actions in the outside world. This view differs from Freud's only in placing the process in the immediate rather than the distant past. Where resistance to, or denial of, psychic reality is strong, where "attention" is diverted from internal processes to the external world, the dream does not appear in memory, but is transformed either inside ("acting in") or outside ("acting out") the analytic situation.

Therefore, when faced with the absence of dream material in the analysis, the analyst is confronted with two important possibilities: either the emotional experiences in the analytical situation are not being transformed into dreams (failure of alpha-function, in Bion's terms, or two-dimensionality: Meltzer et al. 1975; Meltzer 1976), or they are being transformed, but externalized. The analyst must watch for evidences of consequent activity: (1) meaningless behavior and verbalization; (2) group behavior or somatic symptoms in the first instance; or (3) acting in or acting out in the second. The first is a frequent phenomenon in the analysis of borderline and psychotic patients, but is by no means absent with neurotics or patients with character disorders.

On the whole, what we have thus far discussed relates to the patient's inability to remember dreams. We must not omit the instance where the dream is remembered, but not reported. This must be taken as a situation that straddles our differentiation between the patient's resistance to psychic reality and the analyst's resistance to understanding the transference. Failure to report remembered dreams is frequently accompanied by an adolescent type of rationalization for secrecy, namely that "you would only misunderstand," and has its roots not only in the transference, but also in past events in the analysis in which the analyst and patient were at loggerheads. The issue here often rests upon the patient's preconceptions of the analyst's limitations in understanding by reason of sex, culture, education, evident interests, or therapeutic intentions. But such preconceived limitations cannot be assumed to remain unfounded, and this takes us to our second category, the analyst's resistance.

THE ANALYST'S RESISTANCE TO UNDERSTANDING DREAMS

It is not my intention to discuss the general area of an analyst's limitations in understanding certain emotional conflicts because of limitations in his own analysis and residual psychopathology. However, I am not inclined to set this aside, in the manner of Winnicott (1949), as having only one possible answer—that the analyst needs more analysis. In the view of analysis which sees its natural sequel to be a capacity for self-analysis, it is with just those patients who press the analyst into searching areas of his own personality which have remained unrevealed by his personal analysis that his self-analytic struggle is most furthered, if he will rise to the challenge. This is often manifest by the appearance of the particular patient in the analyst's own dreams.

But leaving that general limitation aside, the analyst's resistance to understanding the patient's dreams may be viewed from several points. Assuming that the analyst has both a theoretical respect for dream-analysis as part of his technical equipment, and has developed sufficient skill at the investigation and elucidation of dreams so that a failure to do so in a particular case would impinge upon him as a particular phenomenon in his countertransference, I will discuss the problem under three headings: (1) the fear of invasion; (2) the fear of confusion; and (3) intolerance to impotence.

Fear of Invasion

Since analysts have become accustomed, through their own analysis and through work with patients, to hearing and reciting dreams, hearing another person's dream is an experience of intimacy to which they may have become blasé. They have forgotten that it is a most unusual event in daily life for one person to recite a dream to another, particularly if it is a recent dream, and especially if the listener also appears in the manifest content. They may also have forgotten the embarrassment that this extraordinary intimacy excites, as well as the feeling of invasion that accompanies it. I think it is true that there is no more vivid way of communicating a state of mind than by telling a dream, but by virtue of this vividness the dream image also has little fish hooks from which the listening mind may find it difficult to shake free. In this sense it is like the impact of pornography. Because the dream of a patient tends to remain more vividly in the analyst's mind than any anecdotal material, it is subject to the same tendency in the analyst's mind as it is in the patient's—namely, the tendency to be acted out. This touches on the relationship of dreams not only to pornography, but to art. But the evocative power of a patient's dream is more likely to fall into the latter category because of the operation of anxiety under which it was produced. This is not true of all dreams in analysis by any means. There are certainly dreams of resolution of conflict which have a powerful aesthetic impact, but they are in the minority.

In other words, fear of invasion by the patient's projective identification of a disturbed part of his personality can play a paralyzing role in the analyst's approach to the investigation of a dream. He may find that he has forgotten the manifest content by the time the patient has told some associations, or conversely that the projected material is so powerful that he is unable to direct attention to the associations.

Fear of Confusion

I do not mean to discuss the instances in which a patient uses the format of dream reporting for the specific purpose of generating confusion in the analyst's mind. The technique for doing this is fairly easily recognized; the dream content and associations are so interwoven that a patchwork of dream and reality results which must be painstakingly teased apart. No, I wish to refer to dreams in which the patient's states of confusion are so subtly represented that the analyst is no more able to make the requisite differentiations than is the patient. This particularly refers to confusion between "good" and "bad" figures, and therefore between parts of the self and parental objects, but also to confusions of geography and zones (Meltzer 1972). In such a situation the analyst may find that his mind veers off from the dream and follows only the associations, eventually even seeming to ignore the fact that a dream has been presented.

The problem for the analyst in this situation is one that may be found to reside in a failure to utilize his countertransference fully in comprehending the dream. It is usually the emotionality that inhabits the dream that gives the most sure clues to these differentiations, especially where ethical values are concerned. Too prompt a use of the rational faculty in making differentiations tends to leave the analyst in the lurch, much as the patient is prone to be swayed by his own ethical judgments when these are founded on argument rather than emotion. It is necessary for the analyst, when he finds himself confused by a dream, to wait for his emotional intuition to become firmly established; then he can retrace the evidence of dreams and associations to document his intuition. He is liable otherwise to be in the state equivalent to that of the "hung jury," for whom the evidence is contradictory.

Intolerance to Impotence

One of the pitfalls of the analytical use of dreams arises from the expectation of the so-called mutative interpretation (Strachey), in which the analyst's therapeutic zeal tends to take the form of expecting that the marshaling of evidence will "convince" the patient, much in the spirit of Freud's early work before the paper on working through. Habitual apparent disregard by the patient of the evidential value of dreams can greatly dampen the analyst's interest in working with them. The patient's persistent attitude that "it is only a dream" is, after all, not without its historic status, for Freud himself viewed dreams as having little significance other than as a patchwork of day-residues and distortions that enabled the sleeper to sleep on undisturbed. Patients with a strong tendency to deny psychic reality intuitively agree with this posture and manifest their contempt for the dream and for the analyst's use of dreams. They behave as if the analyst were trying them for a mythical crime, in relation to which they stand protected by habeas corpus.

But analysts also may share this attitude unconsciously even when it is quite foreign to their theoretical frame of reference. The trouble is often found to lie in the problem of attitude toward psycho-analytical responsibility. The specter of lawsuits, coroner's courts, and irate relatives may be found to weigh heavily upon analysts. They may have difficulty in accepting the fundamental impotence of the analyst vis-à-vis the patient's psychic structures. They may find the responsibilities discommensurate with the power to implement their judgments. But after all, this is the role of parents as well, not so clear in early childhood, but shockingly apparent with their adolescent children.

Therefore, it often happens that the patient who denies psychic reality may not manifest this by failing to remember, nor by failing to report his dreams, but rather through his attitude; perhaps he views the procedure as a foible of the analyst, one that will generate information for the analyst, but that is devoid of evidential significance for the patient. If the analyst allows himself to be intimidated by this cavalier attitude, he may easily relinquish the use of this powerful method. Powerful, that is, for penetrating the meaning of unconscious events, even though it is powerless to convince. Freud (1937) himself, in the long run, as "Analysis Terminable and Interminable" testifies, was discouraged by this aspect of analytical work. While the dictum about leading a horse to water may seem identical to Freud's conclusion that in the long run it is the economics of the mind that dictates the outcome, there is a great difference on close examination. When the analytical method is viewed as a process having its origins and format within the patient, only presided over and facilitated by the analyst, his tolerance for the impotence of his position vis-à-vis the patient is likely to be greatly strengthened. The thirsty horse will drink when his anxiety has quietened, and the mind is hungry for the truth about itself even when the lies are evasive of pain or even pleasurable in themselves.

In closing this brief investigation, it seems necessary to mention an aspect of analytical work with dreams that, while implied in what has gone before, needs perhaps to be stated unequivocally. In my experience the emotional situation between analyst and patient at the nontransference level (as two adult people working together at a task with knowledge, skill, and an agreed format of procedure) at no point reaches such heights of pleasure, intimacy, and mutual confidence as in the unique process of dream analysis. I think that the reason for this is the aesthetic level of experience to be found in both participants when they abandon themselves to what Ella Freeman Sharpe called the "poetic diction" of dreams. Dreams bring out artistic creativity in both partners and produce an oeuvre—the dream and its interpretation—which both analyst and patient can experience as generated by their combined creativity.

REFERENCES

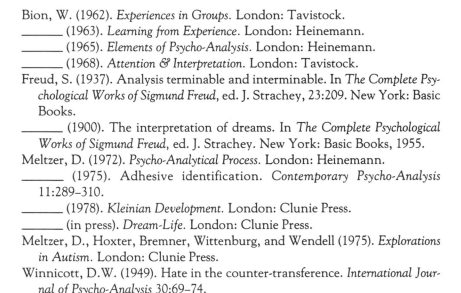

Bion, W. (1962). *Experiences in Groups*. London: Tavistock.

———— (1963). *Learning from Experience*. London: Heinemann.

———— (1965). *Elements of Psycho-Analysis*. London: Heinemann.

———— (1968). *Attention & Interpretation*. London: Tavistock.

Freud, S. (1937). Analysis terminable and interminable. In *The Complete Psychological Works of Sigmund Freud*, ed. J. Strachey, 23:209. New York: Basic Books.

———— (1900). The interpretation of dreams. In *The Complete Psychological Works of Sigmund Freud*, ed. J. Strachey. New York: Basic Books, 1955.

Meltzer, D. (1972). *Psycho-Analytical Process*. London: Heinemann.

———— (1975). Adhesive identification. *Contemporary Psycho-Analysis* 11:289–310.

———— (1978). *Kleinian Development*. London: Clunie Press.

———— (in press). *Dream-Life*. London: Clunie Press.

Meltzer, D., Hoxter, Bremner, Wittenburg, and Wendell (1975). *Explorations in Autism*. London: Clunie Press.

Winnicott, D.W. (1949). Hate in the counter-transference. *International Journal of Psycho-Analysis* 30:69–74.

PART III

Resistance in Specific Diagnostic Categories

CHAPTER 13

Resistance in Character Disorders

Peter L. Giovacchini

As soon as Freud (Breuer and Freud 1895) gave up hypnosis for free association, he discovered the phenomenon of resistance. The overcoming of resistance has remained the chief task of the treatment process and has become the hallmark of the classic psychoanalytic approach. Most analysts consider this struggle an immutable feature of the patient-analyst relationship, and that the battle is finally won by the weapon of transference interpretations.

Contemporary analysts, especially those who are accustomed to working with patients who are much more primitively fixated than these with the oedipal neuroses, do not particularly find the battle metaphor useful and prefer to view treatment as a cooperative venture rather than a continuous tug-of-war. Such a shift in viewpoint requires considerable modification about our attitudes concerning resistance, a phenomenon which unfortunately has a pejorative connotation (Greenson 1969).

Since Freud (1923) postulated the structural hypothesis, clinicians are paying increasing attention to the various layers of the psychic apparatus. The view of the mind as a stratified hierarchy helps us to understand characterological adaptations and how the patient relates in treatment.

If the psychic content of lower levels of the personality cannot be integrated into higher structural levels that are capable of being communicated to an external object, the analyst, we can no longer think in terms of barriers or obstacles either as elements of repression or resistance. Rather, the patient is exhibiting an inherent incapacity that is the outcome of structural defects, and a relative lack of integration of primitive psychic structures into later acquired, more sophisticated adaptive ego states. Unlike a barrier that can be breached, the inability to integrate cannot be dealt with in a similar fashion to the one used by Freud as still used today by many analysts. The patient cannot behave otherwise, and his inability to reveal himself and get in touch with the primitive forces and feelings within is determined by the constrictions of his character structure.

With such patients the overcoming of resistance is the consequence of successful treatment which leads to the acquisition of further psychic structure. The analyst cannot make demands for the patient's cooperation, because his so-called lack of cooperation is an inherent part of his psychopathology and represents a deficit. In fact, the patient may be seeking treatment to free himself from the very same constrictions that do not permit him to be freely open with the therapist.

The differences between resistance and defenses are obscure and they are especially obscure in patients suffering from character disorders. Analysts ordinarily can tolerate defenses and are content with understanding and interpreting them, whereas their attitude to resistance, as already discussed, is somewhat peremptory. Still, it should not surprise us that patients bring the adaptations they use to cope with the external world into the analytic setting. They will, especially at the beginning of treatment, relate to the therapist in the same manner as they have to other significant external objects. If they have needed to be oppositional in the past, they will continue in a similar pattern in the therapeutic present. Rather than trying to overcome this opposition which is known as resistance, it should be analyzed as a defensive adaptation.

Granted there are certain types of defensive adaptations that make analysis difficult if not actually impossible, such as the refusal of the patient to leave at the end of the session (Giovacchini and Boyer 1982). However, if the analyst has an average tolerance for the manifestations of psychopathology, these difficult and impossible patients are comparatively rare. The treatment setting can often be adjusted, perhaps somewhat modified, so that the patient and therapist can work with each other. The patient may initially require certain conditions based upon his needs and anxiety.

RESISTANCE AND THE NEED TO CONTROL

There are certain formal elements to the analytic interaction that are superficially similar to traumatic elements of the infantile past. The analyst has often been imbued with a certain authority and power that is realistically unwarranted but which the analytic setting tends to encourage. This may not be as true today as it was in the past when analysis was considered mysterious, and analysts wore what has now been mockingly referred to as priestly robes. For the most part these esoteric attitudes are no longer as prevalent, but there are a substantial number of opponents of psychoanalysis whose antipathy is based upon the feeling of being threatened by the prestigious position they have attributed to the analyst.

Some patients need to exercise total control and they view the analytic situation as impinging on their capacity to maintain such a position. They often refuse to lie on the couch because they believe they would no longer be in control and are exposing their vulnerability. Technically, this constitutes a resistance inasmuch as the patient is resisting the treatment procedure, but he is behaving as he is because he is terrified of being overwhelmed by inner destructive forces.

A single man in his middle thirties had been hospitalized many times since his adolescence. He was apparently quite bright, had been the valedictorian of his high school class, and had graduated from a prestigious university summa cum laude. He performed very well in a highly technical capacity, but periodically he would become detached and then withdraw completely from his family, friends, and fellow employees. He appeared to be in a fugue state, which in a period of days would change to being agitated and terrified. By that time he would be so disturbed that he had to be hospitalized.

He had seen several therapists on an outpatient basis, but he was always too agitated, literally, to sit still through an entire session. He would ramble on in a hyperactive fashion, either ignoring questions or answering them in a mocking noninformative manner. Not one of the analysts he saw believed he was acting in a psychotic fashion; they viewed him, rather, as being provocatively silly, a wiseacre behaving like a spoiled brat. One therapist described him as an adult version of a minimal-brain-dysfunction child, with some hypomanic features. All the therapists agreed that the strength of his resistance rendered him untreatable. Their conclusion was particularly interesting, given that resistance in this case did not mean resistance to free association, as was described by Freud. On the contrary, this patient always seemed to be free associating in a wild and bizarre fashion. His therapists, in essence, objected to the fact that he *was* so wild and bizarre. He did not present himself in a better-organized, secondary fashion; he did not sit still and let them take an organized history. They believed that the patient had the capacity to control his feelings, and that his choosing not to do so constituted resistance—he was refusing to follow a prescribed sequence that involved diagnostic assessment through history-taking.

When I first saw the patient I also formed the impression that he could behave in a calm, organized manner if he wanted to. However, I had no particular inclination to stop him from rambling in a hypomanic fashion and made no attempt to take a formal history. He remained seated in a chair, and began to revile himself as an odious "festering, polluted" person full of "pus and garbage." He then had a fit of silly laughter and spoke of how successful and creative he could be. He talked about how much he was admired while he was at work and about the numerous innovations he had made. Beside his work, he described his many artistic and musical talents. Still, he could easily return to attacking himself. At the end of the session, which he announced before I could, he stopped abruptly and said that we had accomplished nothing. He quickly left. I had made very few comments, just simply asking an occasional question to clarify something he had just said.

The next session he began by stating that he had nothing to say to me because he was certain that I could not help him. He did not want to reveal himself to me because there was nothing I could offer him. In fact, he was a machine that no one could operate except himself. He continued seeing me as useless, but he alternated in blaming me or himself. He threatened to quit treatment.

I apparently felt fairly comfortable, and gently asked him to lie on the couch. He responded by screaming "No," but despite his vehement refusal he moved to the couch and sat down. In a placating fashion, he said he would sit up but he turned his head the other way so that we did not have to look at each other; however, he maintained a posture in which he could easily keep me within his range of vision. I replied that I would go along with this arrangement for a while because I understood that he had a strong need to remain in control of the situation. I had no wish to intrude upon his autonomy, but sometime in the future for the sake of the analysis he would have to lie down. I added that this was not a personal wish of mine, it was a requirement of the process, although I admitted I felt more comfortable when patients were lying down. He visibly relaxed and became calm.

He sat on the couch for several months and finally lay down, and treatment progressed in a conventional manner.

Refusing to lie down is similar to suppressing associations inasmuch as it represents an opposition to certain rules that have characterized psychoanalytic treatment. Regarding the fundamental rule, as discussed, some analysts do not insist that the patient "tell everything that comes to mind" especially when treating patients suffering from severe or relatively severe characterological problems. In some quarters, there has been a similar flexibility concerning the use of the couch. The relaxation of what had been the immutable requirements of analysis accompanies an extended viewpoint of indications for treatment. Still, the more classically oriented analyst, although he might approve of a modified approach, would be quick to point out that it is not analysis. At best it is psychoanalytically oriented psychotherapy.

This introduces another variable regarding the definition of psychoanalysis. The more a therapist accommodates to resistance, the less resemblance to psychoanalysis the treatment process retains. However, this is a superficial approach; it ignores the deeper factors of therapeutic regression, the transference interaction, and the interpretative modality. If we include the holding environment (Winnicott 1960) as an intrinsic factor of the analytic relationship then the problem becomes further complicated. Accepting the patient's "resistance" may be crucial to the establishment of the holding environment.

With my patient, I firmly believed without deliberately thinking it out that I had to let him sit rather than lie on my couch. I felt it was necessary if I wanted to treat him, and for some reason I did. I can think of other patients who balked at lying down, to whom I would not have given any further appointments if they had absolutely refused to lie down. I wondered what determined my different reactions.

For example, some years ago I saw a successful professional man in his middle forties whose wife had urged him for a long time to seek analysis. She had been successfully analyzed and was, because of changes within herself, unwilling to continue their relationship on the same neurotic basis (Giovacchini 1958, 1965). She had been urging him to get into treatment even before her own analysis, but since being analyzed, she had been firm and unrelenting in her insistence. He finally realized that she would divorce him if he did not acquiesce, and he felt intensely anxious, almost panic-stricken, about losing her. As his anxiety mounted he called me and presented himself as a man desperately in need of treatment. Since he owned his business, he could accommodate himself absolutely to my schedule.

He was in a state of near panic during his first session, being afraid that I would not accept him for treatment and this would mean that his marriage would break up. It was clear that he had very little concept of treatment as something for himself; it was simply a means of appeasing his wife. When I indicated that I was interested in treating him, he became considerably less anxious.

Feeling reassured, he became less compliant. He gave me many reasons why he could not come during certain times of the week. He also told me of several business trips that would keep him away weeks at a time. He was obviously frightened of becoming involved in therapy and was resisting the beginning of treatment. During the second session I had asked him to lie on the couch, and he reluctantly did. We had a special problem arranging a third session, because of his schedule, and I had the definite impression that my putting him on the couch had contributed strongly to our difficulty. Nevertheless, we were finally able to agree on a time.

Before the next session, I had set up a schedule of regular appointments that he would have to be responsible for; at least, he would have to pay for them whether he kept them or not. Immediately upon arriving for his third appointment, he said that he wanted some explanations and he asked that he be allowed to sit up. My response to his request was the diametric opposite to that of the first patient I have briefly discussed. I tried not to show the strength of my reaction, but I firmly refused. If he had been adamant, I was prepared to terminate treatment then and there.

The patient lay down and I discussed, in essence, the analytic setting. He admitted that he did not really want to be analyzed but wanted to be treated by me because he wanted to hold his marriage together. I accepted that this was sufficient reason for analysis, and the treatment relationship continued for many years with a fairly successful outcome.

Looking back at that third session I have wondered why I reacted so differently to these two patients. From a technical viewpoint both were resisting. Each balked at following a procedure that most of us believe is an intrinsic feature of the analytic interaction. As is true of any reaction, however, there are many different underlying factors. These patients' resistance stemmed from different psychic levels. *There are different forms of resistance that cannot be dealt with uniformly.*

The first patient had on occasion been diagnosed as schizophrenic but since he was, for the most part, able to function, the diagnosis was often toned down to schizoid and hypomanic was frequently added. He was conceptualized as having a schizo-affective character structure. Whatever the diagnosis he dramatically displayed the effects of splitting and projective mechanisms, and his sessions, as mentioned, were heavily punctuated with outbursts of both grandiosity and bitter self-incrimination and devaluation.

His life was a constant struggle between good and evil inner forces and he had to somehow control the latter so that he would not be destroyed, or, more aptly, not destroy himself. Basically, he had to be in control of his feelings which also meant he had to control the surrounding world because the boundaries between inner and outer were blurred. At work, he was always on top of the situation, no one telling him what to do. On the contrary, other employees were there to do his bidding. His home was said to be a marvel of electronic wizardry, in perfect harmony, and run simply by pushing buttons.

Very early in treatment he presented me with a revealing dream, one which stressed the polarities of good and evil. He saw two Titans standing in front of him, one dressed in white armor, and the other in black. At first it seemed as if they were going to engage in combat, but suddenly the black Titan moved toward the patient as if he were going to seize him. The patient panicked and ran toward the white Titan, who extended his arms to receive him, to be rescued. He was then carried in the Titan's arms to a cozy warm cave. In spite of being protected and removed from the source of evil danger, his anxiety—although considerably less—did not abate. He felt helpless in his rescuer's arms, and was even aware of a sense of shame. He precipitously jumped out of his benefactor's arms, grabbed his sword, and found himself in the midst of a group of Roman warriors who were slaughtering peasants. The peasants begged him to save them, and he believed he could if he had the "power." Perhaps it was in his sword, but he was not certain. He awakened feeling frightened.

This dream can be studied from many angles. Some readers will immediately recognize that elements of a popular movie *Star Wars* are incorporated in the manifest dream content. The Titans, as figures in both Grecian and Roman mythology, and Roman warriors reveal the transference element of the dream, inasmuch as my name is obviously Italian. However, I wish to stress this patient's fear of losing control and being in the passive position even when he is being rescued, and his need to be actively controlling, as depicted in his running away from his protector and getting in the middle of the melee.

He demonstrated these anxieties and needs in his behavior during sessions, and in his resistance to lying down on the couch. For a long time he was hypomanic, and during the first few sessions he found it difficult to sit still. He would stamp his feet and writhe in the chair. He did not actually get up and pace around but he wanted to. He verbally attacked me because he believed I forced him to stay in one place, and this was to some extent true. Although I never overtly demanded that he not get up and move around, I certainly expected him not to, and I probably conveyed that by my demeanor.

Asking him to lie on the couch I believe was equivalent to being carried in the white Titan's arms. The patient had this dream while he was still sitting on the couch. He felt helpless and vulnerable and in someone else's control, and though he was protected by the Titan he had to relinquish his destiny to someone else. This ultimately meant his destruction.

Thus, resistance was the outcome of fundamental conflicts related to his psychic survival. It was a manifestation of the core of his psychopathology and structural defects. His self-representation had not achieved a cohesive stable integration. It was also being constantly threatened by hostile destructive introjects. He had been able to construct overcompensatory defensive adaptations which protected him from inner invasive destructive forces. These adaptations involved control, mastery, and grandiosity, and his innate talents and creativity helped support them. To insist that he lie down directly threatened his modus operandi, his chief defensive modality.

The situation was different with the businessman. Though his reluctance to begin analysis was also based on intrapsychic factors, they belonged to different levels of the psychic apparatus, higher levels than the first patient. His behavior seemed to be organized on a secondary process basis whereas my other patient's orientation appeared to be primarily following a primary process axis. These distinctions would indicate that the second patient had the capacity to curtail his actions, that he was not so driven to resist in order to survive or to maintain the cohesion of his self-representation. He had much more flexibility.

Resistance as a reaction to the fundamental terror of the dissolution of the self-representation, represents an expression of the deepest elements of the schizoid patient's psychopathology. By contrast, there are other types of resistance that are not connected to basic intrapsychic conflicts or that are the direct outcome of structural defects. The businessman's resistance was a manifestation of a surface defense, but a defense that could continue to exist even if it were prohibited one avenue of expression. It had many others at its disposal.

I strongly believe that if I had not been willing to let the first patient sit on the couch for as long as he needed to, that he would not have been able to continue with me. I conjecture that I would have, in a sense, fed into his delusion by actively assuming the same role as inner destructive evil forces. I would have become the black Titan that he dreamed about. However, not interfering with his need to control and to maintain ascendancy over bad internal objects helped create a safe atmosphere. True, at some point in his treatment he will have to work out his problem in a transference context and deal with me as if I were the black Titan. Still, if he can gain security in the treatment setting, he will acquire the confidence to face his hatred and rage as he begins to understand that the purpose of the analytic setting is to foster maximum autonomy. The delusional qualities of the need to control can be "tamed" to the striving for independence and self-sufficiency as the patient's primary process orientation achieves accretions of secondary process elements. Accepting the patient's resistance helped create a holding environment which made analysis possible.

To have acquiesced to the second patient's request to sit up, and to let him continue dealing with the schedule in cavalier fashion, in my mind, would have made the prospect of analysis impossible. The patient had the propensity to gain his ends by manipulation. His talent for manipulation contributed to his success in business, but it was part of a defensive pattern that protected him from loss of self-esteem based upon a competitive struggle with his father, who recently died, and subsequent guilt. It was a reaction formation and in the analysis also a displacement for both his feeling inferior to his father and his guilt about having wanted to destroy him. He also maintained distance from emotional involvement because he was afraid of intimacy but he was able to manipulate relationships so that on the surface they appeared to be close. Similarly he wanted to appear to have an analytic relationship without becoming emotionally engaged.

In retrospect, I see more clearly that if I had responded to his request to sit up and "talk," I would have been colluding with him and accepting a pseudo-relationship for an analysis. Unlike the situation with my other patient, not accepting his resistance was not threatening to the foundations of his personality. He had many resources, many areas in which he could use the psychic mechanisms of reaction formation and displacement, and innumerable opportunities for forming pseudo-relationships. Furthermore, I felt that I would be doing something out of character if I conformed to his wishes whereas with the schizoid patient I was not particularly uncomfortable when I acceded to his. I will discuss this further later when I review countertransference factors and the loss of the therapist's analytic identity.

RESISTANCE AND THE LOSS OF NARCISSISTIC SUPPLIES

Throughout the years I have encountered with increasing frequency patients who signal at the very outset that they are going to be critical of the analytic method. They implicitly or explicitly criticize analytic neutrality and the relative inactivity of the analyst. They demand feedback and express a need to be "locked" into the relationship. They want an active give-and-take exchange. They also require commentary, questions, and some kind of guiding organization.

If the couch is suggested, they are apt to refuse because they require eye contact. They complain about the anticipated sense of isolation. They need a meaningful relationship and do not want to be abandoned and left talking to themselves. They have to know what the analyst is both thinking and feeling so that patient and therapist can relate to each other as "whole" and "real" persons.

Although the purpose of analysis is to foster the patient's autonomy, the analyst also has to feel that he is autonomous and free to choose how he will relate in the treatment setting. Ideally, the patient's and therapist's autonomy do not clash. When patients make the demands I have just outlined, I experience them as intrusive. Again, the patient's resistance to treatment has to be assessed in terms of the level of psychopathology it represents. Ordinarily, these narcissistic patients can maintain their adaptations outside the treatment relationship and relinquish some of them in order to be analyzed. If they cannot, analysis might not be possible.

I recall two patients whom I handled differently. In one instance, I was able to conduct analysis and in the other I was not. In many ways these two middle-aged married women were similar. Both of them had been popular and attractive in their youth and they received considerable admiration. They were in the center of the stage and one of them earlier in life had been an actress gaining a certain amount of celebrity status. The other patient had been a model, doing mainly cosmetic ads. They sought treatment because of anxiety and depression which were related to the fear of growing old and losing their beauty. Furthermore, their children had grown up and left home. Their husbands seemed to be somewhat indifferent, and the former actress's husband was probably having an affair.

They were quite agitated when I first saw them. The former model found herself "bored to death," and she was furious with her husband although she could not give any specific reasons for feeling so angry at him. He was simply dull and did not relate to her in the vibrant fashion she required. She looked back over her marriage and evaluated it as a failure although her husband seemed content with the way things were. He could not understand why she was unhappy and wanted treatment. In fact, he was opposed to psychoanalysis. She saw his attitudes as further evidence of insensitivity. She insisted that they were not in synchrony and that he had no concept of how to relate to her needs. Analysis was somehow to make up for these deficits in her daily life.

Though she tried to be charming and, to some extent, seductive, there was a peremptory quality to her demeanor. I definitely felt that the sooner we could formally enter analysis the less demanding I would find her, so early in the second session I asked her to lie on the couch. She greeted my request with a storm of protests. She accused me of being as insensitive as her husband, and not understanding her need for eye contact. She was furious at my suggesting a situation where once again she would be just talking to herself. She had discussed classical analysis with friends who were or had been in treatment, and that was not what she wanted. I replied that this was strange because she knew me as an analyst. I added that I could respect her sensitivities but I did not believe I could be of any use to her unless I tried to analyze her, and the process required that she lie on the couch. Of course, it was her choice, but analysis was what I had to offer. She chose to be analyzed, and she resentfully lay down.

For months, she was very angry and saw me as a harsh taskmaster, but she continued coming, was always on time, and never missed an appointment. Briefly, throughout the years, she increasingly revealed how lonely and isolated she felt, how she always had to perform and be attractive in order to receive any attention. She learned to "exist" on the acclaim she received. Without it she viewed herself as an empty void. Narcissistic supplies held together a fragile sense of self.

Her behavior markedly changed; she was no longer histrionic and melodramatic, and did not avidly seek attention and admiration. She became drab and depressed and expressed considerable tension and feelings of intense inadequacy. In other words, she had given up her narcissistic defenses; gradually she began building up self-esteem and received gratification from my interpretations. She found employment which made use of her fine sense of design, divorced her husband and remarried.

I need not discuss further details of her treatment except to emphasize that this highly narcissistic woman presented defensive adaptations that seemed to be at odds with the analytic procedure. She was able to survive the requirements that I consider intrinsic to analysis because, in my opinion, she was able to continue to cope on a narcissistic basis in the external world. If I had accepted her demands, her resistance as I felt it, I do not believe we ever would have achieved an analytic relationship.

The situation with the former actress supports my belief. When I suggested that she lay down on the couch, she adamantly refused. I had concluded that she was extremely fragile and I had no desire to issue ultimatums. I decided I would, at least for a while, let her sit up.

She also wanted to control the frequency of her appointments. Her life was extremely busy, and she really had very little time left in her heavily burdened schedule so she would have to fit me in as best she could. At first, I thought she was devaluing treatment as some narcissistic patients are prone to do in order to enhance themselves. When I indicated that she was being somewhat cavalier in her approach to therapy she vehemently denied that this was the case and wept uncontrollably. She stated that people always misinterpreted her actions and did not understand how overwhelmed she felt. I sensed once again her underlying fragility and viewed her high-handed manner as a desperate attempt to maintain her shaky self-esteem.

As was true for the schizoid patient presented earlier, she had to be in complete control. Regarding analysis this meant that she would determine when to come or not to come. She had to decide how much importance she would give to our relationship because otherwise she would be eclipsed by me if she let me become emotionally significant. Still, she was aware of her intense need for contact.

I had reconciled myself to accepting her conditions for treatment, believing that if I did not she would terminate our relationship. Perhaps that would have happened, but she remained in treatment only for six months. During that time I learned she was terrified of the transference regression which would have led to fusing with me and feeling vulnerable and dependent.

These fears were the outcome of the repetition of a symbiotic relationship with a destructive and devouring mother who exploited her daughter's beauty and talents for her own aggrandizement. During her treatment as well as in her daily life she defended herself against the anxiety of being submerged and destroyed by seemingly attributing little importance to interpersonal relationships. What she was doing with me was typical of her mode of relating.

My acceding to her demands, from another vantage point, giving in to her resistance, represented the acceptance of a defensive stance which she adopted toward the world in general. I was, in effect, reinforcing a psychopathologically determined adaptation, thereby vitiating the opportunity to analyze it. Consequently, the treatment stagnated, leading to unsuccessful termination.

I had thought that this patient's narcissistic defenses were deeply rooted and that I could not prematurely disrupt them. As stated, I was impressed by her fragility but now, in retrospect, I wonder whether I had underestimated her capacity for maintaining integration. She has been skillful in manipulating her environment and achieving her ends. For the moment, her husband had strayed by having an affair. The patient retaliated by having several affairs, and he meekly returned to the fold and gave up his lover.

Treatment had not acquired any specific meaning for this patient. It was simply another facet of her life which became part of her narcissistic adjustment. Her resistance to treatment as I initially wanted to conduct it was an additional manifestation of a general manipulative tendency which made others beholden to her, and that protected her from a destructive merger with emotionally significant external objects. She managed to maintain separateness by not allowing anyone to become, at least from a surface level, emotionally significant.

I still believe that if I had insisted upon certain conditions for treatment, such as a regular appointment schedule and lying on the couch, that she would not have come back. On the other hand, allowing her to exercise her defenses as she demanded in the treatment situation also led nowhere.

The first narcissistic patient did not terminate when I insisted she follow analytic protocol. Now I am inclined to deal with such patients in a standard analytic fashion. Possibly the patient may decide not to pursue analysis but, at least, the therapist would have defined the treatment setting. The patient knows what to expect and can return to a constant analytic environment if he or she so decides.

RESISTANCE AND THE FEAR OF FUSION AND LOSS OF SELF-ESTEEM

There is considerable overlap between the type of patient I am about to describe and the narcissistic woman I have just discussed. Both groups suffer from a traumatic symbiotic phase manifested by a fear of fusion, and have an intense need to be in control of their feelings and lives. The patient I will now present demonstrated some characteristic and common methods of vigorously resisting beginning treatment and shortly thereafter created an impasse which threatened to disrupt therapy (see Giovacchini and Boyer 1982).

This 30-year-old bright single man was full of conflict about starting analysis. This was surprising because he had tried hard for many months to get me to see him for analysis. Since my schedule was full I tried to refer him to various colleagues, but he persistently refused to see them because he was afraid they would reject him because he was "too sick."

When I finally saw him, he spontaneously gave me a long detailed history, obsessionally filling in every detail of past development. Here it is pertinent to mention only that he was doted upon by a beautiful, apparently narcissistic mother, and neglected by a highly successful but passively uninvolved father. The patient was an only child who attracted considerable attention because of his intellectual precocity.

At the beginning of the third session I briefly instructed him about free association and the use of the couch. I knew that I was interrupting his narrative but I saw no purpose in letting him continue as he had been. I had the feeling that he could have gone on giving me a history indefinitely.

He politely listened to me but seemed bewildered. He timidly walked over to the couch and moved the pillow to the other end of the couch. He started speaking in a hesitant fashion and seemed anxious. Five minutes before the end of the session he suddenly sat up and said "I've had enough." He did not leave; he just sat there talking until the end of the session.

He canceled the next four sessions, each time for what appeared to be a "legitimate" reason. For example, he canceled the first appointment because he had the flu with a fever of 103 degrees. He recovered rather quickly but not until after he had missed the second session. Then he was unexpectedly sent out of town by his firm, causing him to miss the last two sessions.

When he returned he walked toward the chair, but I stopped him by motioning toward the couch. Again, he reluctantly walked toward it but he remained sitting up. He looked at me and told me that his problems were current and immediate and he did not want to get lost in the morass of his past. This seemed strange since he had gone into such details of his early history.

I had to resist the impulse to tell him angrily that he should stop wasting my time. Either he would let me analyze him or he could go elsewhere. I knew I was facing intense resistance, but I found it difficult to connect his behavior to his psychopathology. I restrained myself, however, by remembering the fundamental principle of psychic determinism. He had to be reacting to some profound anxiety that prevented him from relaxing and regressing in an analytic context.

I explained that he would determine what he talked about and whether it related to the past or present. However, for technical reasons as well as my personal comfort, I required that he use the couch. If I felt that treatment could progress in any other fashion, one in which he would be more comfortable, I would be glad to conduct therapy on that basis. However, I and the psychoanalytic method had limitations and I knew no other way in which I could comfortably proceed. I also felt that by letting him sit up we might be evading some fundamental problems. He did not seem happy about what I said but he acquiesced. I somehow felt we had avoided a power struggle.

I learned later that the patient's initial reluctance to begin analysis was the outcome of his ambivalence. He desperately wanted analysis but he was frightened. He understood that the aim of analysis is to foster autonomy but he was afraid of losing control. To lie on the couch and not be able to look at me signified that he was helpless and vulnerable. He would feel humiliated and lose the last vestige of self-esteem. Looking at me meant that he was in control as he maintained his vigilance.

Apart from obvious masochistic, homosexual transference elements, the patient was dominated by the fear of fusion, which recapitulated the infantile symbiotic fusion with his mother. The fear of symbiotic merger made it difficult to begin analysis and during treatment he experienced transference regression in a frightened painful fashion, but he had considerable resiliency and integration and had developed sufficient trust in the analytic setting to be able to move in and out of repressed states that corresponded to the symbiotic stage. It was interesting to note how he came out of the regression, that is, how he used certain adaptations to protect himself from fusion.

At these moments, he seemed to have lost his ability to free associate and was outwardly directed. He no longer had any capacity for introspection. He would ask me innumerable questions, the types of questions that are usually directed toward physicians, such as "Are we making progress?," "What is my prognosis?," "Can we summarize what we have accomplished?," and similar queries which I had no inclination to answer. During these periods he had assigned us specific roles. He was the patient and I was the doctor. However, he also viewed himself in terms of his work and various social roles, but his concepts about himself, me, and the world in general were stilted and mechanical.

Clearly, his concrete state manifested itself as a resistance; it was a defensive adaptation to protect him from the dissolution of his self-representation that he feared would occur with symbiotic fusion. This was reflected in his behavior and general functioning; he was inflexible, unfeeling, and inhibited in working creatively (a severe handicap in view of his professional position). However, he was free of anxiety and maintained a modicum of self-esteem.

RESISTANCE AND THE IMMEDIACY OF NEEDS

The resistance of this group of patients tends to be covert rather than obviously expressed. It occurs during sessions and is expressed in an analytic context. It often takes the form of questioning the effectiveness of psychoanalysis, and though it can usually be easily understood in terms of the infantile past and the repetition compulsion, the analyst often reacts adversely and feels as if he is facing a stalemate. These patients frequently succeed in creating a tense atmosphere which seems to interfere with analytic progress.

The patient, a middle-aged successful professional man, spoke in a highly articulate and witty fashion, but after several months of treatment he gradually stopped describing the inner world of his psyche and turned to nagging and complaining about treatment. He had a rigid, obsessive character configuration, which began expressing itself by asking precise, well-organized questions and making very specific demands regarding the goals of treatment.

He had become extremely concrete but unlike other concrete patients he was not persistent. He could easily become psychologically minded and make use of free association, fantasies, and dreams for introspective purposes. Even his nagging and complaining were transient.

Still, I had the feeling that this patient's resistance to gaining access to his mind was intense in spite of his interesting revelations. I finally realized that something was lacking in the transference although the patient had no difficulties in expressing his negative feelings.

Regarding the negative transference, he, in essence, blamed me for his passivity. He drank and smoked too much. He was markedly overweight and his internist was becoming concerned about his cardiac status. Because he was usually tense he was on antianxiety drugs and various other medications to either quiet down his bowels or to prevent constipation. He went into detailed descriptions about the status of his bowels, and the effects of all the drugs he was taking. He had become somatically preoccupied and used me as an audience to listen to his ruminations and, at the same time, to attack me (usually indirectly) because I was not helping him. He meant that he was not giving up his self-destructive behavior and that I was somehow responsible.

Although analytic regression can sometimes be severe, there was something unique about our relationship which had special significance regarding technique and my countertransference responses. I had the impression that he was not aware of me as a person. He made me feel as if I were unidimensional, or lacking depth. I was only a vehicle for his needs, and the external world was simply revolving around him. It was expected to take care of all his needs. This could be interpreted as being the orientation of a highly narcissistic patient who deals with external objects as if they were self-objects. Often the analyst feels as if he does not exist in his own right and apart from the patient. This was not exactly the situation with my patient. He recognized me as a separate person but in a limited way.

I then realized that I was responding to his emotional tone rather than to the content of what he said. Although his material was interesting, the way he presented it was tedious and dull. He never smiled and was totally devoid of humor as an affect although, as stated, he could be witty. He often looked depressed, confused, and perplexed, but never animated, enthusiastic, or happy. At his best he could be calm and mellow. The combination of directing everything back to himself even when he began by focusing on something that interested me, and his humorless mode of presentation, made me uncomfortable. I was able to relax, however, when I understood our relationship in terms of his infantile past.

His mother had been in treatment with a prominent analyst for as long as the patient could remember because of chronic depression. When he was 6 months old, she had been hospitalized for several months. In spite of her severe emotional difficulties he was told that she was a good and devoted mother. He remembered being well taken care of as a child, but he could not recall ever chatting or playing games with her. Apparently she was constantly depressed and never smiled.

She related to his needs with a sense of immediacy, but she could not go beyond the need-gratification level. I was able partially to reconstruct and speculate about the early maternal interaction from the way the patient related to me and from my countertransference responses. I also had the opportunity to gather information about the mother from her analyst who emphasized that she had not been able to recognize her son as a person, but simply as a baby who had to be fed and changed. He confirmed that she never sang or cooed to him. In fact, since he had been interested in her mothering behavior he had asked about the various developmental milestones of her son's life. When questioned, she did not recognize that her child had a smiling response or felt stranger anxiety. Certainly, she had not tried to evoke a smile from him or, as far as her analyst could tell, she had not smiled in his presence. She did not seem to get any pleasure from her son. He was a chore that she conscientiously took care of but not a person whose presence would fill her with pride and a sense of accomplishment.

I experienced his material as resistance. This is not exactly resistance as Freud had described it. He was not putting himself in opposition to any of the formal elements of analysis, such as free associating, lying on the couch, or frequency of appointments. However, I found it difficult to continue analyzing him and the usual analytic tool of interpretation did not seem to work.

Apparently, my countertransference reactions were sufficiently disruptive that the work of analysis bogged down. The patient was producing material that caused me to react adversely and analytic technique was ineffective. I was uncomfortable but it was more than discomfort that was involved. I felt that in some way we were out of synchrony with each other and this created an atmosphere of resistance. In a sense we were resisting each other and this impeded analytic progress. The situation improved when I understood the early maternal relationship, but this led to a modification of technique, something I had previously resisted doing. I will explain this type of modification in the following section.

RESISTANCE, COUNTERTRANSFERENCE, AND THE PSYCHOANALYTIC PARADOX

Resistance has been classically considered to be disruptive to treatment. Traditionally, it emanates from the patient. However, the analyst's reaction to the patient's material is highly significant in determining how effective resistance will be in thwarting the course and purpose of therapy. Thus, countertransference reactions can be incorporated into resistive forces and contribute to therapeutic impasses.

Besides countertransference as a disruptive response, idiosyncratic or otherwise, there are formal elements in the psychoanalytic method and setting that may reinforce the patient's resistance or be experienced as a repetition of the traumatic past. This may intensify the patient's problems rather than provide relief and comfort. I have called this imbrication of treatment method and psychopathology the *psycho-analytic paradox*, a situation that leads to special technical problems (Giovacchini 1969, 1979).

The problems caused by the psychoanalytic paradox and those created by adverse countertransference reactions are related to each other, although they emphasize different facets of the analytic relationship. For example, narcissistic patients, and those who have a profound fear of fusion, by refusing to lie on the couch may threaten the therapist's analytic identity. Apart from technical reasons, allowing the patient to sit up may be disruptive to the analyst because it is contrary to his work style. This is a rather obvious threat to an analyst's modus operandi. There are more subtle interactions.

Narcissistic patients, in particular, complain of the analyst's lack of participation and silence. Either overtly or covertly they may demand responses to their material—for instance, to a dream. The analyst, in turn, feels his professional autonomy threatened, wanting to decide himself when and whether to respond. The treatment may degenerate into a power struggle as the therapist continues to "resist" the patient's demands. This is a form of participation by the analyst which prevents the establishment of an observational frame of reference and an intrapsychic focus.

The analyst's personal orientation is especially important when it comes to choosing an effective approach to treatment, analysis or modified analysis. I find myself reluctant to relinquish my analytic identity, which is part of my ego-ideal, by offering patients something besides analysis. Therapists have to decide whether they want to modify the analytic stance for certain patients, as Eissler (1953) suggested, by introducing parameters. If the therapist feels uncomfortable making such modifications, it will, of course, interfere with the effectiveness of his approach.

Patients who have a constricted view of external objects cause intense strain on the analytic setting. They are extreme examples of the analytic paradox. Their reactions to analytic neutrality and objectivity are especially complex and often create very difficult moments which threaten the integrity of the analytic relationship.

As previously discussed, in this group of patients the maternal relationship was such as to take adequate care of basic biological needs; at the emotional level, however, these mothers were impassive and uninvolved. They did not smile or coo at their children; they did not recognize them as persons in their own right; and after they had met their survival needs, their children did not exist for them. The infant was not related to in terms of his growth potential and sense of aliveness. His need to explore and play, his curiosity about the external world as he tried to move into it, were not reciprocated. Later, as adult patients, children of those mothers may perceive the analytic interaction as being identical to the maternal relationship. They may view it as unidimensional and confined to only a single frame of reference. Indeed, the analyst may want to keep the treatment focused upon only a single frame of reference, the intrapsychic, and purposely not want to enter the patient's external world, striving to avoid emotional involvement. For many such patients urgent needs define intrapsychic processes, and living in the outside world means being accepted and related to as a person. They want the analyst to enter both frames of reference, but the therapist perceives this attitude as resistance.

Under the pressure of the repetition compulsion, they also try to create a situation in treatment that repeats the early mother–infant relationship in the transference. Usually, the reverse of that relationship is recapitulated—the patient treats the analyst the same way his mother treated him and this creates the countertransference problems I have briefly mentioned. The problem is intensified because the analyst, or rather the analytic method, aggravates potential problems and the repetition compulsion is reinforced by the analytic approach. The transference may be impossible to analyze.

Specifically restricting the interaction with the patient to interpretations and the maintenance of a neutral stance is reminiscent of the constricted relationship with the mother who could allow herself no emotional involvement with her child. The analyst is equated with the unavailable mother. The patient suffers the same infantile deprivation in the current treatment setting. This ordinarily happens in the transference relationship, but normally the analyst's neutrality creates a backdrop that causes infantile transference elements to stand out; with these patients, however, infantile reactions blend with the analyst's operational mode. Consequently the patient's transference implications are obscured and he believes he is confronting a reality similar to the one he knew in infancy.

The patient needs to repeat infantile deprivations but he also wants to be gratified, to make up what he lacked in his early object relationships. This is a compensatory attempt, characteristic of patients who have achieved a degree of psychic structure that supports object constancy and allows them to seek segments of the external world that lead to gratification. The patient tries to obtain this compensatory gratification from the analyst. In adult life he is able to make demands he could not make in infancy because then he did not have sufficient ego structure to assert himself; he also felt too vulnerable and helpless.

For the patient, the analyst frequently becomes the aloof mother, and he bitterly resents it, especially because there is some truth in his belief that he is being treated in a fashion similar to the one he experienced as an infantile trauma. An ordinary analytic relationship is characterized by toned down responses and reactions from the therapist. His emotional decibels are comparatively low, and this can be easily interpreted as aloofness. The patient requires something from the analyst to make up for this early deprivation. If the analyst insists upon treating such a patient in a "routine" fashion, impasses most likely will occur.

When I have an awareness of such patients' basic neediness for emotional supplies, I usually find it fairly easy to feel some involvement which goes beyond the need to understand them. My responses become intensified and I develop some degree of excitement. This is not role playing; it is something that happens spontaneously.

An adolescent patient was almost totally withdrawn at the beginning of treatment. He had been hospitalized because he had a complete breakdown in his identity, an "identity diffusion syndrome" (Erikson 1959), and he showed some features of catatonic withdrawal. At the beginning of treatment he was almost totally noncommunicative. His responses to my questions were monosyllabic. I felt I was being intrusive, so I suggested he lie on the couch; he could choose whether he wanted or did not want to share his thoughts with me. He seemed grateful and immediately withdrew to the couch.

Gradually, this young man started asking questions, mundane questions about how to carry on pedestrian activities. He would ask what shoes were appropriate for special occasions; he would even wonder how to make a telephone call to a girl in order to ask her for a date. I became eagerly involved in discussing these issues and it would have been unthinkable for me not to have answered his questions. I rejoiced over the fact that he was producing some material even though he was not free associating in a formal sense. I felt he was no longer withdrawn and was tentatively reaching out toward me.

One day he came to a session looking particularly distraught. He had become upset because the schedule of the train he took as transportation to my office had been slightly changed. He was very anxious as he tried to tell me about the specific changes. I became similarly concerned and if an outsider had been able to see our interaction without hearing the content, he would have thought that we were discussing momentous problems that would affect the fate of our universe. Actually the change in schedule would have no effect on our appointments, but I was nevertheless able to share his anguish.

I have reported the further course of his analysis elsewhere (Giovacchini 1979). It was stormy and had many difficult moments but it had a fairly successful outcome. It could not have progressed to the point that it did if I had not participated in these early exchanges.

This schizoid young man is an example of that group of patients whose needs were well taken care of, but who were not related to as developing persons exploring and knowing the external world. His parents apparently were afraid of their feelings, as evidenced by the fact that they never showed them. They were obsessively oriented and were meticulous in their son's care but what they offered took place in a sterile environment. Winnicott (1958) discussed two types of needs: biologically determined id needs; and those based upon enhancing relationships, which he called ego needs. My patient had his id needs met, but not his ego needs. During the beginning of his analysis I believe I was responding to his ego needs.

Was I permitting a situation to develop that would interfere with the growth of an analytic relationship? I felt I could not have behaved otherwise, being convinced that I would lose the patient if I did. Still, by supposedly stepping out of the analytic stance, I might have been encouraging resistance to analysis which admittedly would have been an expression of deep psychopathology. The subsequent course of his treatment indicated that he could form and maintain an analytic relationship and possibly this could have been achieved if I had remained traditionally analytic from the beginning.

From one viewpoint, I do not believe that what I was doing was nonanalytic. As I have already discussed, if I had not participated by answering questions or sharing his excitement, disruptive or otherwise, I would have created a setting that would have been identical to the infantile traumatic environment. This would have made analysis of the transference impossible because the patient would not be able to separate me from infantile imagos. In analysis we attempt to create a unique setting, one that is different from what the patient has known before, one based upon understanding of the patient's psychic processes as they repeat the adaptations and interactions of the infantile environment. The analytic environment, by setting up a contrast to the infantile environment, makes analysis possible.

The basic principle of analysis is psychic determinism, an intrapsychic focus. The task of analysis is accomplished by recognizing the dominant transference elements which are involved in the repetition of infantile traumatic relationships, the repetition compulsion. This is generally accepted. There are differences of opinion as to how this is accomplished although recently there has been some agreement that the main therapeutic tool is interpretation of the transference.

In order to maintain an intrapsychic focus, and to not become involved in the patient's external world, the analyst is supposed to relate and behave in a certain fashion. He remains neutral in that he is nonjudgmental. He conveys an air of nonanxious calm. He does not give advice and he does not necessarily answer questions. I would agree that these attitudes generally are favorable to maintaining an analytic setting which will form a contrast to the infantile environment. However, there are patients with whom some of these attributes reinforce the infantile environment rather than create an analytic setting.

I regard these attributes as *secondary attributes* of analysis that are not applicable to all patients, in comparison to the primary attributes of an intrapsychic focus — repetition compulsion and transference resolution through interpretation. The therapist has a certain degree of flexibility which is determined by the patient's characterological structure and unique infantile experiences. Every patient has a need for a particular tempo. With my patient I had to increase my tempo to relate to his lowered one.

SUMMARY AND CONCLUSIONS

The phenomenon of resistance in patients suffering from character disorders is considerably more complex than that which Freud described in patients he believed to be examples of hysterical neuroses. The patients I have described often found the treatment process menacing because (1) it threatened to undermine defensive adaptations that compensated for ego defects, or (2) it became associated with the infantile traumatic environment and reinforced it.

Freud's recommendations regarding the handling of resistance were simple and direct. He strove to get rid of it as quickly as possible. Discover the resistance and forbid it, was, in essence, his credo. This method is far from effective for patients suffering from structural defects.

Our main problem as psychoanalytic clinicians is to determine when to adapt ourselves to the manifestations of psychopathology, which in the treatment setting emerge as resistance, and when not to alter the psychoanalytic setting to make such accommodations. I have given several examples in order to illustrate how the therapist may have to respond differently. The general conclusion reached is that if, on the one hand, the resistance is the expression of core psychopathology—that is, the manifestation of a defense against a fundamental ego defect—then to insist on certain formal attributes of psychoanalytic procedure will be counterproductive. If, on the other hand, resistance is the outcome of superficial defenses that can be relinquished in treatment because the patient can continue gaining gratification by exercising them in the external world, the analyst can insist upon maintaining his *analytic modus operandi*. Possibly he may lose the patient, but it is doubtful that he would have been able to analyze him even if he had made concessions.

Schizoid patients who withdraw and need to maintain control may balk at using the couch. They view lying down as being in someone else's power and they are then exposed to their fundamental vulnerability and helplessness. Often, they have not reached a level of psychic integration that permits them to deal with the external world and the treatment setting in a symbolic fashion. They cannot understand the difference between a symbolic submission and the concrete act of lying down. Many other facets of the analytic setting are seen in the same light. Scheduled sessions, payment of fees, and other accoutrements of the analytic action are interpreted literally as expressions of the therapist's destructiveness, a destructiveness that dominated the infantile environment.

Narcissistic patients sometimes need to be constantly replenished. Analytic objectivity may be equated with relative rejection and deprivation. This is also the outcome of a concrete orientation devoid of the capacity for symbolic elaboration. Similarly, vulnerable patients are afraid of being intruded upon, assaulted, or engulfed in a destructive fusion. In all these instances, because of their concreteness these patients cannot separate the current world of treatment from the infantile environment, and this is manifested as resistance.

The patients just discussed may object to one or another aspect of analysis, such as lying on the couch or refusing to free associate. There is another group of patients who are in many ways similar to them but who find the *tempo* of analysis incompatible with their needs. Often these are schizoid patients whose chief defense is withdrawal. However, this group is not confined to schizoid character types; it may include many types of character disorders.

These patients have had emotionally uninvolved mothers who were nevertheless able to relate to their children's biological needs. They did not, however, relate to them after their physical needs were met, such as by playing with them and taking pleasure in their infant's emerging sense of aliveness. Winnicott (1958) would have stated that these mothers could respond to id needs and not ego needs.

Analytic neutrality and the pace of the analytic interaction are equated with the uninvolved mother. This becomes such an exact replica of the tempo of the infantile environment that the analysis faces an impasse. The patient may then become actively resistive by missing sessions or withdrawing into hostile silence. He finds no meaning in treatment and may terminate.

Resistance in patients suffering from character disorders cannot be viewed just in terms of a patient creating a tug-of-war, or pulling away from analytic involvement. There are many subtle interactions between the patient's character structure and ego defects and the analytic procedure that have to be explored before we submit to the label of resistance in a pejorative sense or even as being totally disruptive to treatment. Countertransference remains an important vector in determining whether analysis between a particular analyst and patient is possible. Resistance, therefore, has to be studied in terms of both the patient's and the analyst's character orientations and reactions.

REFERENCES

Breuer, J., and Freud, S. (1895). Studies on hysteria. *Standard Edition* 2:1–307.
Eissler, K. (1953). The effect of the structure of the ego on psychoanalytic technique. *Journal of the American Psychoanalytic Association* 1:104–143.

Erikson, E.H. (1959). *Identity and the Life Cycle.* New York: International Universities Press.

Freud, S. (1900). The interpretation of dreams. *Standard Edition* 4/5:1–361.

―――― (1911–1915). Papers on technique. *Standard Edition* 12:89–170.

―――― (1915). Observations on transference love. *Standard Edition* 12: 157–170.

―――― (1915a). The unconscious. *Standard Edition* 14:159–215.

―――― (1915b). Repression. *Standard Edition* 14:141–159.

―――― (1923). The ego and the id. *Standard Edition* 19:1–60.

―――― (1937). Analysis terminable and interminable. *Standard Edition* 23: 209–255.

Giovacchini, P.L. (1958). Mutual adaptation in various object relationships. In *Psychoanalysis of Character Disorders*, pp. 179–194. New York: Jason Aronson.

―――― (1969). Treatment of marital dysharmonies: the classical approach. In *Character Disorders and Adaptive Mechanisms*, pp. 221–253. New York: Jason Aronson.

―――― (1979). *The Treatment of Primitive Mental States.* New York: Jason Aronson.

Giovacchini, P.L., and Boyer, L.B. (1982). *Technical Factors in the Treatment of the Severely Disturbed Patient.* New York: Jason Aronson.

Greenson, R. (1969). *The Technique and Practice of Psychoanalysis.* New York: International Universities Press.

Winnicott, D.W. (1958). The capacity to be alone. In *The Maturational Process and the Facilitating Environment*, pp. 29–37. New York: International Universities Press.

―――― (1960). The theory of the parent–infant relationship. In *The Maturational Process and the Facilitating Environment*, pp. 37–55. New York: International Universities Press.

CHAPTER 14

An Object Relations Perspective on Resistance in Narcissistic Patients

James S. Grotstein

Resistance is traditionally used in classical analysis to designate patient barriers that arise as a self-imposed censorship on the further flow of spontaneous associations. They are still considered to be variations of ego-defense mechanisms which oppose the free irruptions of id impulses and their derivatives into consciousness. Yet we speak of resistances only in the analytic context. An important distinction should be made, I believe, between mechanisms of defense which inhibit *intrapsychic* communication and those in the analytic dyadic relationship which inhibit *interpersonal* communication. The analytic relationship is a special one in which two people get together to talk about one. Because of the intensity of the feelings which are generated in this atmosphere there seems to ensue: (1) a compulsion to regression on the part of the patient, (2) a predilection toward transference (of present and past experiences), and (3) a development of what Bion (1966) has termed the catastrophic change.

THE OBJECT RELATIONS SCHOOLS AND THEIR BELIEFS

Before exploring the object relations point of view on resistances in narcissistic patients, I should like to comment on the definition of "object relations," and on the object relations point of view. The term object relations, though originally used by Freud (1917), seems to have been formalized by Fairbairn (1952) in a statement of a whole new theory of psychoanalysis that subordinated instinctual drive manifestations into internal objects and internalized egos that come together as "dynamic structures." For Fairbairn the concept of resistance was the reemergence into consciousness of those internalized objects and the subordinated egos attached to them. The Object Relations School became the "Middle Group" of the British Psychoanalytic Institute. Included among its more famous members are Winnicott, Balint, Bowlby, and Khan. Though these latter contributors may not view psychic energy in the extreme way Fairbairn did, they nevertheless seem to eschew the classical notion that the purpose of the object is to facilitate the discharge of the instinct (Winnicott 1958, 1965, 1971; Balint 1968; Bowlby 1969, 1973, 1980; Khan 1974). Instead, they, like Fairbairn, believe that the instincts of the infant are directed toward objects from the very beginning. Hamilton (1982) has recently reviewed the tenets of the British Object Relations School and makes a careful distinction between their usage of the concepts of dependency, object relations, and attachment. She believes that Winnicott and Bowlby fall more into the attachment conception, which is significantly different from dependency (Klein) and object relations (Fairbairn and Balint).

It is interesting to note that Kohut (1966, 1971, 1977) and his followers seem to adhere to the classical notion of instinctual drives aiming toward discharge, and have conceived of selfobjects which are coextensive with the infantile ego as facilitators of discharge to give tension relief, but do not emphasize separated objects which are the direct target of the infant's instinctual drives.

Melanie Klein (1950) had been working with primitive mental states since before 1921 and seems also to have been aiming in the direction of object relations, but her object relations theory differs somewhat from Fairbairn's and other members of the British Middle Group. Because of her propensity to attempt to work within the classical framework she never quite realized that she had arrived at an instinct theory that was significantly different from Freud's. Her instinct theory can be thought of as "object relations" but is significantly different from Fairbairn's, as in the following regard: her conception of instincts allows for discharge rather than for immediate object attachment (as is the case with Fairbairn), but the instincts are instantly reified as objects through projective identification. Just as Freud (1914) said that in narcissism the shadow of the object follows upon the ego, Klein's conception of internal objects can be understood as the shadow of the infant's instincts as it falls upon the object, transforms the perception of that object, and allows for the internalization of that transformed object as an internal object with ego and superego qualities, and also as an internalized dynamic structure (Klein 1932, 1950, 1960).

This latter point about the shadow of the instincts falling upon the object brings us to the next consideration: the differences between the conception of narcissism from the classical, object relations, and Kleinian points of view.

Classical analysis had traditionally considered narcissism as, first, a stage of organization where, following autoeroticism, the id takes the ego as its object. Second, following disappointments in objects, there is a withdrawal of cathexis from the object to the ego, thus the shadow of the object falls upon the ego as secondary identifications within the ego. In essence, then, the classical theory of narcissism is an object-relations theory, although this term has never to my knowledge been applied to it. Fairbairn's conception of narcissism (although he rarely if ever used the term as such) seems to be based upon the "inventory" of one's internal objects. He believes, for instance, that an original unitary ego splits because of disappointing experiences into a central ego which relates to an ideal object. This psychic structure subordinates two endopsychic structures, a rejecting object associated with an antilibidinal ego and an exciting object associated with a libidinal ego, the former secondarily "repressing" the latter. For Fairbairn, narcissism represents the balance among these three psychic structures. The more cohesive the central ego and its relationship to its ideal object, the less powerful is the negative force of the rejecting object and the antilibidinal ego, and the less undermining is the secondarily defensive maneuver of the libidinal ego and its exciting object in its attempt to bypass the persecution of its negative counterpart.

To Winnicott (1965, 1971), narcissism (a term which he also rarely uses) would be the degree to which there has been a "good enough mothering," with a "holding environment" that allows for a maturation of a sense of self so as to preclude the need for the development of a "true self"/"false self" dichotomy. The development of the latter split would foreshadow a narcissistic personality disorder. Balint's point of view would be quite similar. Severe narcissistic disorders, he believes, would be characterized by a "basic fault" in the personality because of a disruptive maternal environment.

The Kleinian conception of narcissism seems to eschew the classical notion of it as a postnatal continuation of primary identification. Klein opts instead for a notion of a separate infantile ego from the very beginning; it interacts with a separate object with primitive mechanisms toward allowing, at first, for splitting, projective identification, magic omnipotent denial, and idealization (schizoid mechanism of the paranoid-schizoid position), and then introjection (depressive position). Narcissism to Klein, therefore, represents the infant's introjection of its experiences with external objects that have been varyingly modified and/or transformed through these primitive mechanisms.

Despite the differences between Klein, Fairbairn, Winnicott, and classical analysis on the issue of narcissism, however, there still seems to be ultimate agreement in the end that the ego feels about itself the way it perceives the object to have felt about it. Thus, narcissism seems to be an object relationship between "I" and self based upon an identification with the way the object related to the self. The main differences between Klein and the others are over the relative reality of the perception; Klein's view is of the projective transformations of the image of the object before internalization and identification.

The term *British Object Relations School* can be loosely applied with the understanding that the Kleinian development does have significant differences which distinguish it in many ways. I have also linked this school with the work of Kohut because he deals with selfobjects that seem to correspond in nature and function to internal objects insofar as the infantile self is thought of as being continuous with or indistinguishable from the object. Whereas Klein and Fairbairn see the infant as separate from the very beginning, they believe that it relates to the external object so that the latter is incorporated through introjection (Fairbairn), or through projective-introjection (Klein), so as to become an internal object with egos attached. Hamilton (1982) implies that the attachment theory employed by Winnicott and Bowlby suggests an infant who is not merely separated and/or fused at the beginning but part of an active interaction with the mother. In other words, there is an instant dyadic interactiveness from the very beginning.

Kohut has evolved a completely different theory of narcissism which is, as I have said, not an object-relations theory of narcissism, but a selfobject conception of the development of the self. In his first theory, Kohut designated two different developmental sequences, one for a separate development of the self, and a second for the development of the relationship with objects (oedipal development) (Kohut 1971). In his later theory he modified the first by subordinating the object relations and drive theory to the development of the self, but maintained and amplified the conception of selfobjects, including mirroring, idealized, and alter ego selfobjects (Kohut 1977). His theory seems to be a cross between Fairbairn's and Winnicott's, on the one hand, and of Klein's, on the other. This can be seen in the following ways: Kohut posits that the smooth development of the normal narcissistic core of the self (the cohesive self) is interrupted by empathic failures on the part of the parental figure, whose function it is to be the selfobject, by which he means an object that is to continue to provide soothing and other functions that the immature infant cannot yet provide for itself. In this regard, he is like Fairbairn and Winnicott, although he does not allow for the internalization of negative or disappointing selfobjects. Kohut also believes in the importance of the idealized object as a protective function, particularly the way Fairbairn and Klein have posited, but he does not, as does Klein, consider idealization as a defense against persecutory anxiety; Klein sees it as a normal as well as a defensive function.

Kohut posits these objects to be external rather than internal and to be coextensive with the self, thus the term "selfobject." Whereas the spatial view differs, the functions seem to be the same. The Classical Object Relations School, on the other hand, has developed a system of object relations based upon the conception of representations of the self and of the object in a representational world. Hartmann (1958, 1964), Jacobson (1964), Sandler and Joffe (1969) seem to be the leading contributors to this school of thought (although the latter two are English). Although Klein, Fairbairn, and Kohut are dealing with primitive object (and/or selfobject) relations based upon partial separation and partial continuation fusion with the object, the Classical Object Relations School deals with selves and objects that have attained representational status; they are separate, are associated with conflict-free spheres of autonomy in the ego, and function with an interrelationship of neutralized libidinal and aggressive energy. This school considers narcissism to be the libidinal cathexis of self-representation by object representations.

The paradigmatic object conceptions of the Classical School of Object Relations and of the British Object Relations School(s) differ in terms of the sophistication and development of the objects involved. The British School and Kohut are describing very early objects for whom the self is partially separated and partially not separated, whereas the Classical School refers to objects at *this* stage of development as "object images," and employs instead an object model based upon the later development of psychical representability of the self, of the objects, and of the instinctual drives. J. O. Wisdom (1961) has tried to bridge the gulf between these various schools by invoking orbital and nuclear objects; the orbital objects correspond to object representations which are seen by him as clustering orbitally around the ego (self-representation), and nuclear objects being objects internalized within the ego (self-representation).

NARCISSISTIC PATIENTS AND THEIR RESISTANCES

It is generally understood that the narcissistic patient has a high degree of immaturity, tends to be grandiose, reacts to events in the world as if they are directed toward him or her personally, and is unusually sensitive to blows to his self-esteem. The Kleinian conception of the narcissistic personality considers a characterological defensive network organized around an envious hatred of dependency upon an object. In order to defend against the awareness of this dependency and of the envy derived from it, the patient institutes a manic defense to deny not only dependency on the object, but also the worthiness of the object itself. Thus the manic defense operates in two sectors: to deny the importance of the object and to deny the experience of the dependent self associated with that object. The worthiness previously attributed to the object is then appropriated to the self, and the worthlessness formerly associated with the dependent self is now transferred to the object. A reversal has seemingly taken place.

Kernberg (1976) has furthered this conception by stating that the grandiose self comprises the ego ideal, the idealized object, and the normal self. From the Kohutian point of view, and by extension the

Winnicottian and Fairbairnian positions, the narcissistic patient is thought to have a false outer grandiose self that may, or may not, be in compliance with the difficulties imposed upon him by the unempathic object world, but that defends against disappointments from this world and protects a withdrawn and enfeebled inner true self. Thus, the Kleinian perspective, like the classical one, ascribes narcissism to the hatred of dependency, whereas the object and selfobject schools assign narcissism to disappointmei.ts and failures on the part of objects in the real world.

Fairbairn (1952) seems to emphasize the importance of the schizoid aspects of narcissism which, according to his scheme, can be understood as the internalization of a grandiose self. This personality is characterized by introversion, relating through *showing* rather than *sharing* (the exhibitionistic defense), and through intellectualization. Winnicott seems to be discussing the same phenomenon when he refers to the distinction between the true self and the false self.

Perhaps we can better understand these two separate trends as manifestations of (1) a failure to achieve satisfactory bonding with the primal object, and (2) a hatred of experiencing weaning from an object with whom the bonding or attachment has been insufficient. Thus the Kleinian view is concerned with the hatred of weaning, probably secondary to insufficient bonding or attachment, and the object relations and selfobject relations schools focus primarily on deficient detachment or bonding. In other words, they are dealing with two sides of the same coin. Furthermore, the principal experience that the narcissistic patient seems to defend against is that of depression. Kohut suggests fragmentation as the underlying affect which appears with the collapse of narcissism, but at times he hints also at depressive despair. Perhaps fragmentation defends against the underlying depression. At the same time, however, it should be noted that Kohut and his followers view the concept of defense quite differently from other psychoanalysts. What are ordinarily called defenses by classical and object-relations analysts are considered by Kohut as "breakdown products."

The resistances which therapists generally experience with narcissistic patients can be classified as follows: (1) resistances to regression and/or regressive disorganization; (2) resistances to the experiences of one's needs, urges, desires, and feelings; (3) resistances to change; and (4) resistances to the development of a new relationship in statu nascendi with the therapist. All these can be considered as resistances that defend against the anticipated danger of a catastrophic change, and/or the anticipation of a blow to their self-esteem and to their equilibrium. The consequences of these types of resistances can be summarized as anticipating the experience of "nameless dread," dissolution of the ego, fragmentation, panic, disruption, disorientation, and depression. It is as if each narcissistic patient has his or her own inner conception of Hooke's law, which states that the amount of strain a solid object experiences when a stress is applied to it is dependent upon its coefficient of elasticity.

All patients fear their lack of resilience, but narcissistic patients do so especially. Thus, the maneuvers of the narcissistic patient in analysis may be resistances deployed against any and all interpretations by the therapist that seek to promote weaning into states of further separation between the self and its object, and he may try stubbornly instead to regain states of union with the object via projective identification, so as to reachieve the state of bonding which he felt was insufficient during infancy. Freud's conception of the erotic transference as a resistance is relevant in this regard. From the object relations point of view one can see the erotic transference as (1) a precocious attempt to get away from the humiliation, dread, and vulnerability of the mouth-breast dependency transference to attain instead a premature genitalization of the relationship between the patient and the therapist so as to equalize the relationship and mitigate the imbalance, or (2) as a way to enter into a state of excitement so as to mitigate or diminish the experience of separateness and thereby achieve a state of exciting fusion between tongue and nipple as if they are one and the same (regaining of primary attachment).

Stated differently, it seems that the narcissistic patient develops resistances to treatment when he feels himself in danger of being overwhelmed by dependency fears. He seeks to employ defensive maneuvers that bypass the awareness and consequences of these dangers, and also to try to institute maneuvers which allow him to relive primitive mental states which were incompletely experienced (primary bonding). The tenacity with which such patients hold on to these positions is sometimes confounding to therapists and causes them to label patients as obstinate, compulsive, stubborn, parasitic, addictive, or perverse. Many narcissistic patients may justify these appellations because of their tendency to "invade" their objects in fantasy and thereby deprive the therapist from having a clear view of his patient.

FEAR OF TRANSFORMATION

Narcissistic patients seem to have a fear of transformation. They fear that their progress in treatment means surrender of their sense of individuality to the therapist and also that the therapist will take them for granted. There also seems to be a fear of progress in analysis based upon a growing disparity which the very progress of analysis causes to develop between the progressive self and the yet remaining immature self. When the schism between these two portions of the personality achieves a critical differentiation, sometimes a negative therapeutic reaction with critical acting out takes place. It is as if the unprogressed portion of the personality undermines the progress of the progressive self in order to call attention to itself.

Some of the issues addressed above can be clearly seen in patients suffering from anorexia nervosa. The patients I have seen with this disorder invariably showed a high narcissistic investment in the anorectic symptomatology; anorexia was personified virtually as an autistic "mothering self" who seemed to protect the enfeebled patient in a state of sanctuary, understood her, and was able to soothe her by the very redoubtability of her disciplining agenda. The therapist was seen as a helpful person on one level, but as an enemy to her "anorectic mother" and self on the other level. In one case, the patient's neurotic personality engaged me in analysis most ably until there was a sufficient differentiation between her normally progressive self and the still lagging anorectic-primitive self. At this time her vomiting became worse and she precipitated a program of such severe weight loss and chemical imbalance that her life was in danger. Her resistances to the analysis subsided only when I acknowledged the positive importance of her anorectic self as a protection for her against her disappointing childhood objects. A peace seemed to emerge which allowed for the gradual transformation of the patient into a non-anorectic agenda.

Of extreme importance in the resistances of narcissistic patients is the differentiation between a virtually autistic self and a normal self. In more severe cases, Bion (1965) has applied the term *transformations in hallucinosis* (− K) to designate those patients who withdraw completely from the external world and, like the women in *The Stepford Wives*, retire instead into a cursorily improvised internal world that is split off from but seemingly reflects the normal external world. This autistic world is characterized by rigid automatisms and stereotypes that hold the patient prisoner.

It is readily apparent, I hope, that this imagery personifies the patient's inner experiences and tends to have a universality among narcissists and borderline patients who have undergone the phenomenon of splitting of the ego and of a repopulation of an altered internal world which seems to be a "mock-up" of the external world but is in fact a rigid and proscribing one.

ATTACKS AGAINST LINKS

Patients of this type may also utilize other defensive resistances, according to Bion (1959). They may not only attack the links between themselves and their dependency objects but may also attack the links in their own thought processes that link up with their feelings. They thus experience internal disconnectedness—as if their minds were filled with cotton wool—or splintering or fragmentary thoughts and feelings. These patients are afraid of the consequences of linking generally, which on the oedipal level is experienced as the fear of the primal scene and/or the fear of losing mother to father, but on the more primitive level is experienced as the fear of catastrophe consequent upon acknowledging a relationship to the dependency object. The nature of this fear is the danger of all the destructive projections the patient may have thrust into the object; the patient then experiences the fear of the object's retaliation on such primitive levels as devouring, demanding, destroying, and usurping.

The therapist treating such patients may experience an attack on his own linking processes in a subtle but striking way so that he experiences difficulties in thinking about the patient. Often the patient may accomplish this feat through elliptical associations which resemble double-talk. If subtle and convincing enough, the therapist may find himself subjected to a dismantling of his own capacity to think about the patient and may even feel that he is being driven crazy.

REVERSIBLE PERSPECTIVES

Bion (1965) has also referred to a variant of this process that he calls "reversible perspectives." This particular resistance is employed by severely narcissistically wounded patients in order to make ambiguous the communicative link between the therapist and the patient. Thus the patient may discuss a matter with the therapist, and the therapist may respond in kind with an interpretation that assumes that he and the patient are talking about the same phenomenon. In fact the patient has secretly withdrawn from the foreground of the discussion to the background but affects that he is attending to the foreground. The common denominator in such resistances is attempts on the part of the narcissistic patient to destroy, alter, or make ambiguous the communicative link between himself and the therapist in order to forestall progress; progress would amount to the expansion of his thinking and the consequences thereof, which are believed to be catastrophic.

COMMUNICATIVE RESISTANCES

The conception of resistances has been considerably broadened by the intervention not only of the school of self-psychology but also by R. J. Langs (1981; see also Chapter 7 of this volume). Lang has employed the term "bi-personal field"—borrowed from the Barangers (1966)—which he has developed into the conception of the communicative field. He now posits resistances as being not just part of the patient, but transactional between the therapist and the patient. He classifies resistances as gross behavior resistances, communicative resistances, and counter-resistances. Of key importance in Langs's conception is that communicative counterresistances (interferences on the part of the therapist) emerge from the therapist's unwarranted interventions into the analytic frame that unites the patient and therapist in their common task. Deviations on the part of the therapist cause resistances in the patient that cannot be considered as transference resistances but rather as understandable responses to the therapist's aberrations. He speaks of the "me/not me" interface in which the patient may internalize aspects of the therapist's deviant behavior as an identification with the aggressor.

Langs (1981) further differentiates resistances according to the nature of the interactive field between the therapist and patient in frameworks which he designates as field type A, field type B, and field type C. Field type A consists of a communicative interaction between the therapist and patient which is on the free associative level, where derivatives are being generated by the patient's free associations that allow for symbolism, displacements, condensations, and the general atmosphere ordinarily considered analysis. Communicative field type

B consists of projective identification by the patient into the therapist, and/or by the therapist into the patient. Langs believes this to be characteristic of narcissistic difficulties on either side of the communication. He believes that the narcissistic aspects of the patient or therapist desire to evacuate mental contents rather than to accept and consider them for meaningful symbolic transformations. Field type C is conceived by him to be associations by the patient (and/or responses by the therapist) in which the material is meaningless and is deprived of meaningful symbolism and coded derivatives. In this situation something like an autistic redoubt, or bastion of an inadmissible me/not me interface, often arises in which the patient feels that the analyst cannot understand him and therefore has to resort to meaningless associations in a "pretend" analysis.

PERSONIFICATION OF DEFENSE AS A CHRONIC RESISTANCE

I alluded previously to the experience of anorectic patients who have split off a portion of their personality and idealized it to such a degree that the newly created structure becomes a formidable resistance. The phenomenon of splitting is very important in resistances, as is projective identification which — in its defensive form — seeks to further the work of splitting by translocating the unwanted cargo of feelings into an object for detoxification. Splitting may be of such intensity that a portion of the personality occupies a separate, dissociated existence, and, once given life, seems to fight for that life and create notable resistances to its resolution in analytic treatment. The following brief case vignette typifies this maneuver:

> The patient is a 42-year-old married physician, father of two children, who has been in treatment for three years. When he first entered analytic treatment he was suffering from an overt manic psychosis. Relevant background material is as follows: He is the eldest of three children in a family where mother suffered from manic-depressive psychotic episodes, was frequently hospitalized, had electric shock treatments, and seemed to suffer from a moderate character deterioration from her illnesses. His father was experienced as a passive, submissive parent who could not help the patient from being "devoured" by the mother's psychosis.

In the course of the analysis a psychotic grandiose self clearly emerged which had "Nazi-like" features in terms of its ruthlessly sadistic fantasies. As the analysis progressed, it became clear that this maniacal self was erected as a veritable clone of his mother's manic self and was employed to defend against being importuned by her. It was also employed to triumph over his father, for whom he held great contempt because of his passivity. As the analysis was able to define and differentiate this self from his normal, dependent self, a battle characterized by great resistances developed. Synoptically, this portion of the personality was constructed as a manic defense to defend against the fear of being unprotected in a psychotic household. In its extremes, however, it seemed to propel the patient to great success in his profession but then became excessive in its demands upon him. A risky geographic move was transacted from one part of the country to the other as one consequence. Once he and I were able to isolate and confront these excesses of personality, his manic self began to fight back in many different ways. The patient would flood me with a torrent of loose associations, attack my way of saying things to him, interrupt me when I was offering interpretations, inconsequentialize the interpretations I offered, and generally conduct "the real analysis" in between sessions under the premise that he was a much better analyst for himself than I.

It slowly emerged that the psychotic portion of his personality was not only an identification with the feared mother, but was also a desperate ploy on his part to ward off catastrophe, as previously mentioned. Further, however, it appeared that this portion of the personality, once given life, was fighting to maintain itself and "had a right to live." A breakthrough came when the patient, in discussing a cancer in one of *his* patients, realized that cancer is like another organism within his patient which also fights for its life under the premise that it has a right to survive.

Personification consequently can be considered as an aspect of splitting and projective identification that devolves into the inner experience of being haunted and controlled by alien selves that seem to have omnipotent control and power of attorney over the will of the hapless patient, whose "innocent," helpless, dependent self is seemingly held hostage within its powerful snare. This configuration also is true for addictive illness as well as for chronic depression. I have seen patients suffering from chronic depressive illness who seemed addicted to their depression and who would ultimately reveal that they were experiencing their depression as a split-off internal persona that was fighting for its own life and that feared the patient having any link with hope, progress, and happiness. I have termed this depressive persona the "Madonna of Sorrows." It is experienced as an autistic self-mother who pities and soothes the narcissistic patient in the presence of ill-treatment by others and in the presence of an unhappy life generally.

At first, therefore, resistance seems to emerge ambiguously as a friendly defense against unbearable mental pain, but later as a formidable obstacle interposed between the agonized self and attempts on the part of the therapist to come to its rescue. On the one hand, the chronic resistance can be thought of as a mechanism, but on the other hand, as a constant companion, a veritable twin self that has stood by the hapless patient through thick and thin, knows the patient best, is his or her best and most trustworthy counselor, and is certainly senior in its role as adviser to the patient. I recall a schizophrenic patient who revealed early on in his analysis that he was guided in most of his ventures in life by "the Advisor," an imaginary companion whom he had had with him since earliest childhood and who continued up through much of the analysis before finally disappearing. The Advisor seemed at times to be my most implacable enemy and always warned the patient that I was not to be trusted since my purpose was to replace him as the patient's principal consultant.

RESISTANCES

Cult Allegiance

I have just described pesonification as a defense but should like to approach this same defense from a different perspective, that of cult allegiance. Cath (1982) has written about the power of cult allegiance as a group resistance in adolescents. One can readily observe the phenomenon of deep bonds of loyalty that many people experience in a group, and how this loyalty becomes focused on a belief system that each member of the group holds in common. The belief system then becomes the organizer of a defense of its continuity, and, simultaneously, of a resistance to any new ideas which threaten it. Bion (1961, 1970) has explored this phenomenon as the group manifestation of the fear of catastrophic change by the container — the Establishment.

Within individuals as well as within groups, however, one frequently begins to realize (often from dreams particularly) that the patient seems to resist progress out of a powerful loyalty to what appears to be an internal family, group, or powerful personages. To get well is equated with disloyalty, disobedience, and a forswearing of vows of eternal bonding (actually bondage) with that highly prized and esteemed group or object; the latter is then believed to either perish or to become dangerously persecutory.

ENCAPSULATION AND CONFUSION

Tustin (1981), in her 30-year study of her analyses of psychotic children, has divided her cases into *encapsulated* and *confusional* categories to indicate the primary nature of the defensive maneuver used to defend against the impingement of the external world. The encapsulated category connotes a walling-off of the embattled self, and the confusion category implies an intertwining with the object. Both maneuvers are designed to defend against the awareness of a premature abruption of primary "at-one-ment," that is, a premature disruption of the narcissistic shield of maternal attachment. Tustin's categories can be viewed as underlying common denominators in all defensive and resistance maneuvers insofar as they address the issues of polarization of defense through encapsulation and distancing of the "not-me" mother, on the one hand, and, on the other, of the inability to defend against the "not-me" mother and therefore being predisposed to an engulfment and incorporation into her substance, in which case the identity of the self seems to one degree or another to vanish. Anorectic patients, as previously stated, seem to personify their encapsulated resistances as autistically protective selves. One finds this maneuver generally in patients who are predisposed toward obsessive-compulsive illnesses, phobias, paranoia, and narcissistic personality disorders. Alternatively, the confusional defense can be seen in hysteria, borderline illness, depression, and in other categories. Personification characterizes the inner experience of the defensive twin in the case of encapsulation whereas, in the confusional case, personification is experienced in terms of the object into whom one has projected oneself for protection — and with whom one has become inextricably bound.

AUTOPOIESIS AND ITS RELATIONSHIP TO RESISTANCE

Recently, Maturana and Varela (1982) have created the concept of autopoiesis to dignify the ultimately indefinable nature of living substances. They espouse the notion that every living entity, whether a cell, a plant, an animal, or a human being, a culture, or a civilization, corresponds to the conception of autopoiesis on each layer of abstraction. Autopoiesis thus seems to imply that every level of living tissue comprises an entity unto itself, seems to have its own "cognition," and is unknowable to its beholder—the beholder being ourselves as scientists who are trying to observe its nature. As a matter of fact, they believe that all we can do as scientists *is* to observe the behavior of living entities and infer conclusions, which, because of our own nature, we must borrow from our preconceptions so as to adduce the nature of our specimen.

The implications that the concept of autopoiesis have for psychoanalysis can only be hinted at, but in terms of its application to the concept of resistance perhaps one can conclude that resistance can be considered as an autopoietic entity that, having "coupled" with the primary autopoietic self as its "client," now becomes a formidable, "living" phantom which fights for its own autopoietic destiny.

RESISTANCE AS A SEMIOTIC

There is another orientation toward resistances in which the very display of resistance can be understood not as a barrier to treatment, but as a dramatic demonstration of a need of the patient that has not been recognized. Silence is a good example of this phenomenon. One often experiences patients who are silent for long periods of time. The first tendency as a therapist is to consider this as a blocking of associations and, as such, a resistance to treatment. Although that may very well be true, especially of neurotic patients, my own experience with narcissistic and other patients suffering from primitive mental disorders is that silence is a sign (semiotic) of a need which is being enacted by the patient because it cannot yet be clearly stated. The experience of silence is indicative of an unconscious need for a barrier, a second skin so to speak, a sense of protective privacy between the patient and the therapist so as to minimize the experience of being overwhelmed, penetrated, or engulfed by the therapist's knowledge of the patient. As one patient told me, "I'm afraid you're going to know me all up!"

CLASSIFICATION OF RESISTANCES OF NARCISSISTIC PATIENTS

From what has been stated it can be generalized that narcissistic patients present resistances in analysis which may *seem* to be impediments to the treatment but can, from another point of view, be understood as semiotic revelations of states of unfulfilled needs, fears, and awarenesses of dangers. From Fairbairn's point of view, and by extension, the points of view of the British Object Relations School, the patient may institute defenses which emerge as a consequence of his belief that his love is bad and therefore is predisposed towards mortification in the transference. This leads to a schizoid defense characterized by a withdrawal into an inner self and the replacement of an outer self as a false self (Winnicott 1965). If the patient believes his hate is bad, then a depressive concern takes place in which the patient internalizes his destructive self and identifies with an internalized rejecting object that oversees an internalized sado-masochistic relationship of eternal penance and contrition.

Fairbairn (1952) characterizes the schizoid and depressive positions as states of infantile dependence. They are developmentally followed by a transitional stage which is characterized by neurotic defenses or techniques that help to keep the split-off parts of self and objects separated. They are the obsessive, paranoid, hysterical, and phobic techniques. They serve to forestall the integration of the polarized objects and egos, a phenomenon which normally takes place when ambivalence can be tolerated in mature dependency.

Klein has hypothesized the paranoid-schizoid position and the depressive position. The first is characterized by persecutory anxiety and the latter by depressive anxiety. The schizoid mechanisms of splitting, projective identification, idealization, and magic omnipotent denial, and the corresponding resistances resulting from them characterize this stage of development. Klein, unlike Fairbairn, believed that destructiveness occurred earlier than the depressive position and therefore has to be split off and projected initially. The depressive position for Klein is the time in which the infant must "recall" his projected experiences so as to integrate them in the stage of ambivalence. The principal resistances emerging at the threshold of the depressive position are the manic defenses and the depressive defenses, the latter being the internalization of the paranoia from the paranoid-schizoid position so that it occupies the self as an internalized paranoid conflict.

Bick (1968) and Meltzer (1975), writing from the Kleinian point of view, have discovered a stage of development earlier than the paranoid-schizoid position that has to do with the development of a skin boundary surface, the failure to achieve which is manifested by "adhesive identification." Perhaps we can see that the failure to develop the experience of a sufficient skin boundary surface as a legacy from the intrauterine environment, and from the postnatal maternal environment, predisposes such infants to a lack of confidence in their capacity to be self-contained, to be able to define themselves between inside and outside, and to withstand difficulties in the external world. Tustin's conception of encapsulation and confusion fall in this category.

Bion (1970) suggested that the postures of resistance can be classified as (1) autistic, (2) symbiotic, and (3) commensal. By autistic, he means all the defensive maneuvers, from schizoid withdrawal to a cursory reconstitution of an altered internal world. By symbiotic, he means those defenses and resistances that emerge at a stage where the infant (and the patient evolving from this infant) experiences himself as being partially separated and partially nonseparated from the object. This experience can be visualized as a Siamese twinship where the separate heads represent separation and the fused body represents the continuation of primary at-one-ment. The defensive struggles against one's self of inner badness, and/or the badness of the object would correspond to this phase of development. Narcissistic resistances per se therefore occupy the autistic and symbiotic levels. Klein's depressive position (though not Fairbairn's) ushers in the awareness of separateness from the object and the allowance for the object's separate agenda. At the same time, there is the institutionalization of cosubjectivity in which the self *and* mother are each subjects in their own right.

The term *commensal* has been employed by Bion (1970) to designate a stage of development and of object relationships in which two separate groups can live in harmony without affecting one another. I think this term can be used to indicate the defenses and resistances of the so-called normal patient whose perception of the external world seems to be relatively clear and unobtruded. The resistances he develops in analysis would be those that are temporary, reasonable, and appropriate in view of the fact that the patient is embarking on a most intimate journey with a stranger who can never truly be totally trusted with such intimacy.

RESISTANCE AND THE REPRESSIVE BARRIER

When Freud (1915) further defined the concept of repression, he referred to the repressive barrier and also to the primal repression of aspects of the unconscious that have never and shall never become conscious. Thus, the repressive barrier seems to be a construct which separates two important systems from each other. The repressive barrier has been considered a defense for the ego against irruptions from the id. In a recent communication I have suggested that the id and ego are two separate systems of consciousness that process the data of experience from separate vantage points, are complementary, normally cooperative, and are not necessarily dialectical (Grotstein 1982). In this newer scheme the repressive barrier would defend the id (and the unconscious generally by extension) from the ego, as well as the reverse. There seems to be a necessity for a protective interface between systems that function from different points of view so as to allow for their individual autonomy, and to permit selective cooperation between them across a "gating" membrane that allows "cross cuing." Over the years psychotherapists have generally observed that dreams, for instance, become more complex and recondite as the analysis progresses and as dreams specifically are subjected to analysis. What this phenomenon suggests is that mental systems seem to function in "privacy" and to react defensively to any attempt to breach their protective boundaries. It is as if every attempt to analyze a dream trespasses on the dream membrane. The same phenomenon might take place when therapists seek to analyze the personality of a patient generally. Thus resistances can be thought of not only as the patient's obstinacy in resisting analysis, but also as an instinctive tendency on the part of his component systems to maintain their pristine integrity. The cooperative venture which ensues in a therapeutic alliance in analysis should not deceive us into a false sense of security that analysis is only benevolent. More research needs to be done on the ultimate instigation of resistance as a necessary protection.

CLASSIFICATION OF RESISTANCES

Klein, Fairbairn, Balint, and Winnicott considered resistances to be due to the infant aspect of the patient instituting resistances to the treatment because of a fear of a dependent object relations to the analyst. Bowlby and Winnicott later spoke of attachment behavior, bonding, and the mother–infant unit. Resistances emerging from this latter paradigm can be thought of in ways significantly different from the separate-infant paradigm. The phenomenon of envy, and its role in instigating analytic resistances, can be seen as a case in point. The Kleinian patient experiences envy because of his hatred of a dependency relationship on a "breast-mother" because of the fear of the power and authority of her goodness in contrast to the littleness and helplessness of the infantile, dependent aspects of the patient. In the attachment paradigm, in contrast, one can view the relationship between the infant and the mother, and by extension the analyst and the patient, as that of a team. In this team the mother and infant have equal status and are intimately cooperating with one another.

The infant's experience of dependency finds its counterpart in mother's total protective concern. Envy in this situation would be experienced by the infant–patient as a breach in this experience of attachment, whether by maternal deviation or neglect, or by physiological or idosyncratic irruptions from the infant. A disturbance in the function of the team would therefore be one in which an affective Siamese twinship disintegrates into two "divorced" partners where the more dependent one, the infant–patient, experiences the humiliation of being left alone and out of the team with his dependency needs. Langs's (1981) conception of communicative resistances closely approximates this newer one of attachment resistances.

REFERENCES

Balint, M. (1968). *The Basic Fault*. London: Tavistock.
Baranger, W., and Baranger, M. (1966). Insight in the analytic situations. In *Psychoanalysis in the Americas*, ed. R. Litman, pp. 56–72. New York: International Universities Press.

Bick, E. (1968). The experience of the skin in early object relations. *International Journal of Psycho-Analysis* 49:484–486.

Bion, W.R. (1959). Attacks on linking. In *Second Thoughts*, pp. 93–109. London: Heinemann, 1967.

―――― (1961). *Experiences in Groups*. London: Tavistock.

―――― (1965). *Transformations*. London: Heinemann.

―――― (1966). Catastrophic change. *Bulletin of the British Psycho-Analytic Society* 5.

―――― (1970). *Attention and Interpretation*. London: Tavistock.

Bowlby, J. (1969). *Attachment and Loss*. Vol. 1. *Attachment*. New York: Basic Books.

―――― (1973). *Attachment and Loss*. Vol. 2. *Separation*. New York: Basic Books.

―――― (1980). *Attachment and Loss*. Vol. 3. *Loss, Sadness, and Depression*. New York: Basic Books.

Cath, S.H. (1982). Adolescence and addiction to alternative belief systems: psychoanalytic and psychophysiological considerations. *Psychoanalytic Inquiry*. Issue on Adolescent Addition: Varieties and Vicissitudes. 2: 619–676.

Fairbairn, W.R.D. (1952). *Psychoanalytic Studies of the Personality. The Object Relations Theory of Personality*. London: Tavistock.

Freud, S. (1914). On narcissism: an introduction. *Standard Edition* 14:67–104.

―――― (1915a). Mourning and melancholia. *Standard Edition* 14:237–258.

―――― (1915b). Repression. *Standard Edition* 14:141–158.

―――― (1917). Libido theory and narcissism. *Standard Edition* 16:412–430.

Grotstein, J.S. (1982). The dual-track theorem. Unpublished manuscript.

Hamilton, V. (1982). *Narcissus and Oedipus*. London: Routledge, Kegan Paul.

Hartmann, H. (1958). *Ego Psychology and the Problem of Adaptation*. New York: International Universities Press.

―――― (1964). *Essays on Ego Psychology*. New York: International Universities Press.

Jacobson, E. (1964). *The Self and the Object World*. New York: International Universities Press.

Kernberg, O. (1976). *Object Relations Theory and Clinical Psychoanalysis*. New York: Jason Aronson.

Khan, M.M.R. (1974). *The Privacy of the Self*. New York: International Universities Press.

Klein, M. (1932). *The Psycho-Analysis of Children*. Trans. Alix Strachey. London: Hogarth Press, 1959.

―――― (1950). *Contributions to Psycho-Analysis 1921–1945*. London: Hogarth Press.

―――― (1960). *Narrative of a Child Analysis*. New York: Basic Books.

Kohut, H. (1966). Forms and transformations of narcissism. *Journal of the American Psychoanalytic Association* 14:243–272.

———— (1971). *The Analysis of the Self.* New York: International Universities Press.

———— (1977). *The Restoration of the Self.* New York: International Universities Press.

Langs, R. (1981). *Resistances and Interventions.* New York: Jason Aronson.

Meltzer, D. (1975). Adhesive identification. *Contemporary Psychoanalysis* 11: 289–310.

Maturana, H., and Varela, F. (1982). *Autopoiesis and Cognition: The Realization of the Living.* Boston: D. Reidel.

Sandler, J., and Joffe, W.G. (1969). Towards a basic psychoanalytic model. *International Journal of Psycho-Analysis* 50:79–90.

Tustin, F. (1981). *Autistic States in Children.* London: Routledge, Kegan Paul.

Winnicott, D.W. (1958). *Collected Papers.* New York: Basic Books.

———— (1965). *The Maturational Processes and the Facilitating Environment.* New York: International Universities Press.

———— (1971). *Playing and Reality.* London: Tavistock.

Wisdom, J.O. (1961). A methodological approach to the problem of hysteria. *The International Journal of Psycho-Analysis* 42:224–237.

CHAPTER 15

Resistance of the Borderline Patient with a False Self

James F. Masterson

Developmental (Mahler 1965, 1968) object-relations theory (Jacobson 1964; Kernberg 1975; Masterson 1972, 1976), which led to a better understanding of the borderline patient, perhaps inevitably did not adequately emphasize the narcissistic psychopathology of such patients.

I began to redress this imbalance in my own perspective with a review of the concept of the false self described by Winnicott (1965). Although Winnicott's clinical descriptions of the syndrome are clear and informative, he did not offer any overarching abstract or theoretical generalizations that would make it possible to apply his observations more widely.

I used this work as a jumping-off point to: (1) reassess his views in the light of subsequent research; (2) devise a crude clinical classification of the narcissistic psychopathology of the borderline (of which the false self was one part); and (3) offer a developmental object-relations theory of the false self that would be useful for treatment. This material, presented in detail elsewhere (Masterson 1981), will be briefly summarized as a prelude to considering the unique qualities of the resistance shown by the borderline patient with a false self.

NARCISSISTIC PSYCHOPATHOLOGY OF THE BORDERLINE

The narcissistic psychopathology of the borderline consists of a collection of complaints that are more or less loosely related to self-expression or individuation. Patients' complaints range from an inability to identify their own individuative thoughts, wishes, and feelings to all degrees of inhibitions and difficulties in activating and implementing those thoughts and wishes reflective of individuation that they can identify. There is always an associated difficulty with self-assertion and a distorted self-image related to a difficulty in autonomously regulating self-esteem. These complaints do not exist in a vacuum, of course, but are presented along with the patient's other complaints such as depression and difficulty with relationships.

A clinical spectrum may be devised showing the degree of self-image distortion, from no self-image at the one end, through false self-image in the middle, to poor self-image at the other end.

"No self-image" refers to those patients whose motivations and behavior were so completely dominated by the need to cling to the object to suppress individuation that few individuative stimuli could break through. Those stimuli that did break through, occasioned great anxiety. The patients were quite unaware of this state of affairs until the need for the clinging defense had been sufficiently reduced and stunted individuation could resume. At this point, they would describe themselves as having been "caretakers of the mother," and as "not being a person" or having "no self."

The false self, although less serious in degree than the no-self image, still reflects severe impairment. It represents a collection of behaviors, thoughts, and feelings that are motivated by the need to cling to the object, with avoidance and suppression of individuative stimuli. The patient comes to identify this pattern as his self, and these encrustations can become so complex that it may not be recognized until well into treatment that it is a false self or collection of defensive behaviors rather than an expression of the true individuated self. As a matter of fact, as some patients improve in treatment, they go through an identity crisis as they begin to lose their false façade and react as if they were losing their true individuated self.

The poor self-image is the least severe of the three conditions, as the patient is aware of and able to report on his poor self-image, his difficulty in articulating his wishes and feelings in reality, and his difficulty with self-assertion. For example, a 21-year-old male, who chose economics as a major in college out of desperation because he was unable to decide what he wanted to do, recently graduated and found himself in the same quandary when it came to getting a job. He articulated clearly his desperation, and his avoidance of this difficulty throughout high school and college by drifting and taking drugs, and by his passivity and reticence about self-assertion.

We can now add this additional vector to the psychopathology of the borderline patient: the self-image distortion and the difficulty in identifying and activating individuative thoughts, wishes, and feelings into reality, and the difficulty with self-assertion. This aspect of the borderline psychopathology was implied in my use of the phrase "a failure to individuate," but its importance was overshadowed by the abandonment depression and the ego and superego fixation. To these must now be added and equally emphasized the parallel failures of self-expression.

A DEVELOPMENTAL OBJECT RELATIONS THEORY

Developmental object relations theory provides a framework for understanding one of the roots that contributes to the development of normal self-expression and some of the later difficulties that can arise as a result of impairments in that root. The base would be the self-representation which emerges from the fused symbiotic self-object representation of the dual mother/child unit as the child passes through the symbiotic phase (3–18 months), through the stages of separation-individuation (18–36 months), to the stage of on-the-way-to-object-constancy (36 months plus).

This emergence of the self occurs probably under the influence of: (1) genetic drives, (2) pleasure in the mastery of new functions, and (3) mother's appropriate cuing and matching to the child's individuation. As the child becomes a toddler and develops the capacity to separate from the mother, the task of separation-individuation ensues during the time that the child develops an image of himself as separate from the mother. This emerges first as two part-images—a good-self and a bad-self representation—which then coalesce into a whole self-representation of both good and bad.

During the rapprochement stage of this process, as a result of phase-appropriate and graduated exposure to frustration and disappointment, the child loses the grandiose image of the self and the omnipotent image of the object-representation preparatory to moving toward whole self- and whole object-representations. In the course of this evolution toward an autonomous self, the child develops a whole self-image (both good and bad), about which he feels adequate esteem, that is based partly but importantly on the achievement of the capacity to utilize self-assertion to identify and activate in reality his own individuative thoughts, wishes, and feelings.

The difficulties with self-expression in the borderline patient are revealed in psychotherapy as being due to the need to avoid the identifying and activating of individuated thoughts and wishes in order to defend against the abandonment depression that such activation would trigger. This sacrifice of self-expression to defense adds an additional negative increment to the already negative self part-image of the borderline patient as a result of the operation of the withdrawing object-relations part-unit (WORU) (Masterson 1976), the experience of the withdrawal of supplies from the maternal object at signs of self-expression.

To compensate for the fact that self-expression is not available for motivation, the patient turns instead to his rewarding object-relations part-unit (RORU) pathologic ego alliance (Masterson 1976) that, while providing him with a defense against the abandonment depression, also provides him with responses to deal with the environment, in other words, a form of adaptation. As these patterns become familiar, stereotyped, and repetitive the patient identifies them as his self. But it is a false self based on a need for a form of adaptation that provides a defense against individuation, rather than one which is an expression of the solutions arrived at by the dynamic experiment and interplay between the evolving individuating self and the environment.

RESISTANCE TO PSYCHOTHERAPY

The resistance to psychoanalytic psychotherapy shown by patients with a false self has a unique tenaciousness which springs from the intensity of their emotional investment in the RORU–pathologic ego alliance to defend against the WORU that is triggered by moves toward individuation. This is further complicated by the fact that they have elevated this defense to a sense of personal identity in the image of the false self.

In psychotherapy we seem to see in microcosm (in the patient's transference acting out) a condensed repetition of the early interactions with the mother. As a child, the patient presumably so incorporated or identified with the expectations of the maternal projections that any filtering through an emerging self-representation was precluded. Thus, the patient's object representations become almost literal replicas of those early expectations that were not altered or modified by further development and interaction with reality, as occurs in normal development. This replica of part object-representations contained both the maternal demands for compliance and the hostility to any separation-individuation.

It is as if, when the self began to emerge from the object, the amount of anxiety and depression experienced was so intense that the infant inhibited and/or gave up the emotional investment of the self-representation as a base for motivation and turned instead to the demands of the object-representation to fill the gap. These patients' experience of an empty self-representation gives a unique flavor of added intensity to their abandonment depression.

The thrust of psychotherapy revives the ashes of this lost battle and becomes a symbol of separation-individuation, as the therapist confronts the patient's RORU-pathological ego defenses. The patient's efforts to grow in psychotherapy now fall prey to all the defenses which he developed originally against the depression associated with his individuation. These are now turned against the work of treatment and become resistances.

The RORU–pathologic ego alliance is in the transference, acted out in therapy through clinging that can be both subtle and pervasive. As the patient moves deeper into treatment, and his clinging to the therapist is confronted more and more, the RORU–pathologic ego resistance now shifts from clinging to the therapist to seeking an opportunity tunity for defense elsewhere, mainly through clinging relationships in the patient's life. The patient now titrates the amount of depression evoked by the therapy, the more the patient acts out through clinging in the outside relationship to relieve it.

The false-self patient is like a chameleon; he is tempted to repeat with the therapist the same defense he erected earlier with the mother (that is, to completely forego or drop his individuation) by sabotaging psychotherapy and incorporating or swallowing whole what he can perceive of the therapist's expectations as a new but equally foreign model to use both for defense against internal anxiety and depression and adaptation to the external world.

The therapist must be careful to avoid conveying by tone, word, or deed any therapeutic expectation other than that expressed by the patient himself; otherwise the therapist can be seduced into resonating with the patient's projections. Of course, to a certain extent this will happen anyway; it is most important that the therapist be on guard against giving the patient fodder for his projections.

CASE ILLUSTRATIONS

Three case illustrations are presented. The first patient, a professional man in his fifties, had had two periods of analysis (of four and nine years, respectively) on the basis of the false self. His identification of his self with the negative, attacking projection of the WORU was so complete that his own individuative stirrings produced mainly anger and counterattack. It was as if he had an internal saboteur in his psyche with whom he was unwittingly colluding. His initial resistance was the transference acting out of the RORU–pathologic ego alliance through clinging or regressive behavior. When these were confronted and his regressive behavior disappeared, his abandonment depression did not emerge as might have been expected. It soon became clear that he was now defending against its emergence by clinging and acting out with his wife. When this was brought under therapeutic control, an intense intrapsychic struggle ensued during which he fought the identification of the feelings of depression and the memories that were emerging. Only emphatic confrontation with the manner in which he colluded with this internal saboteur allowed him to identify, contain, and work through the depression.

The second patient, a young woman, initially transference acted out the RORU–pathologic ego alliance. Confrontation then activated the WORU–pathologic ego alliance, which was also acted out in the transference. After several years of treatment, as the tranference acting-out of both the RORU and WORU–pathologic ego alliance were beginning to be controlled, and the patient's abandonment depression was just beginning to be contained and to make its presence felt, she suddenly and impulsively flung herself into "instant intimacy" with a narcissistic man who required her to forego her self-interest and mirror him. Concurrently, the emerging abandonment depression disappeared from the content of the interviews. She now projected and acted out the RORU on the man and the WORU on me, the therapist, thereby restoring the original defensive balance that had been interrupted by the progress in her treatment. Instead of alternately acting out the RORU and WORU on me, she now projected the former onto the boyfriend and the latter onto me. Another year of therapy helped her to be less self-destructive in the relationship and to gain some intellectual insight into her defenses. However, the integrity of her defenses remained intact, and she was not able to begin to work through her abandonment depression.

The third case is of a young married woman who transference acted out by clinging in the interviews, and with her husband, at great cost to her individuation. After ten years of therapy, as she gave up the clinging and became self-assertive for the first time in her life, she decided to leave her narcissistic husband. However, rather than contain and start to work through her abandonment depression in interviews after she left her husband, she immediately plunged into a frenetic round of sexual acting out, despite and partially because of the fact that her prior sexual life had been minimal. The sexual acting-out was characterized by sex without relationships. Over a period of months, it became clear that the sexual acting-out was based on the same clinging defense she had had with her husband, that is, they both revolved around a deep and pervasive RORU fantasy of: "They want me; I want to be wanted; I don't want me, but they do." When she left her husband she could not contain and face the abandonment depression, so she continued to act out the RORU defense through the sexual relationships and the depression could not emerge.

Case History

A brief summary of the case history is followed by a more detailed presentation of the therapeutic interaction in order to demonstrate the clinical manifestations, the psychodynamics of the resistance and the management. It should be understood that a great deal has been left out to highlight the points of this paper.

The patient, a 50-year-old married writer, came for evaluation of a depression. He had had two periods of analysis based on the false self, the first for four years in his twenties, and the second for nine years in his thirties. He felt despairing and suicidal and was on antidepressants which were not relieving his depression. He reported quite unconsciously but quite accurately: "I am caught between reluctance and pain." He was in his second marriage, had had two children by the first wife, and two by the second. The children all seemed to be doing fairly well, but he was in a more or less continual state of conflict with his wife and felt disappointed and disillusioned with what was realistically considerable success in his profession.

History. He was the first of three children, with a brother and a sister many years younger. He came from the South and described his father as a businessman who had recurrent business failures, was extremely self-centered, was uninterested in him, spent large amounts of time away from home, and was also in constant conflict with the patient's mother. The patient described his mother as demanding, clinging, depressed, and empty, and requiring him to fill in for the absence of the father, although she preferred both the brother and the sister to him. He described himself as being a "good boy." "They never had any trouble with me; I never stepped out of line." The home, he felt, was pervaded with an atmosphere of doom and gloom. He recalled no depression until a move to another city in the third grade when he lost interest in school and his marks went down. He also lost interest in friends and spent all his time sitting around the house. He felt he was rescued in the next grade (fourth) by a teacher who took an interest in him. Thereafter he did quite well in high school, college, and graduate school.

It is striking years later to look back on his initial interview and see how clearly he described his borderline dilemma without any conscious awareness of its significance; for example, his statements that he was caught between reluctance and pain, and was worried about his potential for self-destructive acts, as well as for running away from challenges and taking the easy way out.

The Psychotherapy. The clinical false self of this patient—those external behaviors which were evidence of the rewarding unit pathological ego's defense against the withdrawing unit—was subtle, complicated, and difficult to clearly identify. He had had so much treatment, and as a writer could intellectualize so readily, that he presented an excellent and seemingly convincing intellectual façade. However, over a period of months it became clear — by virtue of the absence of any disturbed affect in the sessions, as well as his inability to assert himself or disagree with me — that he was projecting the omnipotent, rewarding unit onto me and clinging in order to relieve the depression. Thus his initial resistance was transference acting out of the rewarding-unit pathologic-ego alliance in treatment, where he would expect me to direct him, to ask questions, and to take the lead in the investigation, and where he would avoid self-expression and taking responsibility for presenting his thoughts and feelings himself. Confrontation of the destructiveness of this behavior to his therapeutic objectives made him aware that both of his prior analyses had been conducted on this basis. It also demonstrated the difficulties he had with individuation. As he tried to bring to the sessions his thoughts and feelings without clinging, he would block, project, go back to clinging; and over a period of months, a struggle ensued between taking responsibility for sessions and clinging, that is, between individuation and defense.

As he began to get some control over this defense and become more self-expressive in the interviews and in his life, the expected deepening of the abandonment depression did not occur. The reason why soon became apparent. His reports of conflicts with his wife revealed that he tolerated without objection her hostile, inappropriate criticism of his self-expression. When I questioned why he permitted her to be so disparaging and demeaning, he replied that she was simply expressing how he felt about himself, that is, he was incompetent, no good, guilty, and inadequate. It seemed that he did not get more depressed at this point because the withdrawing unit, against which the rewarding unit was a defense, was not internalized and contained but was projected upon his wife. He even provoked her to play the part, to be disparaging, while he acted out the self-representation of the withdrawing unit: he was bad, incompetent, no good. The abandonment depression was not contained and thus could not be experienced internally; it was not available to analysis.

It became necessary to confront the projection of the withdrawing unit onto the wife, and the destructiveness of his compliance with her to his own individuation, in order to enable him to withdraw the projection and contain the depression so that it might be accessible to analysis. Another struggle ensued characterized by confrontation, some efforts at control, some depression, then avoidance, blocking, resistance, further confrontation, and so forth. Slowly, over a period of many months, his control of his compliant behavior gradually improved. His wife's negative, hostile attitude diminished to a great extent, and he became much more self-assertive in his environment as well as in sessions. And as he did so, as expected, the abandonment depression deepened.

Again, however, another defense took over. There was a complete identification of the withdrawing self with the negative projections; that is, the hostile, attacking attitudes of the withdrawing object-relations part-unit to his separation-individuation seemed a reality. These were facts that had to be accepted, not feelings to be analyzed. This emerged as follows: After a discussion of some new writing he had done, he mentioned that I seemed to have had a positive attitude toward his efforts which helped him cope with his own negative self-image. He then reported a dream in which he was in a strange city and felt free, could be on his own, set his own hours, be unhurried and unpressured. His free association was: "It's the opposite of my pressured life. It's the ability to be free and on my own, but I feel that free time is bad news and will get me into trouble. The whole idea of self-expression, being free is like opening the gates of a prison. I feel I'm afraid I'll go out of control, succumbing 'to my own wishes'."

In other words, his identification with the projections of the withdrawing unit impelled him to see his own individuation as evil, bad, and wrong. He continued that to him fun was dangerous; he was both jailer and prisoner, and he kept himself under tight control because letting go brought such enormous anxiety, that is, was so dangerous. He was a toiler or a laborer in life, and many of his so-called choices in life were not choices at all but a result of what he felt was expected.

Again, one might have expected that this setting of limits to his withdrawing-unit projections on reality might have promoted their containment and led to further working through, but instead a new defense of detachment of affect emerged. He reported functioning very well but being very depressed and preoccupied with death without any idea why. At the same time in interviews he appeared to be avoiding efforts to understand why, and he reported feeling detached. I confronted him with the fact that it seemed to me he was trying to individuate without separating; in other words, to be self-expressive without being in touch with or following through with the thoughts and feelings this behavior evoked.

This overcame the avoidance and detachment and led to a marked increase in his depression and massive feelings of hopelessness: "The better things go, the worse I feel." And although he still tended to identify with the negative projections, he now began to question that identification: "Why is it that I can't get to this problem in my head? Why can't I free myself from my parents?" He then reported that he was both anxious and angry that people's demands on him were preventing him from getting where he wanted to be in treatment.

I now interpreted what we came to call "the saboteur" inside him that was so deceptive. I questioned whether his anger was actually due to people's demands interfering with his self-expression, because it was quite clear that at the moment it was not other people who were interfering in his self-expression but rather himself. He was actually avoiding self-expression in interviews, using other people as a smoke screen and rationalization to keep the truth from coming to light in the session. The saboteur who had been in charge for so many years was angry at me and the therapy for interfering with its control and was expressing itself in this manner to deceive both of us. This seemed to do the trick, as there now followed a series of sessions where he was aware of the saboteur, the withdrawing unit, and its projections: "I feel paralyzed; I'm losing the battle with the demons; I'm aware of how terribly poisonous, negative, hostile the controlling saboteur is inside of me, dreams I had as a kid about my mother's face leering and threatening; I used to wake up in terror and feel I needed an exorcist." This led to greater hopelessness: "Life's activities have been just to fill time, the saboteur has been running me, fantasies of having a coronary and dying, the saboteur is strangling me; it's like an alien has possession of me."

He apologized to me in the session for such disturbing feelings, which led to his childhood feeling of not being entitled to feel anything bad around his mother who would not tolerate it. The working through seemed to be consolidated as he had memories of depression in the third and fourth grade; of a feeling that no one cared, that he couldn't go on, that he had been immobilized. The working through was continued dramatically in the next session as he got closer and closer to the feeling of hopelessness he had experienced with his mother, that nothing made any difference with either of his parents, that he had had to be a good boy, that there had been no alternative.

He developed a profound wave of despair, a despair that he had always projected on his capacity to individuate but which he now became aware was his response to the feeling that he would never be able to get what he wanted from his mother, that is, support for separation-individuation. This led to the contemporary awareness that his fantasies about his relationships with women were basically motivated by the need to be taken care of. He wanted to be treated as his mother had not treated him. This working through triggered the saboteur, who made his presence known in the next session. The patient was angry, complaining about life being more difficult, taking too much effort, which I interpreted as the anger of the saboteur at being interfered with. I suggested the working through triggered the saboteur, who reacted by striking down the process and producing resistance. The patient now became fully aware that there were two people in him: the false, compliant self, eager to please, and the saboteur who was really in control with his own agenda for attacking the patient's individuation. He became acutely aware of how he had colluded with that agenda without being aware of it.

Case History

A professional woman in her mid-thirties complained of recurrent depression, difficulty in being alone and managing on her own, a need to be dependent on others, and difficulties with close relationships with men — either falling madly in love and giving up her own identity, or having to maintain too great a distance from them. She did not feel good about herself as a woman, nor did she trust men. She had had four years of psychotherapy twice a week in her early twenties, which "helped me somewhat to assert myself, but it did not change my problems." This was followed by three years of gestalt therapy.

Past and Family History. She described her mother as a professional woman who did not have feminine interests and who was quite overprotective. The mother had a very peculiar outlook on life, tending to direct and overwhelm the patient and, at the same time, indulging her by allowing her to stay home from school and to avoid normal childhood responsibilities. The mother was hospitalized with a psychosis for three months when she was 6. The father, also a professional man, was described as distant, removed, judgmental, critical, highly intellectualized, and a perfectionist. "He seemed to be more interested in his work than in either my mother or myself." The patient had a younger brother and sister, both of whom have serious emotional problems.

She described herself as "having been a good girl in school," doing well except for the fourth grade when she stopped for a third of the year because of her anxiety about conflicts with her friends. She saw a therapist for about six months at this time. She had enuresis until age 11. In adolescence she did well in school, but was isolated socially, and was shy and withdrawn with boys.

She went to college away from home where her shyness dramatically disappeared, and she threw herself into a series of intense emotional and sexual relationships, falling madly in love and then being rejected and feeling depressed. Graduation from college, where she did well academically, coincided with the breakup of a love affair and precipitated a depression, which brought her into treatment. Some time later she gave up treatment and the love relationship and traveled to another part of the country, living with a man for a year and a half, until he rejected her, whereupon she returned to New York City. In the last several years she had been living with a girlfriend and had had no close relationships with men.

The Psychotherapy.   The patient's first transference acted-out behavior was to project the rewarding unit (RORU) onto me, presenting her false self, behaving as an intellectualized little girl who was eager to please and comply with my expectations. However, she showed little or no genuine affect. She manipulated me to give her advice and directions and to provide various kinds of special exceptions for her. My confrontation of her need for these special activities immediately triggered the withdrawing part-unit (WORU), which was punitive, critical, and rigid almost to the point of being paranoid.

She expressed the negative self-image of the WORU by accusing me of being extremely critical, of putting her down, of not being interested in her, of considering her boring and not worth listening to. The issue of manipulation came to a head when she requested a postponement of payment of her bill, as her father had not yet given her the money. I pointed out that that arrangement was between her and her father and not between her and me and, therefore, that I would expect her to pay on time. She was asking me to take over her responsibility; she had to deal with her problems with her father.

This confrontation led to a furious outburst of anger. I was being greedy, rigid, and uncaring; all of her friends were in treatment, and many of them owed their therapists three or four months' worth of bills. By the end of the session, however, as her rage subsided and I questioned the reason for such anger and disappointment, she verbalized her wish to be special. This led to a history of similar maneuvers with her father in order to be special to him.

She freely admitted that this behavior was not spontaneous and self-expressive but was fabricated to get the desired response (the false self), that what she really felt about herself was that she was bad, ugly, disgusting, of no interest, hopeless, and helpless.

At the same time, I pointed out that whenever she expressed a spontaneous thought or feeling in a session (her true self), she would immediately either assume I was critical of it (projection of WORU), or she would adopt the most punitive, critical attitude possible toward her own thoughts and feelings. This patient was able to become aware of the feeling components of her WORU much more readily than the prior patient. In addition, her gross manipulatory acting out in the transference was much more obvious and therefore easier to identify and manage than the prior patient's vague intellectualizations. The self-image of the withdrawing unit now emerged further, with her feelings that her self was dull, vapid, empty.

I anticipated that her projection and acting out having been controlled, she might now begin to remember and revive some of the past history of this negative self-image with mother and father. Instead she presented a dream about rats lodging in her hair that frightened her and that she wanted to be rid of. Her associations led to the idea that the rat's nest was those early relationships with the mother and father that she had attempted to avoid by the transference acting-out.

She now defended against feeling by detachment, and intellectually remembered that her father had been punitive and critical and her mother flat and affectless. As a child she had spent a lot of time with her mother and had felt that she had to stimulate her mother in order to keep her from withdrawing. At the same time, her mother would infantilize her by letting her stay home from school and by not insisting that she take care of her room.

Part of the patient's compact with her psychotic mother had been to substitute the mother's psychotic perceptions of reality for her own reality in order to reinforce the symbiotic tie. This was reflected in treatment a number of times, when the patient insisted that whatever she felt was true objective reality: objective reality did not exist in its own right.

During one of these discussions, for example, she had described asking for another position at her place of work. Her supervisor felt that she was not yet qualified and refused to make the change. The patient was convinced that he did it because "he was out to get me." I suggested some other possibilities, such as that she might not, in fact, be qualified. She began to integrate this confrontation and then in the next session reported a dream: if she went along in any way with my perceptions, she would be attacked by the devil, that is, if she allowed any change in her perception of reality, it would interfere with the symbiotic tie and trigger the WORU, the devil.

As her intellectualized defenses were confronted, and as the intellectualizations and the manipulations to be special disappeared, the patient began to feel more depressed and angry, and the projection of the withdrawing unit onto the therapist became more consistent and more intense: "You do not encourage feeling here. I have no emotion; I can't do it myself; I feel I'm in a vacuum, that all the air has been sucked out."

She then had violent fantasies of destroying me, wanting to have a temper tantrum but not being able to, questioning why she had to do the treatment herself, saying that I was cold and uncaring and asking too much, that I was cruel and even sadistic, that she would like to hurt me as I was hurting her.

Her distorted perception that feeling was tantamount to objective reality was a defense against engulfment by the mother and then by the therapist, as well as reinforcement of the symbiotic compact with the mother to suspend her own reality perception in order to reinforce the symbiotic tie. As these defenses were confronted and the withdrawing-unit self-image began to emerge, her statement that she could not do it herself was a projection onto therapy from the original interaction.

The mother's libidinal unavailability made it impossible for the patient to individuate; this was then reinforced by the extremely negative images taken first from the mother and then condensed and combined with the critical father (that is, to forego self-expression in the service of complete incorporation of the mother's projections as her internalized object).

Feelings of helplessness and hopelessness about herself mounted. She became angry at me and the therapy: "You're intruding, forcing me to do something which is bad." She was crying, feeling that she was wallowing in these feelings, could drown in them, they could take her over, they might drive her crazy: "Real relationships have always been a mirage. There was so much disappointment, I don't want to go back to it again." She described herself in the most abject and derogatory terms and had dreams of being attacked by gorillas or dogs. She would report: "My whole identity is a defense against these bad feelings about myself. I cannot stand them. I cut off my feelings about myself and treat myself as a thing, an object. I cuff it around and allow it to be put down. I am an intellectual computer, very cold. I manipulate to get what I want rather than feel." At the same time she expressed the transference fear of abandonment, that if she allowed herself to go back to these bad feelings about herself with me, I would leave her.

The externalizing and acting out of the rewarding unit pathological ego in the transference having been confronted and contained, the patient was now beginning to experience and analyze the withdrawing unit (WORU). Throughout this period of about 18 months, she had not had any further relationships with men.

However, in the midst of this painful emotional state and on the weekend before the frequency of interviews was to be increased from two to three times a week to work through the abandonment depression, she suddenly and impulsively threw herself into "instant intimacy" with a man, spending the entire weekend with him and having sexual relations. As might be expected, the painful intrapsychic state disappeared as the withdrawing unit (WORU) again was handled by defensive acting out. Now, instead of projecting both part-units onto me, she was projecting and acting out the rewarding unit on the man, and the withdrawing unit on me. As I raised questions about the possible harmful effects of her need for instant intimacy, she felt I was attacking the relationship and nothing I could do would dissuade her. It soon became clear that the man involved was a narcissistic male who required her to forego her self in order to mirror him in the relationship. It was months before she was willing to reveal the degree to which she was throwing herself away in the relationship with him, not supporting her self, not pursuing her own self-interest, but clinging to him, as she had tried initially to cling to me in the therapy. During the next 18 months in treatment, she managed to learn how to assert herself more in the relationship, but the relationship persisted as a defense against the abandonment depression and withdrawing unit, and again she gained some intellectual notions of this, but it was not possible to work through any further.

Case History

The patient was a woman in her late twenties, married with three young children. Her husband was an extremely successful professional man. The chief complaint, rather typically, came not from her but from her husband, that she was sexually frigid. She and her husband had had practically no sexual relations in the last year, She felt no awareness of sexual desire but saw it as an obligation that she resented. When her husband suggested sex therapy, she complied but got so angry in the course of it that she stopped. At this point, she was referred for psychotherapy.

She stressed that as far as she was concerned, her whole life had been one of trying to please other people, that she always placed her husband first, that she was afraid that if people got to know her they would see her as a disaster. She felt that she married her husband because, unlike her father, he was so capable and so competent and could provide her with the image that she was unable to provide for herself. She denied her depression but said that she found life in general dull and boring, and said her only gratifications were from her children, whom she overindulged.

Past History and Family History. The patient's initial reports about her mother were ambivalent. She described her mother as "filling the house." She said her strongest motivation as a child was to do anything to please the mother in order to make up for the mother's disappointment with the father who was not competent and did not make enough money, and her disappointment with her son, who rebelled against the mother's self-centeredness and severe restrictions in the home.

She catered to the mother in every way, not only helping her around the house, but often helping her with her personal hygiene.

Her life revolved around being with the mother. At the same time, she reported that the mother was extremely selfish, did not care about her, did not want to know anything about her that was unpleasant, and would betray her confidences to friends. She said she found all of this quite humiliating.

The father was described as a milquetoast. The mother "did a good job on him," he had failed in business often, and the brother who was four years older was quite unhappy and frequently angry and rebellious in the home. For the first five years of her life, she and her family lived with the paternal grandmother, a woman with whom the patient always was and is in great conflict. The paternal grandmother also favored the brother and waited on the mother hand and foot. When the family moved into its own quarters, the father had business reversals, and the mother was always depressed.

The patient was never encouraged by either parent to achieve in school. Her schoolwork was mediocre, and her personality at school was a replica of that at home; she was happy, eager to please, and socially fairly active.

The patient met her husband in the second year of high school: "He was the only one who paid any attention to me. He was an outstanding achiever but also extremely self-centered." They courted throughout his college career and then got married, much too soon as far as her mother was concerned. The initial years of the marriage were filled with bickering and conflict. The children were unplanned and unwanted.

The Psychotherapy. As treatment began, the ubiquitous function of the patient's false self became quite clear in her relationships with her husband, her children, and her friends, as well as in her relationship with me. With her husband, she acted the role of the pleasing child for his approval, and when this could not penetrate his narcissism, she reacted with rage, projecting the withdrawing unit on him, and sessions were filled with complaints and rage at her husband and his self-centeredness, all the while denying the ways in which she failed to fulfill her responsibilities as a wife. Similarly, as a mother, she projected the rewarding unit onto one child and indulged it, and the withdrawing unit onto the other child and rejected it, at the cost of the development of both. The child to whom she clung developed phobic symptoms that gradually yielded after about a year of treatment.

At the same time, I was confronting her about her avoidance of her own responsibility as a wife with her husband, and as a mother with her daughter. There was a dramatic response with the daughter, for when the patient would respond to the confrontation about the daughter, she would retract the clinging. The daughter's phobia would then disappear.

The same did not occur, however, with the husband. Once the rewarding-unit projection was retracted, she would explode in rages, and it seemed impossible to get through the projections of the rage onto her husband. It was often necessary to make clear to her (without making any argument or brief for her husband) just how intense was her rage, as well as the ways in which she overlooked her failures as a wife. At the same time, she was becoming more and more aware of the conflict with her mother; she would have interactions with her in which she allowed the mother to put her down without any response. This would also occur with her friends. If her good-little-girl behavior did not meet with approval, she would get angry and depressed and say nothing. She began to confront both her husband and her mother with their rejecting behavior, but unfortunately always with an extreme of anger and projection onto the husband. The mother responded by social withdrawal, not speaking to her for weeks and months at a time. The husband came back with attacks about her failures, and eventually he entered psychotherapy himself.

The patient's rage increased, and her depression deepened, but this led not to any kind of working through but to a greater and greater awareness of her total lack of a sense of self, and to feelings of inadequacy and worthlessness. The sexual relationship deteriorated even further, and it became a difficult art to make clear to the patient the extreme projective nature of her rage with her husband, since his narcissistic behavior was such a perfect target for that rage. He was working all the time or sleeping and had little interest in or response to any of her emotional needs. For example, she would say: "We never did have a relationship except for me pleasing him," and her behavior with him amounted to being a slave or a servant. Although she would talk about feeling inadequate about herself, these feelings had a kind of artificial, intellectual quality to them.

As her last child reached school age, she decided to get a job to support herself. Around this point, about seven years into treatment, throughout which she had denied the awareness of any sexual stimuli or responsiveness in herself, she began to have sexual feelings with masturbation and particularly intense sexual fantasies about a member of their social group. These three events signified the slow beginning of the emergence of her true self. It occurred only in response to prolonged, repeated, emphatic confrontations about the degree to which she had permitted herself to be dumped on, the degree to which at all costs she had avoided activating herself to cope with and deal with her intrapsychic problems, as well as her problems with relationships.

She had a number of women friends who regaled her with stories of their sexual acting out. She was, as usual, a passive, detached, nonparticipant listener. She now became more involved in these tales, which reinforced her own sexual fantasies. She played with the idea of having an affair but rejected doing it. As the friction with her husband escalated, she finally acted out sexually at a weekend house party. On return, she was delighted with her first extramarital sexual experience. After a while I attempted to bring to her attention some of the hostility toward her husband that was expressed by the acting out but to no avail. Shortly thereafter, reassured by this episode that she could find other men, she impulsively decided to separate from her husband. She told him that she did not love him and never had, that there was no marriage, that they would be better off apart. My efforts to get her to understand the ramifications of this act were to no avail. The problem, in her view, was her husband. There were lots of other men around who were attracted to her; she would get rid of her husband and her life would be a lot better.

I anticipated that with the separation she might now contain her rage and depression in the interest of working through. However, no sooner did she separate than she impulsively threw herself into a wild spree of sexual acting out characterized by mechanical sex without relationships. She finally carried out the fantasized affair with the member of their social group, which led nowhere. At the same time, she had several other purely sexual relationships with men.

My confrontations met bitter resistance: I was somehow against sex or a prude, and was opposing her new-found sexual freedom. My observation that I thought the emergence of her sexuality was the only good thing coming out of this behavior and my invitations to explore its meaning further were constantly met by resistance. In addition, she denied all possible dangers and consequences of her actions, such as infection or pregnancy.

Finally, after a session of vigorous confrontation of the sexual acting out, she picked up a man in the waiting room and slept with him. The next day she sheepishly reported the event. This enabled me to voice my suspicion that sexual freedom and sexual expression were being used as a rationalization or smokescreen to hide what was really resistance to treatment. In other words, as she lost the one object to cling to, her husband, rather than contain and work through the depression in the sessions she acted out a defense, this time picking purely sexual relationships, rather than an emotional involvement, in order not to have to feel and experience her abandonment depression. She was doing the same thing now that she had with her husband; it was just a different kind of object.

She resisted this interpretation, but eventually the weight of the evidence and character of the men's destructive behavior with her became so obvious that she could no longer deny it. Gradually she cut in on the sexual acting out, and in one dramatic interview said:

> You're absolutely right. I am doing this with them for the exact same reason that I behaved as I did with my husband. I have a fantasy of them wanting me. I want to be wanted by somebody else, that is, by the object; I don't want me. I only have negative, hostile feelings toward myself, and I have to get feelings for myself from somebody else; and when I have to change myself, I don't want to do it. I only have negative feelings; there is no self to change. This fantasy of wanting to be wanted, rather than wanting myself, and the feeling that I do not have to do it myself but that someone else will rescue me is so basic and so deep that when anything you say in the session interferes with it, I just refuse to accept it. Either I argue with you, or I don't hear it, or I try to forget it as soon as possible. It's pathetic. It's as if I want the bad side of me to win. I feel that I am an inadequate, incompetent, unlovable, undeserving nothing. If I don't have somebody else to please in order to get approval, this is the way I feel about myself.

At this point in treatment, the abandonment depression was now being contained rather than defended against, the negative feelings of the withdrawing-unit self-image were contained and expressed. The quality of the interviews changed, the patient now became pervaded with feelings of despair, of inability and unwillingness to accept herself, and for the first time she began to recapture early memories:

> I stayed in touch with my feelings of unwantedness, not wanting my-self, and I got so anxious; it was almost like panic, a loneliness and a panic at the idea of managing myself. . . . My grandmother was the first experience of being unwanted. It all started with her, and I'd rather put my anger at my mother on me than on her. When I was a kid, I would do anything to be wanted. I can remember waking up feeling hopeless. I never got any response or attention for my self-expression. Mother took no pleasure in me, and Father didn't care—almost like a rat in a maze with no passageways open.

The patient exhaustedly stops defending against her abandonment de-pression and begins to reflect on its origins and development, that is, she begins to work through.

CONCLUSIONS

The therapeutic management of the resistances of the borderline pa-tient with a false self can be likened to that of dealing with the tentacles of an octopus: one no sooner gets one tentacle (resistance) under thera-peutic control than several others emerge to take its place and its de-fensive function.

The theme of the patient's behavior to the outside observer seems to be that almost any degree of self-destructiveness is preferable to con-taining and experiencing the affect of abandonment depression. But it cannot be worked through in therapy if it is not contained and experi-enced. If the therapeutic work is successful, every patient eventually becomes utterly amazed and astonished at the extraordinary intensity of his own resistance as well as the degree to which he consciously fos-tered and colluded with that resistance.

REFERENCES

Jacobson, E. (1964). *The Self and the Object World*. New York: International Universities Press.

Kernberg, O. (1975). *Borderline Conditions and Pathological Narcissism.* Pp. 163–177. New York: Science House.

Mahler, M.S. (1965). On the significance of the normal separation-individuation phase. In *Drives, Affects and Behavior,* ed. M. Schur, vol. 2, pp. 161–169. New York: International Universities Press.

―――― (1968). *On Human Symbiosis and the Vicissitudes of Individuation.* New York: International Universities Press.

Masterson, J.F. (1972). *Treatment of the Borderline Adolescent: A Developmental Approach.* New York: John Wiley.

―――― (1976). *Psychotherapy of the Borderline Adult.* New York: Brunner/Mazel.

―――― (1981). *The Narcissistic and Borderline Disorders: An Integrated Developmental Approach.* New York: Brunner/Mazel.

Winnicott, D.W. (1965). Ego distortions in terms of true and false self. In *The Maturational Processes and the Facilitating Environment,* pp. 140–152. New York: International Universities Press.

CHAPTER 16

Resistance in Prestructural (Psychotic) Psychopathology

Robert A. Mednick

Recent advances in developmental psychoanalysis (Stolorow and Lachmann 1980, Blanck and Blanck 1979) and the clinical care of preoedipal early object-relations pathology (A. Freud 1965, Mahler 1968, Giovacchini 1979), have opened up new pathways for understanding and treating resistances in severe psychopathology. In particular, pivotal clinical delineations of Sandler and Rosenblatt's (1962) formulations of the "representational world" (Stolorow et al. 1978, Stolorow 1978), and the new work in the area of "intersubjectivity" (Atwood and Stolorow 1983), offer compelling insights into the phenomenon of resistance, especially as seen in the treatment of psychoses.

Along with this, important controversies have arisen about variant theoretical views of psychoses, especially following Arlow and Brenner's paper "The Psychopathology of the Psychoses: A Proposed Revision" (1969) (London 1973, Grotstein 1977, Pao 1979). The theoretical framework from which this chapter draws its form is not within the structural theory model proposed by Arlow and Brenner (1969). Rather, resistance in psychoses (designated *prestructural* pathology) will be examined based on Kohut's (1971, 1977) work and especially on

---

The author wishes to thank Drs. Frank Lachmann and Robert Stolorow for their helpful suggestions and kind support in this work.

subsequent elaborations in the areas of "developmental arrest" (Stolorow and Lachmann 1980) and "intersubjectivity" (Atwood and Stolorow 1983).

Prestructural psychopathology can be defined as states of subjective experience which have reference pathogenically to very early developmental failures in self-object differentiation, integration, and consolidation. These archaic developmental processes occur *prior* to, and simultaneously with, the consolidation of ego and superego structures. Because these developmental processes are prerequisite to ego and superego structural consolidations, they are called *prestructural*.

The presence of developmental arrests, where self-object differentiation has been impeded, results in the vulnerability to regressive dissolution of the more developmentally advanced representational structures of the personality. The predisposition to profound regression is a cardinal feature of psychosis.

Within this theoretical framework, two central areas of psychopathology have been identified in the psychoses. These include, first, the fragmentation and loss of the archaic selfobject, and, second, the fragmentation of the mind-body-self (Kohut 1971). This latter area in the psychoses has specific reference to what has been called general *structural weakness* (Kohut 1971, Burnham et al. 1969).

The concept of structural weakness as utilized within the theoretical fabric of representational structuralization refers to trauma-impaired developmental processes. As noted, these processes occur prior to irreversible ego and superego consolidations as seen within the structural theory model. Accordingly, and for the purpose of maintaining consistency in this chapter, the concept of structural weakness will be referred to as *prestructural* weakness.

Given these guiding developmental and theoretical viewpoints, *two primary sources* of resistance are proposed and will be elaborated upon. These include resistances whose source is the "dread of repeating" the loss of the archaic selfobject tie,[1] and resistances whose source is prestructural weakness.

---

[1]By "archaic selfobject tie" is meant the *subjective representation* of a primitive object relationship where "self" is not clearly distinguished from "other" within the psychic reality of the person. In addition, the relational tie as experienced performs psychic functions that take the place of undeveloped, missing, or defective psychic structure. The archaic selfobject is therefore a precursor of psychic structure. It is used to maintain both a "sense of self" and "self cohesion" in the wake of missing or precariously developed self-structure.

THE "DREAD OF REPEATING" THE LOSS OF THE ARCHAIC SELFOBJECT TIE

My observations have been consistent with Pao's (1979): the psychotic patient's basic conflict is a wish to be simultaneously close to and distant from others. The question that arises is, what theoretical schema can most adequately account for this phenomenon, especially regarding the understanding and treatment of psychotic resistances?

Kohut (1971) has suggested that it would be fruitful to trace the regression in psychotic psychopathology through particular "way stations." In addressing the question, the most important of these way stations is the fragmentation of the archaic narcissistic positions, including the loss of the narcissistically cathected archaic objects, and thus the disintegration of self and archaic selfobjects. In addition, along this pathway is the "secondary restitutive resurrection of the archaic self and of the archaic narcissistic objects in a manifestly psychotic form" (Kohut 1971, p. 6). Particularly important to the individual who suffers a psychotic regression is the subjectively experienced *loss of the archaic selfobject tie.*

It is following the experienced loss of the archaic selfobject tie that the psychotic restitutive transformations occur. These typically include such manifestations as degeneration of language, concretization of thought, and disturbances in body sensation and self-perception. In addition, hallucinations and delusions can be seen as psychotic efforts to reconstitute the disintegrated self and the lost archaic selfobject tie.

From this background, two basic functions of prestructural resistances whose source is the "dread of repeating" are seen. These include the *avoidance of a repetition of the internal catastrophe experienced during the psychotic regression* (the experience of dissolution of the self); and, genetically, the *avoidance of a repetition of the pathogenic developmental traumata that originally effected the predisposition to regressive dissolution of the "self."*

At this point a central difference between structural and prestructural resistance becomes clear. In structural resistances, due to the repressed instinctual (that is, sexual and/or aggressive) drives of the id that are organized around infantile fantasy-wishes, there is a *compulsion to repeat.* Freud (1939, Vol. 23, p. 75) considered the compulsion to repeat a point that "must be stressed" as a characteristic of neurotic phenomena. The compulsion to repeat in neuroses is in obvious contradistinction to the *dread to repeat*[2] in the psychoses. This factor has significant treatment implications that will be addressed later.

The clinical material and hypotheses that follow regarding a patient called Wendy are intended to illustrate and theoretically organize resisting as an expression of the dread to repeat. The subsequent cases of John and William are intended to illustrate specific forms of resistance whose source is prestructural weaknesses.

CASE HISTORY: WENDY

Wendy was a 19-year-old diagnosed schizophrenic who was receiving substantial doses of neuroleptics and had been hospitalized on a psychiatric ward for three months before the following session took place. Upon initial admission to the hospital, Wendy manifested florid loosening of associations, grandiose delusions, and auditory hallucinations. It should be noted also that for the majority of sessions prior to the one being reported, Wendy ran out of the office following eruptive outbursts.

When I greeted Wendy for this session by saying, "Hello, Wendy," I noticed that she was dressed in a yellow running suit. I invited her into my office where she selected what she termed, for the first time, "the comfortable chair." She sat down and began swinging her crossed legs. She was rapidly chewing gum and seemingly making as much noise as she could from her chews. When I asked her "How are you doing?," Wendy said eruptively and with intense emotional pain, "I don't want doctors no more! I can get along by myself! I belong outside!" At that point she broke into tears, quickly stood up, threw her cigarettes against the chair and said, "I can't take this no more!" She began *repetitiously* pacing in the office, toward the door (touching the door knob) and back again to the comfortable chair, gradually slowing down her pace, tears streaming on her face.

Upon taking her comfortable chair again she said angrily, "You're lucky! When I was at the other hospital I used to spit. You're lucky I didn't spit at you!" Wendy then said, "You look so calm. My father's

---

[2]While the concept "dread to repeat" (Ornstein 1975) is related to the treatment of narcissistic personality disorders, the dynamic formulation of repetition effecting loss of the archaic selfobject has special reference to the more pathological conditions.

like that." (Wendy's father had in fact deserted the family when Wendy was 3 years old.) Then she looked at a small green plastic toy horse on my desk and said, "I've seen green horses before, horse flies. I know horses fly, I've seen them!"

A few weeks later Wendy told me about the experience she had before being hospitalized. She said, "It was real! It was real! I went looking for Henry [her boyfriend]. I went to the beach. The sand turned red. The moon got covered by the clouds, and it got very dark. That was where we were supposed to meet, me and Henry." I asked Wendy, "You had both previously agreed to meet there?," and she replied, "No. It was just with the minds. I knew how certain things happened. I don't know how but I just knew. I knew Henry was at the beach, 'cause I did see him. [Henry in fact had not been there.] He made cat noises. [Wendy's nickname was Kat.] So he was there! I have a great power. God intended it to be that way. It got loud and scary. I went to sleep with one of the cats. In the morning I walked to the train, and everybody there knew that I was the one on the beach who made all the changes happen." Two days later Wendy had been brought to the hospital by police who observed her walking down the middle of the street "directing traffic with my eyes."

I asked Wendy if she had seen her boyfriend Henry after that. She began to cry and said, "I don't remember! It doesn't matter to me 'cause it's over!" When I asked "It's over?" Wendy seemed to go into deep pain again and said, "Go ahead and punch me, kill me!" whereupon she stood up and agitatedly walked again repetitiously back and forth to the door and her comfortable chair.

Discussion of Wendy's Dread to Repeat

As noted, in severe psychopathologies, especially the psychoses, the therapist is not subjectively experienced by the patient as a separate or whole and singularly bounded person, although he or she may verbalize to the contrary. Because of failures in self-object differentiation, the patient's psychic organization is such that the therapist is subjectively indistinguishable from the patient's fragmented and archaically organized "self." The therapist in the patient's mind is innervated within a representational schema where self-from-object are experienced as an undifferentiated amalgamation. A classic example of this is a patient who experienced her body as "a conglomeration of anatomical parts from various other people" (Searles 1965, p. 307).

Using this conceptual framework, we see that Wendy first selected what she called the "comfortable chair." This action was significant since it followed Wendy's earlier repetitive resistive behaviors of storming out of sessions. When I questioned her, asking, "How are *you* doing?" while she was in her comfortable chair, an eruption occurred. It is hypothesized that my question imposed a sense of separateness, that is, "me" as distinguished from "her." Accordingly, it ruptured the momentarily reestablished archaic selfobject tie equilibrium. This equilibrium had been felt just moments earlier in the psychic position represented by the comfortable chair.

It is also proposed that the dread of repeating the loss of the selfobject tie was seen in Wendy's intense vulnerability to any communication that even slightly delimited my function as a selfobject within her experience. In Wendy's world, any delimitation of my function as a selfobject brought with it an intensified dread of repeating the loss of the selfobject. Wendy's wearing of her running suit and the fact that she repeatedly stormed out of prior sessions highlighted this form of prestructural resistance. Paradoxically, by running out, she strove to avoid the dread of repeating.

Wendy eventually began to describe her anger, which she related to the intense anxiety she experienced when I asked "separateness imposing" questions. She later said venomously, "You're supposed to *automatically know* how I feel!"

In exploring Wendy's rage and anxiety at my not knowing automatically, it became clear that she needed to experience with me her wish to communicate "just with the minds." To feel this, as Wendy later said, was to be assured that we were indeed "like one." Remarkably, in a session two months later, Wendy brought in a string. She began to tie two of her fingers together. Rather than my asking "What are you doing?" which in the past had been so upsetting to her, I asked instead, "What's that?" She said, "It's us. I'm tying us together." I found out later that this session had followed an incident on the hospital unit a few hours earlier where Wendy had panicked and cried out desperately, "Where's Henry! I have to call him!"

Wendy's tying her two fingers together was seen as concretely representing her struggle against the dreaded loss of the selfobject bond. We recall that Wendy's nickname was Kat, and that in the emergence of her psychosis she said she knew Henry "was there" because she heard "cat noises." These data could now be understood as an expression of Wendy's search for her lost self, or at least the significant part of it experienced in the representational form of "Henry."

The repetitive pacings from her comfortable chair to the door demonstrated Wendy's intense conflict from which her dread to repeat emanated. On the one hand, she experienced the developmental remobilization and revival of a reestablished archaic selfobject tie, a substitute for missing and precariously formed psychic structure. On the other hand, she experienced the terrifying dread of its reexperienced loss.

Wendy's agitated pacings back and forth from her comfortable chair to the door also reflected the *function* of her resistances. Wendy was attempting to use action as an *organizing metaphor* (not as an "acting in" in the service of denial) to relieve her terror of self-dissolution should the selfobject tie again be obliterated. Failures on my part either to empathically acknowledge Wendy's dread, accurately understand the function of her resistances, or assist in reestablishing the selfobject tie, added further to her dread. This left Wendy anticipating all the more that once again what she so desperately needed for psychic survival would be lost. At the same time, Wendy craved a reactivation of the selfobject tie. This was seen in her repetitive returns to the comfortable chair. It was this tie, as subjectively experienced, that provided relief from the intense anguish which Wendy's precipitous self-dissolving condition created.

Looked at from this perspective, Wendy's resistances can be seen as serving a unique *intersubjective* function. Wendy's resistances were efforts to avoid the self-extinguishing impacts that occurred when my presence as a selfobject failed in its needed function. At the same time, my understanding of the *meanings* and *functions* of Wendy's resistances, from her developmentally archaic frame of reference, facilitated the diminishment of her dread to repeat.

PRESTRUCTURAL WEAKNESSES AS A PRIMARY SOURCE OF RESISTANCE

The concept of *psychic deficiency* in the psychoses has traditionally been a central theoretical tenet and point of reference for therapeutic treatment. In line with the structural theory model, particular deficits in ego functioning have been emphasized. Such ego deficits have been conceptualized in terms of ego deviations and structural weakness (Arlow and Brenner 1969, Bellak et al. 1973).

From a prestructural framework, resistances in psychoses are not seen clinically as expressions of an experienced subjective danger vis-à-vis ego and superego conflicts. The psychic danger in psychoses that effect resistances is *not* fundamentally a conflict between sexual and/or aggressive drive derivatives organized around specific unconscious wishes and fantasies that are opposed by prohibitions against such wishes. Rather, the dangers in psychoses, from a prestructural viewpoint, stem from experiential eruptions that threaten significant *alterations in the organization and equilibria of the representational world.*

While the manifest varieties of the resistances may vary widely, it is postulated that they are based on two processes intrinsic to prestructural weaknesses. The first refers to *threats of self-extinction through disequilibrating "mergers" with the selfobject.* The second process refers to dangers posed by traumatogenic and shattering disappointments, or other empathic failures, that effect a *subjective "separation" from the archaic selfobject bond.* The following clinical material is intended to demonstrate these two strains of resistance whose source is prestructural weakness.

Resistances Effected by Separation from the Selfobject Bond

John is a 33-year-old black man who has been hospitalized eight times over the course of the last ten years. His first hospitalization lasted for eighteen months, and he was catatonic for the initial three-month period of that hospitalization.

During the acute episodes of his illness, John exhibited florid hallucinations of audition and intense paranoid delusions in which he was terrified of being attacked. Over the last four years of his treatment he has increasingly stabilized. This increasing stabilization, along with his superior intelligence, has made it possible for him to attend college. He has been managed on prophylactic doses of neuroleptics and has been in psychotherapeutic treatment on the basis of two sessions per week. John has had a long-time interest in psychology, and has shown a particular interest in psychological concepts.

Significant features of John's early history include his mother's chronic depression and sadistic responses to John's demonstrations of emergent capacity. In addition, his parents' marriage was stormy with frequent violent separations prior to John's third year. When John was age four his father committed suicide. John's first psychotic break occurred in the context of his returning from a brief trip to Chicago to find, totally unknown and unexpectedly, his mother residing with a man she had just married.

During the third year of his treatment a particular set of events unfolded. They occurred in the context of unusual strides being made in John's level of psychic organization, spontaneity, and contextually apppropriate humor with the therapist. These events are seen as illustrating resistances prompted by John's subjective experience of *separation from the selfobject bond*.

John's level of functioning had improved markedly over the course of a three-month period. During this period of rapid organization, he demonstrated increased interpersonal acuity and clarity in communication. This accelerated period of organization, however, was followed by a change that occurred over the course of six sessions. It was marked by a flooding of despair where he voiced "I'm helpless to change," and "what's the use anymore."

During this despairing period John came to sessions disheveled and emitting an intense body odor. When the therapist broached the issue of John's body odor, making every effort to be sensitive, John seemed to be unaffected. However, very uncharacteristically, he canceled the next two sessions. In addition, one hour prior to the third session, John called to say that he no longer wanted to come to sessions twice per week.

When John came for the next session, the therapist made every effort to restore the rupture of the selfobject bond that was seen as being brought on by the therapist's broaching the topic of John's body odor. John reacted with relief, and appeared to be soothed by the therapist's empathic efforts to articulate what John undoubtedly experienced when the therapist called attention to his body odor. At the close of the session John voluntarily requested that he resume sessions twice a week. However, questions remained regarding the appearing despair, the apparent "need" for the body odor, and the therapist's failure to understand the meaning of these experiences from the patient's subjective frame of reference.

During the next session John demonstrated a renewed and heightened level of functioning and spontaneity. The theme of the session began to quickly evolve around John's concerns about wanting to feel "solid," "like a single person," "together." He then questioned in an intense manner, "What's that word that means you're all together? Con. . .sol. . .a. . .date? No. [Silence.]" Then he came up with his discovery and declared, "Oh yeh! *Differentiate!* That word *scares me to death!* It's so scary. It means to be different! To be different at one time and then be different the next time. It's so scary!"

Exploring what was scaring John revealed that he had endured a particular repetitive anxiety experience that had evolved with increasing intensity during the earlier three-month period of his increased organization within sessions. About this experience, John said, "I don't know what it was. I'd get afraid after leaving here, then go home and have to stay in cause of being so afraid." John said that what had prevented him from mentioning this was, "It was like it never happened when I was here with you."

John's repetitive anxiety was theoretically seen as an accompaniment of his experience of rapidly increasing representational differentiation. Rapid psychic organization and differentiation brought with it separation from the selfobject bond, and his representational equilibrium was altered. In addition to his depressive reaction to this separation, John manifested specific resistances in order to preserve what he felt was being lost. For example, one of the multiple functions served by his refraining from bathing was the avoidance of change in bodily sense and integrity; it was a concrete effort to maintain his fragile sense of self in the wake of subjective separation from the selfobject bond. Because of John's prestructural weakness, threats of self-dissolution were posed when he began to experience too rapid separation from the selfobject bond prompted by rapid differentiation. These threats paralleled John's early life experiences where change, especially demonstrations of mastery, were met by his mother's sadism and withdrawal.

Paradoxically, by canceling sessions John could delimit the threat of subjective separation from the selfobject. He could avoid the representational alterations that occurred when he experienced rapid differentiation and organization. Also, he could avoid the intense anxiety that followed immediately after leaving sessions. These resistances were seen as responses to the psychic danger of rapid separation from the selfobject bond, and the accompanying threat of self-loss and psychotic regression.

Resistances Effected by Disequilibrating Mergers with the Selfobject

Two developmental prototypes for the merger experience have been identified. One occurs in the phase of symbiosis at four months of age where infants alternate between melting into, in contrast to stiffening against, the mother's body (Mahler et al. 1975). A second prototype has been seen as originating in the rapprochement subphase of separation individuation during ages 15 to 24 months. Here, the infant deliberately searches for, or tries to avoid, intimate bodily contact with the mother (Mahler et al. 1975). The fear of merging which prompts resistances can have its inception at thse early stages of psychic development.

The symbiosis experience has been seen as necessary in the treatment of psychoses (Searles 1965) because the development of psychic structure proceeds from this position. The therapist must become established as an archaic selfobject in the mental life of the psychotic patient in order to substitute for missing psychic structure, and in order to promote the remobilization of early developmentally arrested psychic processes, including the transmuting internalization of the selfobject (Kohut 1971, Stolorow 1982).

The patient called William, who is described in the discussion that follows, was treated by a female therapist who was under my supervision. The following material is seen as demonstrating specific resistances to merger whose source is prestructural weakness.

William is a verbal and bright 32-year-old man who has been hospitalized twice over the course of the past seven years. He carried the diagnosis paranoid schizophrenia, and upon each admission exhibited florid psychotic symptoms, including grandiose delusions of omnipotent powers regarding "knowing what is in their minds." The following session occurred in this patient's first year of treatment during a time when he was obsessively preoccupied with redecorating and wallpapering his mother's home, where he lived. In the session that preceded, William had exclaimed his fury and contempt for his mother because, when on the telephone, she had let the telephone cord rub against the newly papered wall.

William came to his session angry and commented, "I'm bored." When the therapist asked, "Do you think you might be angry?" William altered his affect immediately, smiled, and said "No, maybe irritated, but not really." The therapist tried to pursue what William may have been "bored" about, but as she did the patient quickly turned the focus to another topic. He began to discuss his interest in "having a car," and followed this with his obsessions about wall-papering.

The therapist conceptualized William's responses as "diversions." As she persisted in focusing on William's aggressive affect, he increased his diversions, adding florid embellishments that included the detailing of vivid colors and spiraling aggrandizements of the "magnificent job" he had done in "covering the walls."

As William elaborated his ideas about covering walls, he began to disorganize markedly. While his therapist correctly articulated how William experienced himself emotionally, the patient became increasingly disassociated from what the therapist was saying. He stayed fixed on descriptions of covering walls and his ideas jumped chaotically and frantically from description to description.

William's experience of the therapist being synchronous with his aggressive affects had a boundary-dissolving impact. His increasingly frantic descriptions of vividly colored painted and papered walls was later seen as concretely symbolic of his efforts to counter the erosion of internal self-object boundaries. From this frame of reference, his resistances—initially seen by the therapist as diversions—were now seen as psychic attempts to preserve a particular representational equilibrium. The boundary-dissolving merger that William experienced when the therapist accurately articulated his feelings threatened self-extinction. The resistance expressed by the patient's becoming "lost," as the therapist put it, in regressive disorganization served the function of limiting the pursuing therapist's capacity to articulate William's "self state" in the service of halting the merger.

TREATMENT APPROACHES TO PRESTRUCTURAL RESISTANCES

A central aim in the treatment of the psychoses is the accurate recognition of the patient's subjective psychic reality and intentionality. Two therapeutic processes that bear directly on this task have special reference to the understanding and treatment of resistances in psychoses. These include the *therapeutic alliance* and *transference.*

In contrast to structural conflict pathology, as in neuroses where the patient is developmentally capable of forming a therapeutic alliance, the psychotic patient is incapable of such an achievement. A prerequisite for the attainment of a therapeutic alliance is that self and object representations have in large part become differentiated and integrated. Since the therapist is not subjectively experienced as a separate and whole person within the psychic organization of the patient, a mutually collaborative self-and-object-bounded relationship is not present. Under these circumstances, the therapist's empathic communications serve the crucial function of acting as a precursor or *prestage* of a therapeutic alliance (Stolorow 1982).

The therapist, in addition, is needed by the patient as a selfobject that serves as a substitute for the patient's missing or precariously formed self-structure. This therapeutic achievement allows the drive-regulating, integrating, and adaptive functions of the self-structure to proceed and be maintained (Kohut 1971). This therapeutic condition allows for the reactivation of arrested development.

In the classical transference neurosis where structural conflict prevails, the therapist's neutrality allows the patient—and therapist—to observe the defensive revival, wishful reproduction, and anxiety-arousing repetition of early conflicts. These replicative revivals occur in a manner in which mental contents are transposed across *consolidated boundaries* from the patient as a whole-and-bounded "self" to the therapist as a whole-and-bounded "object." Therefore, what prevails in the treatment of psychoses is a prestage of transference. The meaning, function, and treatment of resistances in psychoses must include the therapeutic implications of these conditions.

Two psychic patterns have been proposed as primary sources of resistance in psychoses. First, the dread of repeating the loss of the archaic selfobject refers to interferences in treatment that may come into play as the therapist is becoming established as a selfobject in the mental life of the patient. The second form of resistance recognizes the patient's *prestructural weaknesses*, and requires the therapist's attunement to alterations in the patient's representational schema and equilibria. When the patient experiences intense or too rapid *mergers* with or *separations* from the selfobject bond, resistances occur. Resistances therefore serve to avoid threats of self-dissolution or loss of the selfobject bond. Looked at from an intersubjective perspective, resistances are seen as responses to the therapist-as-selfobject within the patient's representational world.

Treating these forms of resistance also necessitates the clinical recognition of *developmental arrests*, which refers to early interferences in the formation of self-structure and allied processes of ego development. Since an ego defense is considered to represent an endpoint in a series of developmental achievements (Stolorow and Lachmann 1980), prerequisites for the operation of ego defenses include a particular level of ego articulation, self-development, and other necessary developmental tasks.

The presence of consolidated ego defensive activity is not the predominant state of affairs in psychotic pathology. Defensive activity in psychoses is founded instead on threats of self-extinction originating from what has been elaborated as the dread of repeating and prestructural weaknesses. For example, distortions in reality that occur in treatment, such as denial, do not typically stem from intersystemic structural conflict. Rather, they are based on developmental inabilities and arrests, and are therefore considered prestages of ego defenses.

Resistances that occur in treating a developmental inability require very different approaches from resistances arising out of structural (object-instinctual) conflict. In structural pathology such as neuroses, the therapist generally interprets what the patient is endeavoring to defensively *ward off*. In prestructural pathology, the therapist focuses instead on the state which the undifferentiated person is *striving to achieve* (Stolorow and Lachmann 1980). Using this model in the clinical illustration with Wendy, for example, the therapist had incorrectly emphasized Wendy's loss of her boyfriend by asking "It's over?" He did not focus on the state that Wendy was struggling to achieve. As we saw, this resulted in the patient's disorganization and intensified anxiety.

Adhering to the prestructural model, the therapist should have focused instead on the importance of Wendy's relationship to Henry as a selfobject that was necessary in order to survive psychotic regression. If the therapist had been attuned to Wendy's archaic selfobject strivings, instead of asking "It's over?" he might have said simply, "Henry is very important to you."

In working through prestructural resistances whose source is the dread of repeating the loss of the selfobject tie, the essential task is to *make the selfobject tie more of a source of strength than a source of danger* (Mednick 1984). This task requires analyzing and working through the dread so that the patient can be *hopeful of a new beginning* (Balint 1968) in the reestablishment of the needed selfobject bond.

Two primary obstacles to the accomplishment of this task are *representational disjunctions*, and (especially) the *failures in empathy* that emanate from these disjunctions. "Representational disjunction" is a process whereby the therapist mistakenly assimilates the patient's material into representational configurations and imagery that—while holding for the psychic organization of the therapist—significantly distort the material's actual subjective meaning within the patient's psychic world (Stolorow et al. 1981).

Failures to accurately understand the psychotic patient's archaic strivings from his or her psychic reality (because of representational disjunctions or because of conceptualizing prestructural pathology in structural conflict terms) limit the therapist's capacity for empathy. Such empathic failures may not only incite or maintain paralyzing resistances, they also impede the patient's desperate struggles to reawaken traumatically arrested development and overcome the predisposition to regression. Empathic failures and misunderstandings of psychic intentions and strivings leave the psychotic person tormented by a "hopelessness for a new beginning," and subject to the terrors of psychic oblivion in regressive dissolution and self-extinction.

REFERENCES

Arlow, J., and Brenner, C. (1969). The psychotherapy of the psychoses: a proposed revision. *International Journal of Psycho-Analysis* 50:5–14.

Atwood, G.E., and Stolorow, R.D. (1983). *Structures in Subjectivity: Explorations in Psychoanalytic Phenomenology.* Hillsdale, NJ: Analytic Press.

Balint, M. (1968). *The Basic Fault: Therapeutic Aspects of Regression.* New York: Brunner/Mazel.

Bellak, L., Hurvich, M., and Gediman, H.K. (1973). *Ego Functions in Schizophrenics, Neurotics, and Normals.* New York: John Wiley.

Blanck, G., and Blanck, R. (1979). *Ego Psychology II: Psychoanalytic Developmental Psychology.* New York: Columbia University Press.

Burnham, D.L., Gladstone, A.I., and Gibson, R.W. (1969). *Schizophrenia and the Need-Fear Dilemma*. New York: International Universities Press.

Freud, A. (1965). *Normality and Pathology in Childhood*. New York: International Universities Press.

Freud, S. (1939). Moses and monotheism: three essays. *Standard Edition* 23: 3–137.

Giovacchini, P.L. (1979). *Treatment of Primitive Mental States*. New York: Jason Aronson.

Grotstein, J. (1977). The psychoanalytic concept of schizophrenia: II. reconciliation. *International Journal of Psycho-Analysis*. 58:427–452.

Kohut, H. (1971). *The Analysis of the Self*. New York: International Universities Press.

————— (1977). *The Restoration of the Self*. New York: International Universities Press.

London, N. (1973). An essay on psychoanalytic theory: two theories of schizophrenia. Part I: review and critical assessment of the development of the two theories. *International Journal of Psycho-Analysis* 54:169–178.

Mahler, M.S. (1968). *On Human Symbiosis and the Vicissitudes of Individuation*. New York: International Universities Press.

Mahler, M.S., Pine, F., and Bergman, A. (1975). *The Psychological Birth of the Human Infant*. New York: Basic Books.

Mednick, R.A. (1984). Theoretical scaffoldings toward a "new beginning" in the ontogenesis of subjectivity: discussion of Dr. Magid's paper. In *Dynamic Psychotherapy*, Vol. II, No. 2, pp. 112–115. New York: Brunner/Mazel.

Ornstein, A. (1975). The dread to repeat and the new beginning: a contribution to the psychoanalysis of the narcissistic personality disorders. In *Annual of Psychoanalysis*, Vol. 2, pp. 231–248. New York: International Universities Press.

Pao, P. (1979). *Schizophrenic Disorders: Theory and Treatment from a Psychodynamic Point of View*. New York: International Universities Press.

Sandler, J., and Rosenblatt, B. (1962). The concept of the representational world. *Psychoanalytic Study of the Child* 17:128–145.

Searles, H.F. (1965). *Collected Papers on Schizophrenia and Related Subjects*. New York: International Universities Press.

Stolorow, R.D. (1978). The concept of psychic structure: its metapsychological and clinical psychoanalytic meanings. *International Review of Psycho-Analysis* 5:313–320.

————— (1982). On feeling understood. Discussion of Galatzer-Levy's (1982) paper, "The opening phase of the psychotherapy of hypochondriacal states." Unpublished.

Stolorow, R.D., Atwood, G.E., and Lachmann, F.M. (1981). Transference and countertransference in the analysis of developmental arrests. *Bulletin of the Menninger Clinic* 45:20–28.

Stolorow, R.D., Atwood, G.E., and Ross, J. (1978). The representational world in psychoanalytic therapy. *International Review of Psycho-Analysis,* 5: 247–256.

Stolorow, R.D., and Lachmann, F.M. (1980). *Psychoanalysis of Developmental Arrests: Theory and Treatment.* New York: International Universities Press.

CHAPTER 17

The Reluctance to Experience Positive Affects

Morton Kissen

Repeatedly in clinical practice patients are seen who have a great deal of difficulty in tolerating positive affective experiences. These patients cut across the spectrum of psychopathology, stemming from the largely neurotic forms of personality difficulty at one end, to the more clearly narcissistic and borderline types of problems at the other end. It is the central thesis of this paper that a characterological form of difficulty, frequently expressed as a resistance to the treatment, is fundamentally involved in such difficulties. The use of the term *reluctance* to describe this form of resistance maintains the *action language* frame of reference suggested by Schafer (1976), as an antidote to the relatively passive implications of both the classical analytic and ego psychological approaches to the conceptualization and technical handling of this clinical syndrome.

A series of clinical phenomena will document the reluctance to experience positive affects and associated object-relational experiences manifested by certain patients. The resistive aspects of such behavior will be emphasized and some technical suggestions for dealing with them in the context of psychoanalytic psychotherapy will be offered. Finally, the subtle shifts in our metapsychological model for understanding resistive behavior stemming from clinical experiences with these characterologically impaired patients will be described.

CLINICAL EXAMPLES OF THE RELUCTANCE TO EXPERIENCE POSITIVE AFFECTS

Certainly discomfort with positive emotional states is a common enough form of psychological expression. Many neurotic patients express this difficulty in the form of relatively inhibited reactions to opportunities for self-actualization. A good example is the patient who develops a case of stage fright when faced with the opportunity to have center stage in some form of theatrical performance, following an extended period of rigorous preparation and disciplined practice of a particular musical skill or talent. The psychodynamic implications of such a relatively temporary inhibition of talents and exhibitionistic strivings has frequently been conceptualized as a response to unconscious oedipal fantasies and wishes that conflict with conscious and preconscious values, ego ideal, and rules for proper social conduct. At a more behavioral level, an attitude of shyness seems to be observable that does not allow for a smooth and comfortable expression of various exhibitionistic strivings in such patients.

A similar form of reluctance can be seen in patients manifesting more severe forms of character pathology. Many depressed patients become extremely uncomfortable when confronted with some complimentary or potentially positive ego experience. One patient, in particular, expressed this discomfort in her mode of dress by wearing the most frumpy and unappealing clothes possible. It seemed as though her choice of clothing was designed to least accentuate her various feminine attributes and potential sexual appeal. She clearly needed to protect herself against some positive regard or seductive approach by a man. This reluctance to experience positive sexual affects was manifested as a transference resistance in her interaction with her therapist and formed a central metaphorical theme which needed to be worked through during her treatment. Another patient recoiled at the possibility that she might be considered an interesting or worthwhile patient by her analyst. She frequently criticized the paltry nature of her free associations and was very critical toward any dreams that did not seem worthy of her analyst's interpretive interest or attention. Her reluctance to experience herself as an interesting, valuable sort of person was an important manifestation of her depression and needed to be explored as a resistance during the course of her psychotherapy.

Patients manifesting severe weight disturbances most commonly express this form of resistance during their treatment. An anorexic patient could not enjoy a meal without punishing himself by vomiting afterwards. But this self-punitive gesture was not deemed sufficient. He subsequently had to swim consecutive laps at a local olympic pool for three hours straight, until he was reassured that he had not gained a single pound as a result of ingesting the food. He feebly attempted to rationalize his compulsively ritualistic behavior by citing the intense athlete's high and spiritual feeling of uplift that he experienced at the end of his exercise. His intolerance for the pleasures of food was evidently camouflaged by a severely compulsive and self-punitive anhedonic regimen of physical exercise.

Bulimic patients, too, frequently manifest an incapacity to tolerate potentially pleasurable activities, particularly those centering on experiences with food. Thus, a young woman tended to go through an elaborate ritual of preparing her food in a special way, putting on the television and getting under her bed covers for a relaxing eating experience. However, subsequently she had to pay for the pleasurable nature of the experience by expelling the contents of her stomach via violent vomiting episodes. She would frequently do this until her face became chalky white and ghost-like in appearance. The pleasures of food were, paradoxically, quite intolerable to this patient. She had to pay a very high price indeed for her various enjoyments in this area. A number of themes were evident in the story of her life that contributed to at least some clarification of the psychodynamic significance of her bulimic intolerance for the pleasures of food.

Her mother had died after a chronic period of illness when she was five years of age, and she had never had the opportunity to adequately mourn her loss. Indeed, she recalled coming home from a pleasurable play activity with a friend on the day her mother died. A crowd of sad mourners had gathered at the home. She could not comprehend why they seemed so sad but specifically recalled their frowning reactions to her seeming gaiety and unawareness of the tragic event that had just occurred. She was clearly made to feel guilty for her emotional spontaneity and playfulness. She was subsequently sent away from the home to stay with an uncle and aunt, while her father attempted to deal with his deep sense of depression and loss. She returned to her home two years later. Her father had, during this period of time, remarried. Her relationship with her stepmother was a very stormy one that centered largely on the stepmother's explosive rage reactions to the patient's food binges and tendency to forage through the refrigerator in a seemingly excessive fashion. The stepmother's efforts to curtail her evidently compulsive eating pleasures were experienced in a very harsh fashion by the patient. She always felt in conflict with her stepmother, at least in part as a result of those eating interactions; she viewed her father with a great deal of resentment because she felt he was too weak to intercede actively and effectively on her behalf.

The patient gradually became more and more resentful of the stepmother's presence within the home, the same home that her father had previously lived in with her mother. Any effort on the part of the stepmother to change some decorative aspect of the home was met with deep feelings of resentment by the patient. She felt, probably correctly, that the stepmother was attempting to erase her natural mother's presence from the home. The stepmother's very great enjoyment in homemaking and decorating activities only increased her resentment and rage. She began to hoard souvenirs and memorabilia of her own mother in a desperate effort to preserve her presence as a factor in her life, and to ward off her stepmother's intrusive presence.

Her need to protectively maintain introjects and identifications with her natural mother became a central psychodynamic theme in her life. This identification process became increasingly pathological; she felt impelled, for instance, to identify with the depressed, chronically pain-ridden, and dying mother of her early childhood as a means of warding off any potential identification with her seemingly unacceptable stepmother. Even the stepmother's more positive and competent aspects could not be effectively internalized as a result of this resistive pattern, of course.

Although the patient attempted rather feebly to idealize her natural mother and to depreciate her stepmother, the effort even further curtailed any possibility of more benign object-relational experiences and identification interactions with her stepmother, a woman who was, in many ways, a very competent and emotionally healthy sort of person. The need to protect, guiltily, the idealized mother's memory increasingly led to the maintenance of pathological, depressive, and extraordinarily anhedonic behavioral attitudes. Her guilty reluctance and incapacity to sustain any enjoyment in eating became the most prevalent expression of this pathological identification process. Her expressive behavior was thus permeated by a guilty, depressive anhedonia that became the psychodynamic bulwark of her bulimic symptomatology. Her tendency to expel the food that she had voraciously gorged herself with was unconsciously linked to a need to undo any of the pleasures that food symbolically represented to her.

Thus, this pathological introjective process was the dynamic core underlying her psychopathology and was manifested in the form of a very pervasive resistance during the course of her treatment. The resistance had characterological features that made it relatively intractable and certainly very difficult to permeate therapeutically. She could not tolerate the pleasures of food or pleasures of any other nature over a sustained period due to an unconscious association of such pleasures with the loss of her depressive, chronically pain-ridden natural mother. She too had to keep herself in a chronically deprived, depressed, and pain-ridden state as an unconscious act of loyalty to this natural mother whose loss she had never had the opportunity to effectively mourn. She was pathologically identified with a dying mother whose ego and affective functioning had been severely impaired as a result of a chronically debilitating physical illness. This severely constrictive identification process had object-relational characteristics that interfered pervasively with her capacity to be competent and her ability to enhance her self-esteem through appropriate forms of competitiveness and self-assertion.

She could not internalize and identify with some of the very healthy, competitive, and self-assertive aspects of her stepmother due to a frozen sort of introjective process that was associated with the genetically grounded failure to mourn and to become psychologically separate from her natural mother. The bulk of the transference work during the course of her psychotherapy, therefore, involved a repeated analysis of her characterologically ingrained resistance to the pleasurable affects associated with food experiences. She was given many interpretations, frequently in the form of dynamic reconstructions of the painful object-relational experiences she must have had as a young child faced with the loss of a pain-ridden but much beloved mother. The identification with her natural mother was repeatedly stressed as the dynamic core underlying her anhedonic difficulties. Her reluctance to form a maturationally higher level identification attachment with her stepmother was also repeatedly clarified.

Her ultimate resistance, of course, was to the powerful and maturationally facilitative aspects of the therapy process itself. Her therapist by continually empathizing with her incapacity to tolerate the pleasur-

able affects associated with the ingestion of food and by interpreting repeatedly the dynamic roots of this resistance pattern, was eventually
able to offer her a more benign containing experience than was possible during her childhood. She attempted to resist the therapist's more
permissive attitude toward the pleasures of food in many ways and
thereby was able to rigidly hold on to her bulimic psychopathology.

The therapy could only become effective via an extensive analysis of
her resistance to pleasurable experiences (symbolically contained in
her bulimic symptom) that eventually crystallized itself in the form of a
transference resistance. She needed to be made aware of how frightened she was of yielding to the maturational pulls of the therapist and
his therapeutic environment. His optimistic expectation that she
might one day give up her pathological identification with a depressed,
pain-ridden, and dying mother was felt by her as very threatening. Indeed, the interpretive exploration of her early experiences of maternal
loss, that she had for so long kept out of her awareness, was initially
very difficult for her to internalize. She repeatedly returned to an acting out of her depressive tendencies via her rigidly ingrained bulimic
behavior patterns.

The therapist's seeming resiliency and comfort with such symptomatic regressions, however, had a benign and ego-supportive effect.
Despite the patient's pessimism about the possibility of ever curbing
her symptoms, the therapist remained undaunted and convinced that
the interpretive model being utilized would eventually have a benign
effect. Continual reminders with regard to her incapacity to tolerate
pleasurable experiences (particularly those involved in eating) also had
a clearly ego supportive and maturationally facilitative impact. Following each bulimic symptomatic recurrence, the therapist repeatedly reminded the patient of her dread of the pleasurable experience involved
in incorporating food into her body.

The patient's various protests with regard to the unpleasant dis-
torting effects that the food might have on her body image were duly
noted but were not accepted by the therapist as sufficient cause for the
patient's compulsive need to immediately rid herself of the ingested
food by vomiting. Her dread that she might gain weight and look ugly,
one of her rationalizations for the vomiting that always followed the
ingestion of large quantities of food, was gradually seen as a superficial defensive cover for her more basic resistance to pleasurable
experiences.

The patient rigidly held on to a dream that her symptom might be incurable. The therapist, on the other hand, continually made her focus on the possibility that she might have a much greater fear of pleasurable experiences. Should she allow herself to retain and thereby enjoy her food, she might then begin to allow herself to contain other enjoyable and maturationally beneficial experiences. The therapist repeatedly emphasized the patient's seeming incapacity to tolerate and internalize a more benign environmental milieu. Her home environment had to be as unpleasant as the hospital-like environment that her mother probably had to continuously face during the course of her childhood. The patient felt guilty whenever she began to experience a more benign, less chronically ill and ego-incapacitating sort of milieu. Her paradoxical incapacity to allow herself benign object-relational experiences was the primary resistance that needed to be explored in treatment. Indeed, the central transference resistance was manifested in the form of a reluctance to experience optimism in the therapeutic environment. She needed to hold on to the dread that she might never be able to give up her bulimic symptom. Her recurrent bulimic regressions ultimately involved a need to inject the pessimism she experienced during the course of the symbiotic attachment with her natural mother into her relationship with the therapist.

The containing task for the therapist was to tolerate the pessimism engendered by the patient's repeated symptomatic regressions without himself becoming unduly pessimistic. Ego resiliency needed to somehow be incorporated into the therapeutic environment in the form of a continuing optimism with regard to the patient's eventual potential for sustained positive experiences. Each protest by the patient that she was essentially incurable had to be met with a therapeutic clarification and reminder about her dread of positive object-relational experiences. The patient's insistence that her symptom was intolerable and anxiety producing (an implicit statement with regard to its ego-dystonic character) had to be repeatedly translated into a formulation of her much more basic fear of the possibility for sustained ego resiliency and more benign and maturationally facilitative object-relational experiences. The therapist's repeated reminders with regard to this very central resistance pattern eventually had a beneficial effect. An internalization process began to be evident both in her relationship to the therapist and to her stepmother.

Whereas she had previously always become embroiled in essentially masochistic sorts of sexual relationships, she met a young man who was able to treat her more positively. Her capacity to tolerate and sustain a nonmasochistic relationship occurred simultaneously with a decision to go back to school. She chose a very difficult scientific field involving a need for great intellectual discipline and scientific rigor. She also chose a field requiring that she compete with men rather than idealize them in a submissive and masochistic fashion. Her increasing self-confidence at school (where she had previously felt a sense of failure due to intense experiences of test anxiety) spilled over into an intense desire to redecorate her apartment. She began to compulsively reorganize and reshape the depressing and morbid environment in which she had been living.

Her intense decorating efforts paralleled the home reshaping activities performed by her stepmother earlier in her life and up to the present. Her capacity to tolerate the identification aspects of this behavior allowed a furthering of her ego development and a new experience of both attachment to and competition with her stepmother. She began to shift from a preoedipal attachment to her depressed mother to an oedipal level conflictual identification relationship with her stepmother. She was able to markedly increase her self-esteem due to this new receptivity to identification with the adaptive behavior of her stepmother.

In conceptualizing the marked ego enhancement and maturational growth that occurred in this case, it is important to emphasize the primary ego restorative effects of the continued analysis of the patient's seemingly intractable resistance to positive affects. At an object-relational level, this patient repeatedly manifested a reluctance to internalize beneficial and maturationally facilitative sorts of interpersonal experiences. She dreaded benign and maturationally high-level experiences in a similar fashion to the way that the neurotic patient dreads and becomes inhibited by unconscious signal anxiety. In contrast to the more neurotic sort of patient who may become inhibited due to an unconscious castration fantasy, this patient and others like her tend to unconsciously dread the giving up of primitive, essentially toxic introjects and object attachments. A primary ego ameliorative benefit can be attained from a continuous analysis of that dread and the way it expresses itself in a reluctance to tolerate positive affective experiences.

Various patients manifest in subtle and not so subtle ways their dread of positive affective experience. Some patients cannot tolerate a compliment about an aspect of their personality or an ego attribute. These patients tend to blush and communicate an intense discomfort with such benign affective experiences. Most depressed patients are involved in primitive object-relational attachments that can be conceptualized as toxic introjects. These introjects radically distort their ego functioning and capacity to internalize more benign affective experiences. The anhedonic features of the symptoms manifested by such patients can be seen as characterologically ingrained and essentially structural forms of resistance.

Quite often, the reluctance to internalize positive affects can be noted in a sequence analysis of the themes introduced during a psychotherapy session. Many patients manifest their intolerance for positive object-relational experiences via a subtle shift in the mood and affective tone of the session. One patient, a chronically depressed woman, exhibited this tendency when she began a session by describing a very exciting and pleasurable day she had recently experienced. She noted that on that particular day she felt alive in a way she had not felt for a long time. She ended the day by going to a movie that she had been looking forward to seeing for some time. She thoroughly enjoyed the movie and was so excited when it was over that she absentmindedly stumbled on the balcony steps, severely twisting her ankle in the process. She then went on to describe more typical laments and complaints about the thoroughly intolerable and unpleasurable nature of her current life situation. Her mood shifted to a sadder note at that point. The therapist suggested that she might be feeling discomfort over having experienced such an exciting and mood-uplifting sort of day. She therefore needed to punish herself and to get in touch with the far more familiar feelings of sadness and pessimism with regard to her life. She was very uncomfortable about the buoyant start of her session and therefore had to shift to a much more familiar plaintive and lamenting tone.

Another patient manifested the resistance to positive experiences via a similar sort of sequential shift in the thematic content and affective tone of a session. He began his session by noting that he had really been feeling *on a roll* lately. He had been making a number of successful sales at work and everyone at his place of employment had been responding to his seemingly boundless energy and enthusiasm. He felt very handsome and was receiving continuous seductive offers from the secretaries. He went on to note that he had been very vigorous and sexually potent with his wife for the first time in a long while. His very buoyant, excited mood continued for some time during the session but began gradually to diminish and to shift into a subtly sadder and more worried sort of affective tone. He brought up once again his concern about going crazy and having to be hospitalized. The dynamics of this concern had been analyzed many times during previous sessions. He became visibly sadder and less excited as the session progressed. The sequential affective shifts in the patient's session, as in the case of the previous patient, reflected his incapacity to tolerate and effectively internalize benign and maturationally ego-enhancing experiences. He actually feared, and hence had to avoid, the maintenance of a buoyant and self-confident frame of mind over an extended period of time.

Many paranoid transferential reactions to the therapist also convey this form of resistance pattern. One young woman who had finally been able to rid herself of her undesired virginity via a very enjoyable sexual experience began a therapy session with the conviction that the therapist quite clearly frowned upon her recent behavior. The therapist seemed like a moralistic stuffed shirt who almost certainly judged her behavior in a negative fashion. When the therapist noted the similarity of this "judgmental behavior" to the frowning face of her father throughout her childhood, however, it could not be completely overlooked by the patient.

The unconscious wish to avoid positive affective experiences is a pervasive one in the therapeutic process and can be seen in patients across the diagnostic spectrum of character pathology. It can be seen in neurotic patients, and in patients with higher and lower level character disorders. It is a quite familiar pattern to most therapists, discernible in the painful communications of a great variety of patients. However, the object-relational and resistance implications of these communications have not been focused upon sufficiently. The therapeutic technique for dealing with these resistances has not yet been clarified and fully elaborated.

SOME TECHNICAL SUGGESTIONS FOR DEALING WITH THE RESISTANCE TO POSITIVE AFFECTS

Reich's therapeutic model for exploring and resolving characterological resistances has been clearly articulated in his classic book, *Character Analysis* (1933). His basic model for resistance analysis is well incorporated in the treatment model practiced by most dynamically oriented psychotherapists. His essential recommendations stress the importance of focusing upon characterological resistance prior to more dynamic interpretive exploration and genetic reconstructions. He specifically suggests that genetic interpretations be held back from the patient, at least until partial exploration and resolution of the patient's main resistances have been initiated.

Reich stresses the centrality of characterological resistances and notes that they are hierarchically organized within a given patient's personality structure. Resistances are seen as structural features of personality and ego organization. The essential technical recommendation of Reich, therefore, is that ego structural features such as resistances need to be focused upon prior to a deeper, more dynamic interpretive exploration of the genetic antecedents underlying these characterological resistances. He stresses the essentially hierarchical organizational structure of these resistances and notes that the more basic, cardinal resistances need to be explored and resolved prior to working with the more peripheral and less primary resistances.

Once a very basic or cardinal resistance has been discerned by the therapist, it needs to be focused upon in a repeated fashion with the patient. Reich notes that the typical sequence of characterological resistance analysis is a three-step process. First, the patient is told that he has a particular resistance. Second, he is informed *how* he is resisting, that is, the particular defensive maneuvers that he is utilizing in order to resist the therapeutic process. Finally, the patient is involved in an exploration of the dynamic issues underlying his resistances. Interpretations are offered of a genetic and more reconstructive nature.

This was the basic therapeutic model utilized with the bulimic patient described previously. Her resistances were explored in accordance with the three-step approach recommended by Reich. One difference, however, was the fact that a continuous interweaving of genetic-dynamic interpretation and more structural and characterological confrontations occurred during the course of her treatment.

The genetic and object-relational features underlying the patient's symptomatic behavior were interpreted continuously from the very beginning phase of her treatment. The more characterological and structural sorts of observations with regard to her reluctance to experience and internalize positive affects were also made from the beginning of treatment.

Indeed, in this particular patient's treatment, the object-relational and reconstructive interpretations were repeatedly offered at the earliest phases of her treatment and gradually were diminished and replaced by an almost sole focus upon her cardinal characterological resistance to experiencing positive affects. At an intermediate phase in her treatment, the genetic and object-relational dynamics underlying her symptoms were repeatedly linked to her primary characterological resistance. Her reluctance to enjoy the pleasurable experiences of eating were linked repeatedly through genetic interpretations to the early toxic environmental milieu she had experienced with her natural mother. As the treatment progressed, these object-relational interpretive connections, particularly their impact on her identifications, did not have to be made for the patient quite as often. She began to internalize an understanding of the impact that her natural mother's death had had upon her. She gained an emotional grasp of the toxic frozen nature of her maternal introject and its impeding effect upon her capacity to make healthier, more functional identifications with her stepmother. Subsequently, the therapeutic focus shifted to a repeated exploration of the various symptomatic and behavioral manifestations of her incapacity to tolerate pleasurable affects. In the latter phases of the treatment, the therapist was continually forced to contain the optimistic affects that the patient could obviously not tolerate very well. This containing effect took the shape of constant reminders about the reluctance to experience positive affects that underlay the patient's pessimism and dread that she might never fully recover from her bulimic symptom.

It is thus being suggested that Reich's model for analyzing characterological resistances can be directly applied to the exploration and resolution of the reluctance to experience positive affects. His emphasis upon the need to always precede genetic and dynamic interpretations with a more structural focus upon characterological resistances, however, need not be followed too rigidly. Ultimately, an interweaving of the object-relational features underlying the patient's psychopathology with the more structural and characterological resistance aspects will need to be interpretively presented to the patient. The pathological identifications underlying the resistance to positive affective experiences need to be interpretively explored in a solidly object-relational fashion. Once the patient has a solid emotional and cognitive grasp of the deleterious impact of his reluctance to experience positive affects, he has begun to effectively work through the characterological aspects of the resistance.

Just as in other forms of character and resistance analysis, a great deal of patience is required on the part of the therapist. There are certain repetitious features to the technical handling of this very well-entrenched and characterologically engrained form of resistance. The therapist's task is to continually remind the patient who is experiencing and reporting feelings of painful self-awareness and disappointment, of the defensive and resistive nature of these feelings. The patient makes it quite clear that she has never even considered the possibility that her depressive affects might be a resistive, anhedonic avoidance of more positive and pleasurable affects. The therapist's continual reminders with regard to the reluctance to internalize benign emotional experiences are most often met with reactions of surprise and disbelief. The process of continual resistance analysis, however, eventually allows for a suspension of disbelief and a gradual internalization of the therapist's more optimistic attitudes and beliefs with regard to the patient's ego and maturational potentialities.

The therapist can and should maintain the position of technical neutrality recommended by Kernberg (1976) during the course of this process of resistance exploration and resolution. Although empathically aware of the patient's depressive suffering and sense of despair, the therapist is most effective when he or she maintains a degree of objectivity with regard to the dynamic and structural factors underlying the patient's sense of pain. The repeated reminders to the patient that this sense of pain actually involves a preferred and unconsciously chosen defensive maneuver eventually allows the patient to work through the resistance to positive experience.

Nydes, in his brilliant clinical contribution to the treatment issues involved in working with a group of patients that he labeled paranoid-masochistic characters (1963), makes a number of technical suggestions similar to the ones being made in this paper. After articulating some of the dynamics underlying both paranoid and masochistic forms of psychopathology, Nydes notes, however, that the paranoid patient also has a deep dread of the successful actualizing of unconscious oedipal wishes. The various paranoid doubts and worries continuously expressed by such patients convey their fear of potentiating phallic ambitions.

The ultimate dilemma for both sorts of patients is that any inner

sense of effectiveness is linked to an aggressive attack on an oedipal figure. Thus a male patient who successfully marries unconsciously feels
that he has aggressively attacked and defeated his father. He may
therefore conceal his sense of victory by developing paranoid preoccu-
pations that interfere with his sexual gratifications. He may become
worried over his potency or masculinity as a means of punishing himself for an unconscious oedipal victory. Masochistic patients may continually sabotage themselves through a depressive depletion of energy
and thereby avoid any competitive or assertive behavior that might
lead to unconsciously dreaded phallic achievements.

Nydes recommends that both types of patients need to be continually made aware of the unconscious guilt feelings that underlie their expressive behavior. The therapist's objectivity with regard to the
characterological features of these patients' psychopathology is his
most effective tool. Nydes sums up his treatment recommmendations
with the following statement:

> It is clear that one of the major therapeutic problems in dealing with
> the paranoid-masochistic character is to avoid the temptation to yield
> to the patient's diversionary tactics. The analyst's inner emotional reac-
> tion serves as a clue to the patient's intention. To express such reactions
> often serves only to fortify the mechanism rather than to undermine it.
> In the predominantly masochistic phase an attempt is made to excite in
> the analyst a sense of great compassion for the hardship which the pa-
> tient is enduring but to extend pity serves only to add to the patient's in-
> vestment in suffering as a means of demonstrating his innocence. What
> may appear to be a ruthless denial of pity to the suffering masochist, is in
> effect a genuine respect of his strength. To extend pity where none is
> needed is to join the patient in his demonstration of inadequacy. To
> withhold pity tends to frustrate his need to be the victim and to con-
> front him with his real effectiveness. Often it is necessary to be sensitive
> to the patient's tone of voice, rather than to the context of what he is at-
> tempting to convey. He may speak of happy events with a subdued
> mournful affect as if to say, "Even though good things have happened,
> don't blame me: I'm really not happy." On the other hand, he may
> sound quite forceful and even exuberant when discussing the injustices
> and hardships to which he has been subjected. It is essential that the an-
> alyst understand the dynamics underlying the patient's mood rather
> than yield to the temptation to adopt the same mood while relating to
> the patient. (1963, pp. 246–247)

Nydes recommends certain paradigmatic sorts of interventions that can be effectively utilized with such patients. Paradigmatic techniques mesh well with the contemporary object relations model of psychotherapy. In a recent paper (Kissen 1980) the present author has traced some of the overlapping features both of the paradigmatic and object relations models of psychotherapy. The common feature underlying both Nydes's approach to treating paranoid-masochistic characters and the approach being espoused in this paper, is that resistance analysis is central to the therapeutic task. The sort of patients being described in this paper are quite similar to the help-rejecting complainers described by Nydes. The need to speak of happy events in a subdued, mournful tone or to apologize for happy occurrences by undoing them in various self-defeating ways, is a primary resistance pattern that can be focused upon during the course of the psychotherapy process. Paradigmatic interventions of a humorous, playful, or ironic nature can also be effectively utilized to resolve these resistances.

The paradigmatic approach fits quite well with object relations conceptualizations and is a direct outgrowth of Reich's early recommendations of an irritative, therapeutic approach to exploring and resolving character resistances. Paradigmatic modes of resistance analysis have been clearly articulated in the contributions of Nelson (1957, 1962), Spotnitz (1976), and Strean (1970). They offer a useful adjunct to the therapist struggling with the need to find a constructive means of utilizing countertransference feelings induced via the projective identifications of characterologically impaired patients. The intolerance for positive affects often expressed by such patients induces many unpleasant feelings in the therapist that can be partially contained via paradigmatic interventions. Ultimately the therapist's optimism about the patient's capacity to internalize positive affective experience and to attain a higher maturational level of character functioning will provide the most effective form of containing experience for these patients.

CONCLUSIONS

Clinical experience with patients manifesting a reluctance to experience positive affects suggests the need for a reconsideration of Freud's original proposals with regard to the theory of anxiety and resistance. Both his original toxic theory of discharge (1895, 1896) and his later updating of resistance theory in the form of proposals with regard to the signal functions of anxiety (1926) imply a struggle by the ego to cope with either consciously felt negative affects or some preconscious awareness of the potential for such negative affects. Anxiety is theoretically depicted as a negative affect that operates as a signal to the ego that it must inhibit some course of action. Spontaneous and potentially pleasurable forms of expressive behavior are inhibited as a result of the dangers they unconsciously portend to the ego which, according to Freud's structural theory, must continually monitor the external environment for such dangers.

Affective states of anxiety, and the inhibitory processes that they initiate, are both felt to be extremely noxious and unpleasant experiential conditions. They have adaptive potential in that they allow the ego to defend itself against the variety of inner and outer stressors alluded to by Anna Freud in her classic work on the ego and mechanisms of defense (1936). They also, however, have a debilitating effect on the ego in its search for realistic and effective means of pleasure gratification. Inhibitions, by their very nature, restrict the possibility for pleasurable, self-actualizing forms of affective experience. It is the very unpleasant nature of the affects arising out of these inhibitory processes that ultimately leads to the possibility of a psychoanalytic treatment approach to the neuroses.

The viability of a psychoanalytic model for treating neurotic symptoms stems at least in part from Freud's theories of signal anxiety and inhibition. The basic notion is that neurotic inhibitions are felt to be unpleasant ego-restrictive states. It is the affectively unpleasant, essentially ego-dystonic nature of these inhibitions and neurotic symptoms that eventually allows the patient to establish a therapeutic alliance with his analyst. The subsequently successful analysis and resolution of resistances to the therapeutic process can be performed thanks to the establishment of such a therapeutic alliance.

Freud's metapsychological concepts of anxiety and inhibition are nicely applicable to the theory of psychoanalytic treatment of the neuroses. They are not, however, sufficient explanations of the various complications seen in therapeutic work with more disturbed and ego damaged patients.

Treatment experiences with patients manifesting character disorders, narcissistic or borderline conditions, have led to observations that do not quite jibe with Freud's structural theory of anxiety.

Giovacchini (1975) reports the interesting case of a woman who suffered from pervasive experiences of anxiety. Although her anxiety symptoms consisted of extremely unpleasant affective states, they were not truly ego dystonic.

She needed these anxiety states to firm up her shaky sense of ego identity and to feel a greater sense of inner aliveness. For this woman, anxiety did not have the signal function alluded to by Freud. Her anxiety did not initiate processes of ego defense. Rather, it was a primitive form of defense maneuver in its own right. Giovacchini concludes his case discussion with the following statement, "From [previous remarks] one can see that the adaptive significance of anxiety is considered also as a positive factor in its own right, one that can lead directly to a better equilibrium by enhancing ego feeling or narcissism" (1975, p. 17). This is a paradoxical statement, when viewed in light of Freud's signal anxiety theory. Anxiety is not seen by Giovacchini as being either a noxious state of affect discharge or as an unpleasant affect signaling the need for ego defenses or other forms of inhibitory behavior. It is rather depicted as a positive factor allowing for a greater sense of self-articulation and narcissistic gain in a primitively fixated patient.

Anxiety evidently has a different structural and functional character within the psychic economy of more primitively organized and ego damaged patients than it has in neurotic and higher level patients. The paradoxical need to seek out anxiety and other forms of unpleasant affective experience can frequently be discerned in these patients. This paradoxical tendency to seek out unpleasant affects and to avoid more pleasant affects is particularly evident in the approach many such patients have to feelings of depressive anxiety. The need to defend against, and the relative incapacity to tolerate, feelings of depressive anxiety that Zetzel (1949) describes as a typical feature of certain neurotic patients, is not as evident in many primitively fixated patients. Rather these patients tend to defend against potentially positive affective experiences. Their inhibitory tendencies and resistances seem, ironically, to get set off by the dangers posed by positive affects to their primitively organized egos.

There is often an anhedonic quality to the defensive and resistive tendencies of patients manifesting serious character disorders. The reliance by such patients on more primitive defensive maneuvers such as denial, idealization, splitting, and projective identification tends to be associated (on an experiential and object relations level) with a reluctance to experience more benign and potentially maturational self and object representations. This discomfort with more benign object-relational encounters, and seeming comfort with less pleasant forms of affective experience, does not mesh very well with Freud's original or subsequent metapsychological formulations with regard to neurotic inhibitory processes. Thus, the reluctance to experience positive affects tends to be an ego-syntonic and characterological form of resistance in more primitively fixated patients. A different metapsychological conception of anxiety is required to explain this form of resistance. The capacity of anxiety states (particularly of depressive anxiety) to have a functional and structural utility for certain ego-impaired patients needs to be incorporated in a revised theory of anxiety and the inhibitory process.

There can be no doubt that the resistance to positive affects is linked to a form of superego pathology. In accordance with Freud's structural theory and its metapsychological elaboration in the work of the later ego psychologists (Hartmann and Loewenstein 1962), the superego is envisioned as a precipitate consisting of ego ideals, values, and moral prohibitions. These evaluative tendencies are largely derived from authority figures who serve as role models. The severity and inhibitory restrictiveness of a given individual's superego is directly related to the severity of the superego of his or her role models.

The superego, in accordance with Freud's early formulations, is one end product of an effective resolution of the oedipal developmental crisis. The more severe the original oedipal conflict, the more severe is the superego structure resulting from the eventual resolution of that conflict. Schafer (1960) has alerted us to the potentially more loving features of the superego in healthier and better integrated individuals. One attainment from an effective psychoanalysis, according to Sandler (1960), is the ultimate dissolution of the infantile superego and its primitive injunctions against pleasure. This dissolution of primitive superego structures allows for the substitution of a more benign, permissive, and self-loving sort of superego structure.

Given their quite primitive and rigid superego structures, many severely disturbed patients are initially threatened by the therapist's efforts at exploring their reluctance to experience positive affects. They perceive the therapist's interventions as an endorsement of a hedonistic and excessively permissive lifestyle. The therapist has no such interest in imposing a hedonistic orientation upon his basically anhedonic patients. Quite to the contrary, his interest is in supporting viable superego structures and in replacing only those that inhibit the patient's potential for a maturationally higher level of experience and affective flexibility. The therapist's interest in resisted pleasurable affects is related to the maturational and object-relational goals of the psychotherapy process. Ultimately, effective psychotherapy should broaden the range of affective experiences available to a given patient. It should also increase the object-relational maturity of these affects.

The splitting mechanisms that Kernberg (1975) has so convincingly delineated as basic to the defensive organization of narcissistic and borderline patients are, in part, a reflection of the primitive organization of their superego structures. Many borderline patients idealize and envy the self-actualizing and pleasure attainment capacities of others around them, while at the same time depreciating their own capabilities for such ego attainments. These patients are basically fixated at the rapprochement developmental stage. They seldom attain object-relational experiences of an individuated nature, nor can they allow themselves the pleasures often associated with such benign affective experiences. The difficulty in attaining a solid sense of separation and individuation is one major object-relational feature of severe character disorders. This difficulty has been repeatedly noted in the theory of psychotherapy articulated by Winnicott (1965), Giovacchini (1967, 1975, 1979), and Kernberg (1975, 1976). The developmental theory underlying the contemporary object relations approach to psychotherapy owes a great deal to the contributions of Mahler (1952). Horner (1979) has recently contributed a systematic elaboration of the developmental stages underlying various forms of severe character pathology.

We now commonly accept the fact that a major difficulty in primitively fixated patients is their incapacity to attain a true state of separateness and ego identity. Many characterological manifestations of psychopathology can be linked to such separation-individuation difficulties. The incapacity to tolerate pleasurable experiences is a manifestation of both a structural ego defect and an object-relational impairment. Searles (1975) has poignantly described the inherent loyalty with which schizophrenic patients maintain their pathological object relationships and disorganized thought processes. He argues that a failure in the unconscious quest to cure a damaged parental introject is one major object-relational feature in schizophrenic and other forms of severe character pathology. The schizophrenic patient, according to Searles, cannot allow himself a higher level of object-relational attainment due to an unconsciously felt failure at curing a significantly ego damaged parent. There is so much unconscious guilt associated with the psychic act of separation-individuation that it becomes virtually impossible. There is a paradoxical sense of disloyalty associated with states of psychic health for such primitively organized patients.

A similar sense of disloyalty to damaged parental introjects can be noted in the characterological manifestations of nonschizophrenic patients. Colson (1982) has recently described the need to protect the structurally damaged parental environment as basic to the difficulties of transference resistances and countertransferences often experienced in therapeutic work with borderline patients. He makes the following points about the negative therapeutic reactions typically manifested by such patients:

1. In the initial phase, the opportunity that psychotherapy offers for growth threatens much that the patient holds most dear; in particular, it poses the prospect of eventual independence, fantasized by the patient to be destructive to both himself and his family.

2. As the patient begins to recognize all that he has sacrificed to ensure the family homeostasis and his "special" role in the family, he feels increasingly resentful, angry, and depressed.

3. As he takes steps toward individuation, he is confronted with a series of identity crises. That is, as he considers the promise of more mature functioning, he is also confronted with a loss of old, familiar, and predictable patterns of self-experience and of relating to others. The patient may panic in response to the uncertainty about where these changes will lead.

4. The patient experiences depressive emotion and a profound narcissistic injury after discovering the possibility that he can discontinue playing his protective, caretaking role. He comes to feel far less "important," which is accompanied by a loss in the sense of purpose in his life and questions of a despairing nature about whether life is worth living. This phase may be accompanied by concerns about suicide or other forms of nihilism and self-destruction.

5. At times, the treatment process becomes a major obstacle to change. In an effort to save the pathological family from destruction,

the patient employs treatment in a self-defeating way or talks interminably of the risks of making constructive changes in his life. (1982, pp. 318–319)

Whereas neurotic patients manifest such negative therapeutic reactions at a definite point toward the end of psychotherapy, more primitive patients manifest such reactions fairly continuously throughout treatment. They basically resist treatment due to an unconscious appreciation of its capacity to enhance their object-relational experience. The reluctance to experience positive affective experiences is a pervasive resistance feature noticeable during the course of the psychotherapy process with all patients. Oedipal dynamics are almost certainly involved in the paranoid-masochistic sort of transference reactions manifested by many patients to the therapist's efforts to explore and ultimately resolve this resistance. Nydes (1963) has emphasized these oedipal dynamics in explicating his theory of psychotherapy with neurotic characters. More primitive character disorders, however, tend to be fixated at a largely preoedipal level of object-relational development. The fear of separation from a damaged and largely anhedonic infantile milieu is evident in the resistances of preoedipal patients. The psychotherapy process itself, from the very start, poses a dreaded danger to such patients due to the maturational potential unconsciously perceived as inherent in that process.

More primitive patients dread, at an unconscious level, the benign and maturationally higher internalization potential of the psychotherapy process. They sense that they will be asked during the therapeutic experience to give up anhedonic and pathological—yet, nevertheless, loyally maintained—introjects. The fact that they can substitute more benign, pleasurable, and maturationally ego enhancing identifications for these damaged introjects is not very reassuring to such patients. The therapist's task, therefore, is to continually monitor and interactively explore this characterological form of resistance, particularly as it manifests itself in the reluctance to experience positive affects.

REFERENCES

Colson, D. (1982). Protectiveness in borderline states: a neglected object-relations paradigm. *Bulletin of the Menninger Clinic* 46: 305–319.

Freud, A. (1936). *The Ego and the Mechanisms of Defense.* New York: International Universities Press, 1966.

Freud, S. (1895). *Project for a Scientific Psychology. The Origins of Psychoanalysis Letters to Wilhelm Fliess, Drafts and Notes.* 1877–1902. New York: Basic Books, 1954.

———— (1896). Further remarks on the defense neuro-psychoses. In *Collected Papers*, vol. 1, pp. 15–185.

———— (1926). *The Problem of Anxiety.* New York: Norton, 1936.

Giovacchini, P., and Boyer, B.L. (1980). *Psychoanalytic Treatment of Schizophrenic, Borderline and Characterological Disorders.* New York: Jason Aronson.

———— (1975). *Psychoanalysis of Character Disorders.* New York: Jason Aronson.

———— (1979). *Treatment of Primitive Mental States.* New York: Jason Aronson.

Hartmann, H., and Loewenstein, R.M. (1962). Notes on the superego. *Psychoanalytic Study of the Child* 17:42–81.

Horner, A. (1979). *Object Relations and the Developing Ego in Therapy.* New York: Jason Aronson.

Kernberg, O. (1975). *Borderline Conditions and Pathological Narcissism.* New York: Jason Aronson.

———— (1976). Technical considerations in the treatment of borderline personality organization. *Journal of the American Psychoanalytic Association* 24: 795–829.

Kissen, M. (1980). Therapeutic use of self and object representations in the treatment of character disorders. Unpublished manuscript, Adelphi University, Garden City, New York.

Mahler, M. (1952). On child psychosis and schizophrenia: autistic and symbiotic infantile psychoses. *Psychoanalytic Study of the Child* 7:286–305.

Nelson, M.C. (1962). *Paradigmatic Approaches to Psychoanalysis: Four Papers.* New York: Department of Psychology, Stuyvesant Polyclinic Reports in Medical and Clinical Psychology.

Nelson, M.C., and Nelson, B. (1957). Paradigmatic psychotherapy in borderline treatment. *Psychoanalysis* 5:28–44.

Nydes, J. (1963). The paranoid-masochistic character. *Psychoanalytic Review* 50: 215–251.

Reich, W. (1933). *Character Analysis.* New York: Simon and Schuster, 1972.

Sandler, J. (1960). On the concept of the superego. *Psychoanalytic Study of the Child* 15: 128–162.

Schafer, R. (1960). The loving and beloved superego in Freud's structural theory. *Psychoanalytic Study of the Child* 15:163–188.

———— (1976). *A New Language for Psychoanalysis.* New Haven: Yale University Press.

Searles, H. (1975). The patient as therapist to the analyst. In *Tactics and Techniques in Psychoanalytic Therapy*, vol. 2, ed. P. L. Giovacchini, pp. 95–151. New York: Jason Aronson.

Spotnitz, H. (1976). *Psychotherapy of Pre-oedipal Conditions*. New York: Jason Aronson.

Strean, H. (Ed.) (1970). *New Approaches in Child Guidance*. Metuchen, NJ: Scarecrow Press.

Winnicott, D.W. (1965). *The Maturational Processes and the Facilitating Environment*. New York: International Universities Press.

Zetzel, E. (1949). Anxiety and the capacity to bear it. *International Journal of Psycho-Analysis* 30:1–12.

Index

Action language, 381
Adler, Alfred, 211
Affects. *See also* Positive affects
   and analytic technique, 129–130
   defense against, 126–127
Ainsworth, M., 211
"Analysis Terminable and
   Interminable," 5, 285
Analyst. *See also* Therapeutic
   interaction
   and control, need for, 291
   and dream analysis, 282–284
   and narcissistic resistance,
     170–172
Analytic interpretations, 43
Analytic technique, 129–132
Anorexic patients, 383
Anticathexis, 36–40
Arlow, J., 363, 370
Atwood, G. E., 363–364
Autism, 188–189
Autobiographical Study, 35–36
Autopoiesis, 332

Balint, M.
   and classifications of resistances,
     336
   and object relations, 318
   and prestructural psychology, 377

Baranger, M., 327
Baranger, W., 327
Barash, D., 210
Basch, M., 235
Behavioral resistances. *See* Gross
   behavioral resistances
Bellak, L., 370
Bergman, A., 230
Beyond the Pleasure Principle, 5
Bick, E., 334
Billow, R. M., 273, 276
Bion, Wilfred
   and autism, 189
   and dream analysis, 17, 279–281
   and object relations, 317, 325–327,
     330, 334
   and relatedness between patient
     and therapist, 202
Bird, B., 154, 161
Blanck, G., 363
Blanck, R., 363
Borderline patients
   clinical examples of, 344–360
   and emotions, 222–223
   Masterson's theory of, 20
   narcissistic psychopathology of,
     340–341
   and object relations, 341–342
   resistance of, 342–344

Borderline patients (*continued*)
  summary of, 360
  Winnicott's work on, 339
Bornstein, Berta, 145
Bowlby, J.
  and classification of resistances,
    336
  and mother-infant interaction,
    211
  and object relations, 318
Boyer, L. B., 290, 302
Brenner, C., 363, 370
Breuer, J.
  and character disorders, 289
  and hypnosis, 31–33
British Object Relations School,
  318–322, 333
Bulimic patients, 383
Burnham, D. L., 364

Cath, S. H., 330
Character analysis
  and abundance of recall, 82–83
  clinical example of, 48–50
  and formation of character, 51–53
  and impediment of recall, 81–82
  in inferiority case, 58, 65, 68–69
  and neuroses, 44–47
  process of, 9
  and resistance, 51–52
  sequence of, 10
Character Analysis, 9, 250, 390–391
Character armor
  and narcissistic character, 77–79
  and neurotic character, 47
  and resistance, 50
Character disorders
  and control, need for, 291–298
  and countertransference, 307–312
  Freud's, Sigmund, theory of,
    289–290
  and fusion, fear of, 302–304

Giovacchini's theory of, 18–19
  and narcissism, 298–302
  and needs, immediacy of, 305–307
  and positive affects, 382
  and psychoanalytic paradox,
    307–312
  and self-esteem, loss of, 302–304
  summary of, 312–314
Character neuroses, 44–47
Character resistance. *See also*
    Resistance
  analyzing, 47–55
  and basic rules, 42–44
  clinical example of, 55–69
  in individual situations, 55
  of passive-feminine type, 49–50, 53
  of phallic-aggressive type, 48–49,
    53
  Reich's concept of, 9–10
  Sources of, 44–47
Chertok, L., 260–261
Classical school of object relations,
  319–322
Classical transference neuroses
  diagnosis of, 172–173
  and infantile situation, 173
  and narcissistic personality
    disorder, 174–175
  resistance in, 176–178
Cohen, D., 211
Colson, D., 400
Commensal, 334–335
Communication, 192–193, 202, 317
Communicative approach
  clinical example of, 198–205
  and communication resistance
    versus behavioral resistance,
    181–182
  and defenses, 196–197
  description of, 181–182
  findings of, 182–184
  hypothesis of, 182–184

summary of, 205–206
and technique, 197–198
and therapeutic interaction,
185–196
Communicative resistances. *See also*
Communicative approach
and communicative approach,
183, 192
definition of, 13
and object relations, 327–328
Compulsion to repeat, 365–366
Confusion, 284, 331
Conscious, 264–267
Control, need for
and analyst, 291
clinical example of, 291–298
and patient, 291
and resistance, 292–293, 296–298
Countertransference
change in view of, 272–273
and character disorders, 307–312
clinical example of, 273–276
concept of, 269–272
Mendelsohn's theory of, 16
protection against treatment-
destructive, 276–277
and psychoanalytic paradox,
307–312
resistance to, 269–272
summary of, 277
and transference resistance,
258–261
Cult allegiance, 330–331

Dahl, Hartvig, 222
Dare,C., 3
Darwin, Charles, 210–211, 213–214
Defenses
against affects, 126–127, 129–132
against instinct, 125–126, 129–132
against symptom-formation,
127–128

Freud's, Anna, theory of, 396
Greenson's concept of, 135–136
interpersonal, 184, 196–197
intrapsychic, 184, 196–197
permanent, 127
personification of, 328–329
and resistance, 134–140
transference of, 121–123
and transference reactions,
146–150
de Saussure, R., 260–261
Deutsch, H., 6
Developmental arrests, 376
Development of Psychoanalysis, 250
"Difficulty in the Path of Psycho-
Analysis, A," 167
"Discussion of Certain Forms of
Resistance, A," 6
Dora case, 5, 152
Dread of repeating, 365–366
Dream analysis
analyst's resistance to, 282–286
and ego, 119–120
Freud's, Anna, theory of, 119–120
Freud's, Sigmund, theory of, 26,
281, 285
Meltzer's theory of, 17–18
patient's resistance to, 280–282
and psychotherapy, 26
view of, 279–280
Dream interpretation. *See* Dream
analysis

Edel, A., 210
Edel, M., 210
Ego. *See also* Ego defenses
and dream interpretation,
119–120
and free association, 117–119
and resistance, 39–40
*Ego and the Mechanisms of Defense,
The,* 10, 117–132

Ego defenses. *See also* Ego
  Freud's, Anna, theory of, 11
  in inferiority case, 65–68
  and object relations, 230
Ego-resistances, 125
Eissler, K. R., 270
Ekman, P., 213
Ekstein, R., 154
Elisabeth von R., 4–5
Ellsworth, P., 213
Emotions
  clinical examples of, 216–225
  Freud's theory of, 212–216
Empathy, failures in, 377
Encapsulation, 331
Epstein, L., 269, 271–272, 277
Eroticized transference, 146, 324

Failures in empathy, 377
Fairbairn, W. R. D.
  and definition of object relations,
    318
  and Kohut, 321
  and narcissism, 319–320, 323,
    333–334
  and psychic structure, 229
  and resistance, 336
False self
  Masterson's theory of, 20
  and transference resistance,
    232–233, 240–242
False-self patients. *See* Borderline
  patients
Feiner, A. H., 269, 271–272, 277
Fenichel, O.
  and resistance analysis, 134–138,
    141, 164
  and transference reactions, 147,
    151–152
Ferenczi, S., 250, 261
Field, T., 211

Fleiss, R., 269
"Fragment of an Analysis of a Case of
  Hysteria," 5
Frame breaks, 185–186
Framework deviation cures, 185–186
Free association, 117–119
Freeman, T., 135
Freud, Anna
  and analysis of resistance, 10–11
  and classifications of resistance,
    7–8
  and defenses, 396
  and emotions, 214
  and id-ego defense, 251, 261
  and prestructural psychology, 363
  and Reich, 10
  and resistance analysis, 134–135,
    138
  and theory of resistance, 10–11
  and transference reactions, 146,
    150
Freud, Sigmund
  and anticathexis, 36–40
  and character disorders, 289–290
  and classifications of resistance, 6,
    8–9
  and communication, 182
  and compulsion to repeat,
    365–366
  and countertransference, 259–260
  and Dora case, 5
  and dream interpretation, 26, 281,
    285
  and Elisabeth von R. case, 4–5
  and emotions theory, 212–216
  and guilt, 210
  and identifications, 230–231
  and indifference of patient, 222
  and initial resistance, 25–28
  instinct theory of, 197
  and intellectual resistance, 28–29
  metapsychology of, 209–210

and narcissistic resistance, 167–168
and neurotics, 28, 31–33, 37
and object relations, 318–321, 323, 335
and positive affects, 395–396
and primary process, 212
and psychoanalysis, 249
and Rat-Man case, 182, 216–221
and repression, 33–35, 335
and resistance analysis, 134–136, 138–139
and sources of resistance, 5–6
and theory of resistance, 8–9
and transference, 29–30, 35–36
and transference reactions, 140, 144, 152–153, 157, 164
and treatment of illness, 227
and unconscious fantasy, 228
and unconscious transference, 265
and Wolf-Man case, 221–223
Friedman, S. W., 154
Friesen, W., 213
Fromm, Erich, 211
Fromm-Reichmann, F., 251
Frosch, J., 144
Fusion, fear of, 302–304

Gains from illness, 8, 39
Gero, G., 136–137
Gill, Merton, 136–138
Giovacchini, Peter L.
and character disorders, 290, 293, 302, 308, 311
and object relations, 234
and positive affects, 397, 399
and prestructural psychology, 363
and theory of resistance, 18–19
Gitelson, M., 147, 150
Glover, E.
and character resistance, 44
and classification of resistances, 6

and countertransference, 182
Goldman, G. D., 269–270, 272
Greenacre, P., 153
Greenberg, R., 211
Greenson, Ralph
and character disorders, 289
and classifications of resistance, 6–8
and communicative approach, 182
and countertransference, 269, 271
and resistance analysis, 164
and theory of resistance, 3, 6–8, 11–12
and transference reactions, 154
Gross behavioral resistances
and communicative approach, 182, 185, 192
definition of, 13
Grotstein, James S., 19, 363
Guilt, 14, 210. See also Emotions

Haizmann, Christopher, 212, 214–215
Hamilton, V., 318
Harlow, H. F., 211
Harlow, M. K., 211
Hartmann, H.
and id-ego defense, 251, 261
and object relations, 229–230, 321
and positive affects, 398
and resistance analysis, 138
Healthy autism, 188–189
Healthy symbiosis, 187
Hoffman, M., 211
Hogan, R., 211
Holder, A., 3
Hooke's law, 324
Horner, Althea J., 14–15, 233
Horney, Karen, 211, 251, 261
Hypnosis, 31–33
Hysteria
character analysis of, 46

Hysteria (*continued*)
and rationalization, 45
and resistance, 37–38

Id, 39
Identifications, 230–231
Identity, 194–195, 230–231
Identity diffusion syndrome, 310
Id-impulses, 121–122
Id-resistances, 8–9
Impotence, intolerance to, 284–286
Infantile situation
classical transference neuroses in,
173
and contemporary situation,
79–81
in passive feminine character case,
93–114
Inferiority, case of
case history of, 55–60
and character analysis, 58, 65,
68–69
and ego defense, 65–69
explanation for feelings in, 60–64
resistance in, 63–64
Inhibitions, Symptoms and Anxiety, 6,
8, 36–40
Instinct
and analytic technique, 129–132
defense against, 125–126
Freud's, Sigmund, theory of, 197
Intellectual resistance, 28–29
Interactional resistance, 183
Interpersonal communication, 317
Interpretation of Dreams, The, 5, 266
Intrapsychic communication, 317
*Introductory Lectures on Psycho-
Analysis*, 25–35, 251, 261
Invasion, fear of, 283
Issacharoff, A., 271, 276
Izard, C., 213, 215

Jacobson, E.
and borderline patients, 339
and object relations, 321
and self, 230
James, W., 211
Joffe, W. G., 321

Kernberg, O.
and borderline patients, 339
and countertransference, 269
and narcissistic patients, 322
and positive affects, 393, 399
Khan, M. M. R., 235–236, 318
Kissen, Morton, 22–23
Klein, G., 255
Klein, Melanie
and countertransference, 261
and dream analysis, 17, 279–281
and object relations, 318–321, 323,
333–334, 336
Knight, R. P., 134
Kohut, Heinz
and Mednick, 21
and Mr. A, 223–225
and object relations, 318, 321–322
and prestructural psychology,
363–365, 373, 375
and theory of resistance, 12–13
Kris, E., 251
Krystal, H., 235–236

La Barre, W., 210
Lachmann, F. M., 363–364, 376
Laforgue, 38
Langs, Robert
and classification of resistances,
336
and communicative resistances,
327–328
and countertransference, 269
and identity, 194

and listening-formulating-
   intervening process, 198, 202
and relatedness between patient
   and therapist, 187–191
and theory of resistance, 13
Leeper, R., 213
Lewin, B. D., 154
Lewis, Helen Block
   and theory of resistance, 14,
   221–222
Libidinal impulses, 120–121
Links, attacks against, 326
Little, Margaret, 270
Loewenstein, R. M.
   and id-ego defense, 251
   and positive affects, 398
   and resistance analysis, 145
London, N., 363

MacKinnon, R. A., 273
Madness, 195–196
Mahler, M. S.
   and borderline patients, 339
   and identifications, 230
   and positive affects, 399
   and prestructural
   psychopathology, 363, 377
Masterson, James F.
   and borderline patients, 339, 342
   and theory of resistance, 20
Maturana, H., 332
Mednick, Robert A., 21, 377
Meltzer, Donald
   and confusion, 284
   and dream analysis, 279–282
   and narcissistic patients, 334
   and theory of resistance, 17–18
Mendelsohn, Robert
   and countertransference,
   272–273, 276
   and theory of resistance, 16

Menninger, K., 269–271, 273
Metapsychology, 209, 255–258, 279
Michels, R., 273
Milman, D. S., 269–270, 272
Mr. A, 223–225
Murphy, H., 212

Narcissism. See also Narcissistic
   patients
   and character disorders, 298–302
   and dream analysis, 279
   as driving force in psychoanalysis,
   172–178
   and emotions, 222–223
   Grotstein's theory of, 19
   Kohut's theory of, 12–13
   loss of supplies of, 298–302
   primary, 211
   and psychopathology of
   borderline patients, 340–341
   as resistance in psychoanalysis,
   167–172
   and shame, 224
Narcissistic barrier
   breaking down, 69–79
   definition of, 42
   methods of dealing with, 42–43
Narcissistic defense, case of
   analysis of technique in, 74–77
   case history of, 69–73
   character armor in, loosening of,
   77–79
   and infantile fear, 73–74
Narcissistic patients. See also
   Narcissism
   and attacks against links, 326
   and autopoiesis, 332
   classifications of resistances of,
   333–336
   communicative resistances of,
   327–328

Narcissistic patients (*continued*)
  and confusion, 331
  and cult allegiance, 330–331
  and encapsulation, 331
  and personification of defense,
    328–330
  and repressive barrier, 335–336
  resistances of, 322–324
  and reversible perspectives,
    326–327
  and silence, 332–333
  and transformation, fear of,
    325–326
Narcissistic personality disorders,
    174–175
Narcissistic resistance
  and analyst, 170–172
  chronic, 172
  and Freud, Sigmund, 167–168
  nonspecific, 168–170
  and Reich, 167–168
  specific, 176–178
Needs, immediacy of, 305–307
Negative transference, 170
Nelson, M. C., 395
Neurotic patients
  character analysis of, 44–47
  and character resistance, 42–43
  and repression, 28, 31–33
  and resistance, 37
Nontransference-based resistances,
    184
"Note on the Unconscious in
    Psychoanalysis, A," 265
Nunberg, H., 141
Nydes, J., 393–395, 401

Object-relational model, 19. *See also*
    Object relations
Object relations. *See also* Narcissistic
    patients
  and borderline patients, 341–342

clinical examples of, 236–240
definition of, 227
and dream analysis, 279
and false self, 240–242
Freud's, Sigmund, theory of,
    227–228
Grotstein's theory of, 19
Horner's theory of, 14–15
and identification, 230–231
and identity, 230–231
and interpretation of resistance,
    timing of, 245–246
and perfection, need for, 242–245
schools, 317–322
and self, threat to, 235–236
theoretical considerations of,
    229–230
and transfer resistance, 231–235

Pao, P., 363, 365
Parasitism, 189–190
Passive-feminine character, case of
  case history of, 83–86
  character resistance in, 49–50, 53,
    86–93
  infantile situation in, 93–114
  summary of, 114–115
Pathological autism, 189
Pathological symbiosis, 188
Patients. *See* Anorexic patients;
    Borderline patients; Bulimic
    patients; Narcissistic patients;
    Neurotic patients; Therapeutic
    interaction
Perfection, need for, 242–245
Permanent defence-phenomena, 127
Personification of defense, 328–329
Piaget, J., 229
Pine, F., 230
Poetic diction, 286
Positive affects, reluctance to
    experience. *See also* Affects

aspects of, 381
clinical examples of, 382–390
Freud's theory of, 395–396
Kissen's theory of, 22–23
suggestions for dealing with,
390–395
summary of, 395–401
Positive transference, 42–43, 242
Preconscious, 35, 264–267
Prestructural psychology
clinical example of, 366–369
controversies of, 363–364
and repetition, dread of, 365–366
as resistance source, 369–374
treatment approaches to, 374–377
views of, 363–365
Prestructural weaknesses, 374–377
Primary narcissism, 211
Primary process, 211
Psychic deficiency, 369–370
Psychoanalysis, 249. See also
Communicative approach;
Psychoanalytical thought;
Psychotherapy
Psychoanalytic paradox, 307–312
Psychoanalytic thought, in 1930s,
261–264
Psychology, 255–258
"Psychopathology of the Psychoses:
A Proposed Revision, The" 363
Psychoses, 21
Psychotherapeutic situation. See
Therapeutic interaction
Psychotherapy. See also
Communicative approach
borderline patient's resistance to,
342–344
and dream interpretation, 26
and resistance, 3–4, 13
Psychotherapy: A Basic Text, 194
Psychotic psychology. See
Prestructural psychology

Racker, H., 269, 271, 274
Rank, O., 250, 261
Rapaport, D., 215, 255
Rappaport, E. A., 146
Rationalizations, 45
Rat-Man case, 182, 216–221
Reich, Wilhelm
and characterological resistances,
390–392, 395
and classifications of resistance,
7–8
and defense phenomena, 127
and Freud, Anna, 10
and human nature, 211
and narcissistic resistance,
167–168
and resistance-impulse
analyzation, 138
and study of resistance, 250, 261
and submissive feminine-
masochistic attitude, 121
and theory of resistance, 9–10
and transference reactions,
150–151
Reider, N., 150
Reik, T., 224
Relationship resistance, 183
"Remembering, Repeating and
Working Through," 5
Repetition, avoidance of, 365–366
Repression
and energy, 36–37
Freud's, Sigmund, concept of, 5,
33–35
and hysteria, 37–38
of instincts, 125
process of, 33
Repression resistance, 8, 39
Repressive barrier, 335–336
Resistance. See also Character
resistance; Resistance analysis;
and specific types of resistance

Resistance (*continued*)
  and acting in transference,
    123–124
  and affects, 126–127, 129–132
  and anticathexis, 36–40
  autopoiesis, 332
  of borderline patients, 342–344
  and character analysis, 51–52
  in children, 11
  chronic, 328–329
  in classical transference neuroses,
    176–178
  clinical example of, 198–205
  confusion, 331
  and conscious, 264–267
  and control, need for, 292–293,
    296–298
  and countertransference,
    258–261, 269–272
  cult allegiance, 330–331
  and defenses, 121–123, 196–197
  definition of, 3–4
  Deutsch's theory of, 6
  and ego, 38–39
  and emotions, Freud's theory of,
    212–216
  Freud's, Anna, theory of, 7–8,
    10–11
  Freud's, Sigmund, theory of, 4–6,
    8–9
  and fusion, fear of, 302–304
  Giovacchini's theory of, 18–19
  Glover's theory of, 6
  Greenson's theory of, 6–8, 11–12
  Grotstein's theory of, 19
  historical considerations of,
    209–212
  Horner's theory of, 14–15
  and hysteria, 37–38
  and id, 39
  in infantile situation, 80–81
  in inferiority case, 63–64

  initial, 25–28
  and instinct, 125–126, 129–132
  intellectual, 28–29
  Kissen's theory of, 22
  Kohut's theory of, 12–13
  Langs' theory of, 13
  Lewis' theory of, 14
  and libidinal impulses, 120–121
  Masterson's theory of, 20
  Mednick's theory of, 21
  Meltzer's theory of, 17–18
  Mendelsohn's theory of, 16
  and mergers with selfobject,
    disequilibrating, 373–374
  motivation of, 4
  of narcissistic patients, 333–336
  and narcissistic supplies, loss of,
    298–302
  and needs, immediacy of, 305–307
  of neurotics, 28, 31–33, 37
  in passive-feminine character case,
    49–50, 53, 86–93
  to positive affects, 390–395
  and preconscious, 264–267
  and prestructural weakness,
    369–374
  and psychoanalytic paradox,
    307–312
  and psychoanalytic thought of
    1930s, 261–264
  and psychology versus
    metapsychology, 255–258
  in psychoses, 21
  and repressive barrier, 335–336
  and self-esteem, loss of, 302–304
  and selfobject bond, 370–372
  as semiotic, 332–333
  study of, as psychic experience,
    249–252
  and successful treatment, 4
  and super-ego, 40
  and symptom-formation, 127–128